INTERNATIONAL ENCYCLOPEDIA OF PHARMACOLOGY AND THERAPEUTICS

Sponsored by the International Union of Pharmacology (IUPHAR)

(Chairman: B. UVNÄS, Stockholm)

Executive Editor: G. PETERS, Lausanne

Section 36

HEMATOPOIETIC AGENTS

Section Editor

J. C. DREYFUS

Paris, France

VOLUME I

HEMATINIC AGENTS

ii

TERNATIONAL ENCYCLOPEDIA OF
ARMACOLOGY AND THERAPEUTICS

Hematopoietic Agents

VOLUME I

Hematinic Agents

CONTRIBUTORS

A. ASCHKENASY
I. CHANARIN
E. A. DEISS
B. DREYFUS
J. C. DREYFUS

G. R. LEE
D. MOLLIN
J. P. NAETS
H. ROCHANT
C. SULTAN

A. H. WATERS

PERGAMON PRESS

OXFORD · NEW YORK · TORONTO
SYDNEY · BRAUNSCHWEIG

Pergamon Press Ltd., Headington Hill Hall, Oxford

Pergamon Press Inc., Maxwell House, Fairview Park, Elmsford, New York 10523

Pergamon of Canada Ltd., 207 Queen's Quay West, Toronto 1

Pergamon Press (Aust.) Pty. Ltd., 19a Boundary Street, Rushcutters Bay, N.S.W. 2011, Australia

Vieweg & Sohn GmbH, Burgplatz 1, Braunschweig

First edition 1971

Library of Congress Catalog Card No. 70–126124

Printed in Great Britain by Bell & Bain Ltd., Glasgow

08 016211 8

CONTENTS

v

CONTENTS OF VOLUME II

LIST OF CONTRIBUTORS

ASCHKENASY, A., Centre National de la Recherche Scientifique, Laboratoire d'Hématologie Nutritionelle, 45-Orléans-La Source, France

CHANARIN, I., Department of Haematology, Northwick Park Hospital and Clinical Research Centre, Harrow, Middlesex, England

DEISS, E. A., Division of Haematology, Department of Medicine, University Medical Center, Salt Lake City, Utah, U.S.A.

DREYFUS, B., Unité de Recherche sur les Anemies (I.N.S.E.R.M.), UER de Creteil 94, France

DREYFUS, J. C., Université de Paris, Institut de Pathologie Moléculaire, Groupe I.N.S.E.R.M., Associé au C.N.R.S., 24 rue du Faubourg-Saint-Jacques, Paris (XIVe), France

LEE, G. R., Division of Hematology, Department of Medicine, University Medical Center, Salt Lake City, Utah, U.S.A.

MOLLIN, D., Department of Haematology, St. Bartholomew's Hospital, London, E.C.1, England

NAETS, J. P., Laboratoire de Médecine Experimentale, 1, Avenue Jean Crocq, Bruxelles, Belgium

ROCHANT, H., Unité de Recherche sur les Anemies (I.N.S.E.R.M.), UER de Creteil 94, France

SULTAN, C., Unité de Recherche sur les Anemies (I.N.S.E.R.M.), UER de Creteil 94, France

WATERS, A. H., Department of Haematology, St. Bartholomew's Hospital, London E.C.1, England

A*

PREFACE

THE section of the Encyclopedia devoted to Hematology that we present here can be divided into two parts. In the first are described the different factors which are necessary for proper hematopoiesis. These comprise the constituent stones of the structure: iron and proteins, which make up the first two chapters, and then the catalysts necessary to hematopoiesis, each of which is the object of a chapter: vitamin B_6, folic acid derivatives, vitamin B_{12}, and erythropoietin. The second part consists in a description of the agents which are destined to prevent an overproduction of red and white cells. One chapter is devoted to the physical agents, another chapter to chemical agents. Between these two sections, we have inserted an attempt at a discussion on generalized medullary insufficiency and its treatment.

The factors of hematopoiesis have all been reviewed, and none has been neglected. It is evident that these factors are for the most part more directly involved in the biosynthesis of erythrocytes than in the manufacture of leucocytes and platelets. This predominance merely reflects our current understanding of the subject. In addition, two comments must be made regarding two voluntary omissions:

(1) The section does not include a study of methods in the use (Radioisotopes, since these questions have been covered in Section 78 of radioisotopes in Pharmacology), edited by M. Y. Cohen de Saclay.

(2) The section does not include an explicit discussion on the comparative pharmacology of hematinic agents, since this matter has been reserved for Section 85 (Comparative Pharmacology), edited by Mr. Michelson of Leningrad.

Within the limits of the chosen subject matter, all the chapters were indispensable. The necessity of obtaining them all, and also of replacing an author who withdrew at the last minute, has made it difficult for the editor to complete the preparation of this volume.

For the undertaking of the preparation of this work on Hematology, the Board of the Encyclopedia has turned to an editor who is not a pharmacologist, but a biochemist. This is probably why many of the

articles in this volume describe in detail the metabolic pathways and biochemical aspects of hematology, as well as the pharmacology and
therapeutics.

This approach can be justified by the fact that much of the progress in
our understanding of the mechanisms of hematopoiesis and of the pharmacology of hematinics is to be found in the realms of biochemistry, as will
probably remain the case in the future. We hope therefore that the omissions and imperfections of this work will be forgiven, and that the efforts
of the editor and the contributors will have succeeded in producing a
useful work.

CHAPTER 1

VITAMIN B_{12}

A. H. Waters, M.B., B.S., Ph.D., M.R.C.Path., M.C.P.A.,

and

D. L. Mollin, B.Sc., M.B., B.S., F.R.C.Path., M.R.C.P.

Department of Haematology,
St. Bartholomew's Hospital and Medical College,
London, E.C.1

INTRODUCTION

VITAMIN B_{12} deficiency, like folate deficiency, causes megaloblastic anemia in man. The classical B_{12} deficiency state is Addisonian pernicious anemia and much of our knowledge of the role of vitamin B_{12} in human metabolism is derived from the study of the pathogenesis of this condition. Research in this field stems from the experiments of Whipple *et al.* (1920), who demonstrated the effect of dietary factors on blood regeneration in severe anemia. This was followed in 1926 by Minot and Murphy's observation that large amounts of liver in the diet would produce a hematological response in patients suffering from pernicious anemia.

Isolation of vitamin B_{12}

More than twenty years elapsed after Minot and Murphy's discovery before the "anti-pernicious anemia factor" in liver was isolated. The delay was due largely to the difficulties involved in extracting the minute amounts of the hematopoietic factor in liver, and to the absence of a suitable biological assay for guiding the fractionation work. The various stages in this work have been reviewed by Lester Smith (1965) and Castle (1966)

1

both of whom were personally involved in this outstanding piece of research. Finally, in 1948 the hematopoietic factor was isolated almost simultaneously by Rickes *et al.* (1948) in the U.S.A., and by Lester Smith and Parker (1948) in England. It was a red, cystalline, cobalt-containing compound, which was given the name vitamin B_{12}. The hematopoietic activity of vitamin B_{12} was soon confirmed by many other workers, and subsequent clinical experience has established its efficacy in the treatment of pernicious anemia and other B_{12} deficiency syndromes.

Castle's theory of the "intrinsic" and "extrinsic" factors

By the end of the nineteenth century it was well established that the stomach is abnormal in pernicious anemia. Fenwick (1870) described the typical atrophy of the gastric mucous membrane in pernicious anemia, and in 1886 Cahn and von Mering recorded the achlorhydria that is now recognized as characteristic of the disease. It was also shown that achlorhydria might precede the onset of pernicious anemia by as long as ten years (Riley 1925), and even after successful treatment with liver the achlorhydria persists (Johanson, 1929).

These observations led Castle, among others, to suspect that there might be some relationship between gastric achylia and the pathogenesis of pernicious anemia. There followed in 1929 the first of a series of brilliant papers entitled, "Observations on the Etiologic Relationship of Achylia Gastrica to Pernicious Anemia", in which Castle* put forward the theory that an "extrinsic factor" in the normal diet reacts with an "intrinsic factor" secreted by the stomach, to produce a "hematopoietic principle" which is necessary for blood formation. This principle was presumably absorbed in the small intestine.

Castle's theory was not, however, accepted in its original form. Wintrobe (1939, 1951), for instance, suspected that there might be a close relationship between the "extrinsic factor" and the "hematopoietic principle"; and since the isolation of vitamin B_{12} it has been established that these factors are identical. It has therefore been necessary to modify Castle's original theory, for it now seems likely that the "intrinsic factor" secreted by the normal stomach merely facilitates the absorption of the "extrinsic factor", vitamin B_{12} (Berk *et al.*, 1948; Castle 1953).

---

*See Castle (1929); Castle and Townsend (1929); Castle *et al.* (1930); Castle (1953).

CHEMISTRY AND BIOCHEMICAL ROLE OF VITAMIN B$_{12}$

Not long after the isolation of vitamin B$_{12}$ a group of factors with closely related chemical and physiological activity was discovered (for a review, see Lester Smith (1951)). The term "cobalamin" was suggested for these compounds by Kaczka *et al.* (1950), and vitamin B$_{12}$ was referred to as cyanocobalamin. Other cobalamins isolated at this time include vitamin B$_{12a}$ (hydroxocobalamin) and the closely related vitamin B$_{12b}$ (aquo-cobalamin), which are interchangeable in solution depending on pH, and vitamin B$_{12c}$ (nitrocobalamin), which was isolated from the fermentation liquor of *Streptomyces griseus*.

A fourth cobalamin, vitamin B$_{12d}$ also isolated from this latter source, was subsequently shown to be the same as vitamin B$_{12b}$. These cobalamins were shown to have the same therapeutic value as vitamin B$_{12}$ in patients with pernicious anemia (for a review, see Ungley (1951)). The inter-relationship of these various forms of B$_{12}$ was clarified when the structure of vitamin B$_{12}$ was determined by Hodgkin *et al.* (1955) at Oxford. The structural formula of cyanocobalamin is shown in Fig. 1, and the other cobalamins differ only in the nature of the anionic group attached to the central cobalt atom (see also Fig. 3).

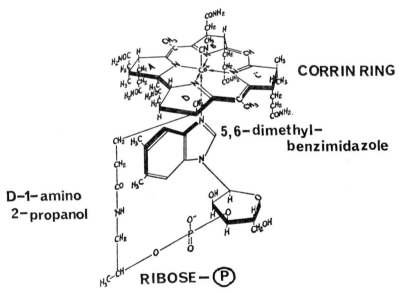

FIG. 1.   Structural formula of vitamin B$_{12}$ (cyanocobalamin).   From Lester Smith (1965).

No sooner had the structure of vitamin B_{12} been determined, than Barker *et al.* (1958) showed that an entirely new form of B_{12} was probably the active form of the vitamin in biological systems. The structure of the coenzyme was determined by Lenhert and Hodgkin (1961), who showed that a 5-deoxyadenosyl group replaced the CN–group of cyanocobalamin (Fig. 2). The explanation for the delayed discovery of coenzyme B_{12} is simple enough, as Lester Smith (1965) has pointed out. The coenzyme is highly sensitive to light and to cyanide, and moderately sensitive to acid (Weissbach *et al.*, 1960); consequently, during all earlier isolation procedures one or other of these agents would have converted the coenzyme to another chemical form.

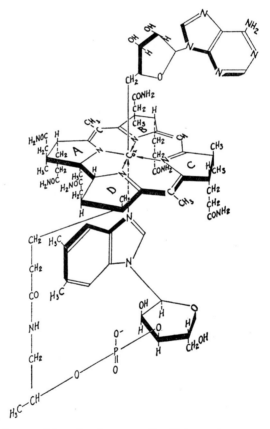

FIG. 2. Structural formula of coenzyme B_{12} (5-deoxyadenosyl-cobalamin). From Lester Smith (1965).

In addition to the cobalamins already mentioned there is a large family of natural and synthetic analogs of vitamin B$_{12}$ (see reviews by Coates and Kon (1957) and Lester Smith (1965)). Many of these are micro-bioligically active, but with some variation from one organism to another, and some are therapeutically active in patients with pernicious anemia although they have not been used in routine clinical practice.

The physical and chemical characteristics of vitamin B$_{12}$ and its analogs have been summarized in recent reviews (Perlman, 1964; Lester Smith, 1965; Wagner, 1966), and will not be dealt with in the present chapter, except in so far as they have a direct bearing on the clinical and biochemical aspects of B$_{12}$ metabolism.

NOMENCLATURE

Vitamin B$_{12}$ is one of a family of compounds containing the corrin nucleus called "corrinoids". A systematic nomenclature for vitamin B$_{12}$ and its derivatives has been adopted by the Commission on Nomenclature of Organic Chemistry of the International Union of Pure and Applied Chemistry (Lester Smith, 1962). The systematic names are in general too cumbersome for routine use, and in practice a simplified nomenclature is used. The term cyanocobalamin applies to the vitamin B$_{12}$ molecule as shown in Fig. 1 with a CN— group attached to the cobalt atom. For descriptive purposes the B$_{12}$ molecule can be represented diagrammatically as in Fig. 3. There is a "planar" group of four pyrrole rings linked together as a corrin nucleus with a central cobalt atom. The cobalt atom forms two other links with groups situated "above" and "below" the planar group. The CN— group may be considered to be "above" and the parent base (most commonly 5,6-dimethylbenzimidazole) "below" the plane. The parent base is also linked to the corrin ring via ribose-phosphate and amino-propanol in sequence. The term "cobalamin" (or B$_{12}$) is a general term for the molecule without the CN— group, and is prefixed by the name of the attached anionic group, R (Fig. 3). The term "cobamide" refers to the cobalamin portion of the molecule without the base (Fig. 3).

Naturally occurring forms of B$_{12}$ *in human liver and plasma*

The liver is the main site of B$_{12}$ storage, containing about 1 mg per kg, and liver B$_{12}$ stores are depleted in severe B$_{12}$ deficiency (Girdwood, 1952;

Ross and Mollin, 1957; Nelson and Doctor, 1958; Anderson, 1965). The major B_{12} component is coenzyme B_{12}, 5-deoxyadenosyl-B_{12} (Toohey and Barker, 1961; Stahlberg, 1965, 1967). However, Stahlberg *et al.* (Stahlberg, 1965, 1967; Stahlberg *et al.*, 1967) also demonstrated the presence of methyl-B_{12} in liver, and showed that this form may predominate when the total B_{12} stores are depleted in pernicious anemia. The significance of the latter observation is not clear, but may be related to the accumulation of methyl-folate in severe B_{12} deficiency (p. 12).

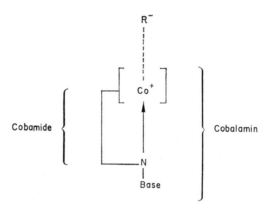

FIG. 3. Diagrammatic representation of the B_{12} molecule (after Huennekens, 1966). The cobalt atom (Co) is enclosed within the corrin ring ([ ]); the anionic group (R) is attached ionically (– – –) to Co; a nitrogen atom (N) of the parent base DMB (5,6-dimethylbenzimidazole) is linked to Co by a coordinate bond (→), and to the corrin ring by an amide bond via ribose-phosphate and amino-propanol (see Fig. 1). Changes in the anionic group R give rise to a family of cobalamins (R-DMBC):

R = CN—	: cyanocobalamin (B_{12})
= OH—	: hydroxocobalamin (B_{12a})
= H_2O—	: aquocobalamin (B_{12b})
= NO_2—	: nitrocobalamin (B_{12c})
= CH_3—	: methylcobalamin (methyl-B_{12})
= 5-deoxyadenosyl—	: coenzyme B_{12} (adenosyl-B_{12})

In contrast to liver, the major portion of B_{12} in plasma is methyl-B_{12}, with only traces of adenosyl-B_{12} and hydroxo-B_{12} (Lindstrand and Stahlberg, 1963; Lindstrand *et al.*, 1966; Stahlberg, 1964, 1967). Stahlberg (1964) showed that methyl-B_{12} is also the main compound in patients with pernicious anemia, and in patients with chronic myeloid leukemia or acute hepatitis who had higher than normal serum B_{12} levels.

None of the B_{12} analogs have been detected in human tissues and only traces of cyano-B_{12} were demonstrated in liver and plasma in the above studies. It has also been shown by other workers that cyano-B_{12} given by parenteral or oral routes is either converted to cyanide-free forms or excreted (Rosenblum *et al.*, 1963; Rosenblum, 1965; Reizenstein, 1967).

Vitamin B$_{12}$ *binders in plasma*

One of the characteristics of B_{12} is that it binds readily to proteins. Early experience with the assay of B_{12} in serum showed that most of the B_{12} was unavailable to *Euglena gracilis* unless the serum was first boiled (Ross, 1952). This served to "free" the B_{12} from a protein binder which migrated in the α-globulin region on electrophoresis (Latner *et al.*, 1952; Pitney *et al.*, 1954). Subsequent studies have shown that there is a second B_{12} binding protein in plasma in the β-globulin region (Hall and Finkler, 1962, 1963; Simons, 1964), and it has been proposed by Hall and Finkler (1963) that these two B_{12} binders be referred to as "Transcobalamin I", TC I, (α-binder) and "Transcobalamin II", TC II, (β-binder). Recent observations by Hom *et al.* (1966) show that TC I has a molecular weight of the order of 121,000, and TC II 36,000, or a polymer of this (Finkler *et al.*, 1970).

When physiological amounts of radioactive B_{12} are given by mouth or by injection, B_{12} is at first bound mainly to TC II, but after some hours the major portion of B_{12} remaining in the plasma is bound to TC I (Hall and Finkler, 1965). On the other hand, when small amounts of radioactive B_{12} are added to the plasma of patients with pernicious anemia or chronic myeloid leukemia, most of the B_{12} is bound to the α-binder, TC I (Hall and Finkler, 1966; Retief *et al.*, 1966). These changes in B_{12} binding help to explain the previously observed slower than normal plasma clearance of injected B_{12} in pernicious anemia and chronic myeloid leukemia (Mollin *et al.*, 1956; Mollin and Booth, 1959; Miller *et al.*, 1957a; Brody *et al.*, 1960; Ritz and Meyer, 1960; Hall, 1961), since radioactive B_{12} bound to the α-binder disappears from the plasma much more slowly than when bound to the β-binder (Hall and Finkler, 1965; Hom, 1967). This may be due to a more efficient transfer of B_{12} to the tissues by the β-binder (TC II) than by the α-binder (TC I) (Finkler *et al.*, 1965; Finkler and Hall, 1967; Retief *et al.*, 1966, 1967).

These observations suggest that the β-binder (TC II) may pick up B_{12}

on absorption into the portal circulation and transport it to the liver and possibly other tissues, whereas the α-binder (TC I) carries the bulk of the circulating B_{12} (Hall and Finkler, 1965; Lindstrand, personal communication). While it is possible that the β-binder is related to, or perhaps derived from intrinsic factor, there is no definite evidence for this (Simons, 1964; Hall and Finkler, 1965; Cooper and White, 1968). The origin of the B_{12} α-binder complex is uncertain, but it has been suggested that it may be derived, in part at least, from effete granulocytes (Mollin and Ross, 1955; Meyer *et al.*, 1962; Gottlieb *et al.*, 1966).

In liver, on the other hand, B_{12} appears to be bound to a protein which has the same electrophoretic mobility as the β-binder in serum (Pitney *et al.*, 1955). Liver B_{12} is available to *Euglena gracilis* without the preliminary heating necessary in the assay of serum. In conditions associated with hepatocellular damage the serum B_{12} level is elevated, owing to release into the circulation of B_{12} loosely bound to "liver protein" (Rachmilewitz *et al.*, 1956 1958; Grosswicz *et al.*, 1957; Jones *et al.*, 1957; Neale *et al.*, 1966).

*Distribution of B_{12} in subcellular fractions**

The localization of B_{12} within the cell has been investigated in several tissues of experimental animals. Swendseid *et al.* (1954a) showed that in mouse liver the mitochondrial fraction had the greatest concentration of B_{12} as determined by microbiological assay. Since then a similar distribution has been found in rat liver (Newman *et al.*, 1962a), brain (Newman *et al.*, 1962b), heart and kidney (Newmark *et al.*, unpublished observations), both for endogenous B_{12} and for physiological doses of radioactive cyanocobalamin in equilibrium with the endogenous stores. Not all workers have found this mitochondrial concentration of B_{12}, but it is possible that their methods of homogenization and subcellular fractionation were at fault. This may also apply to the one published investigation of subcellular B_{12} distribution in human liver (Rachmilewitz *et al.*, 1959), which showed the greatest concentration of B_{12} in the nuclear and soluble protein fractions. Even, if we accept the mitochondrial fraction as the site of B_{12} occurrence in the cell, it should be pointed out that most mitochondrial fractions contain lysosomes and peroxisomes, in addition to mitochondria, and it is therefore impossible as yet to be certain with which subcellular particle B_{12} is primarily associated.

---

*The authors wish to acknowledge the assistance of Dr. P. Newmark with this section.

Biochemical functions of B$_{12}$

The major interest in this field centres around the role of B$_{12}$ in the pathogenesis of megaloblastic anemia in man, and the relationship of B$_{12}$ deficiency to subacute combined degeneration of the cord. The literature on this subject is extensive, and the reader is referred to a number of recent reviews (Beck, 1962, 1964; Herbert and Zalusky, 1962; Mollin *et al.*, 1962; Waters, 1963; Waters and Mollin, 1963; Arnstein, 1964; Buchanan, 1964; Weissbach and Dickerman, 1965; Huennekens, 1966).

Two B$_{12}$ compounds, adenosyl-B$_{12}$ and methyl-B$_{12}$, have been shown to act as coenzymes, and these have now been identified in human liver and plasma (p. 5), as well as in a number of other mammalian and bacterial systems. The different biochemical reactions involving these co-enzymes are summarized in Table 1, from which it can be seen that our knowledge of the biochemical functions of B$_{12}$ is derived largely from studies with bacterial systems.

Of the several reactions involving B$_{12}$ co-enzymes in bacteria, only two have so far been established for animal systems—methylmalonyl-CoA isomerase requiring adenosyl-B$_{12}$ (Table 1, Reaction 2), which is the basis of the urinary methylmalonic acid excretion test for B$_{12}$ deficiency (p. 34 Fig. 13), and homocysteine transmethylase requiring methyl-B$_{12}$ (Table 1 Reaction 5). This latter reaction also requires methyl-tetrahydrofolate as the methyl donor, and is a focal point for the possible interaction of B$_{12}$ and folate in the pathogenesis of megaloblastic anemia. This will be discussed more fully in the next section, together with a discussion of the possible role of B$_{12}$ in the formation of deoxyribonucleotides from ribonucleotides (Table 1, Reaction 6).

Biochemical basis of megaloblastic anemia

The underlying biochemical abnormality in megaloblastic anemia due to either B$_{12}$ or folate deficiency appears to be a defect in nucleoprotein synthesis. In 1947 Thorell showed that there was an abnormal persistence of cytoplasmic RNA in the megaloblast during hemoglobinization, and subsequent biochemical studies showed that the RNA/DNA and uracil/thymine ratios of bone marrow cells were increased in megaloblastic anemia, but returned to normal after specific therapy with B$_{12}$ or folic acid (Davidson *et al.*, 1951; Mueller *et al.*, 1952; White *et al.*, 1953; Glazer *et al.*, 1954; Mueller and Will, 1955). These and more recent observations (Wickramasinghe *et al.*, 1967) suggest that the morphological and nucleo-

TABLE 1. BIOCHEMICAL REACTIONS REQUIRING B_{12}

Reaction	Active form of B_{12}	Occurrence	References
(1) Glutamate isomerase	Adenosyl-B_{12}	Bacteria	Barker et al., 1958
(2) Methylmalonyl-CoA isomerase	Adenosyl-B_{12}	Bacteria and animals	Lengyel et al., 1960; Stern and Friedman, 1960; Stadtman et al., 1960; Gurnani et al., 1960; Marston et al., 1961
(3) Glycol dehydrase	Adenosyl-B_{12}	Bacteria	Abeles and Lee, 1961
(4) Sulfhydryl reduction	Unknown (? Non-enzymatic)	Bacteria and animals	Dubnoff, 1950; Register, 1954; O'Dell et al., 1961; Peel, 1962
(5) Methionine synthetase (Homocysteine transmethylase)	Methyl-B_{12}	Bacteria and animals	Kisliuk and Woods, 1960; Guest et al., 1960; Hatch et al., 1961; Takeyama et al., 1961; Buchanan et al., 1964; Loughlin et al., 1964; Foster, 1966
(6) Ribonucleotide reductase (Thioredoxin)	Adenosyl-B_{12}	Bacteria and animals	Downing and Schweigert, 1956; Spell and Dinning, 1959; Floyd and Whitehead, 1960; Manson, 1960, 1962; Reichard, 1962; Blakley and Barker, 1964; Blakley et al., 1965; Beck et al., 1966

protein abnormalities in megaloblastic anemia are due to a failure to synthesize DNA.

This focused attention on the possible role of B$_{12}$ and folic acid in the methylation of deoxyuridylic to thymidylic acid, a key reaction in DNA synthesis, which had been described by Friedkin and Wood (1956) Subsequent *in vitro* studies have shown that a folate coenzyme is essential in this reaction, but that B$_{12}$ is not directly involved (Wahba and Friedkin, 1961; Greenberg *et al.*, 1961). These observations provide a ready biochemical explanation for the development of megaloblastic anemia in folate deficiency, but do not indicate the way in which B$_{12}$ deficiency interferes with DNA synthesis.

A possible explanation is that B$_{12}$ deficiency exerts its effects by interfering with folate metabolism, and thereby has an indirect effect on DNA synthesis. The introduction of the *Lactobacillus casei* assay for the naturally occurring folate in serum (Baker *et al.*, 1959; Herbert, 1961; Waters and Mollin, 1961) has made it possible to study the interaction of B$_{12}$ and folate metabolism in man. It was shown that there is an accumulation of folate in the serum of patients with pernicious anemia, and that the level of this material falls after B$_{12}$ therapy (Waters and Mollin, 1961, 1963; Herbert and Zalusky, 1962). The accumulation of serum folate in these patients is inversely proportional to the severity of B$_{12}$ deficiency (Fig. 4). Furthermore, after an intravenous injection of folic acid, the serum folate (*L. casei*) activity of patients with pernicious anemia tends to persist at higher levels than normal (Herbert and Zalusky, 1962; Mollin *et al.*, 1962; Waters, 1963). However, this can be prevented by the simultaneous administration of B$_{12}$ with the injection of folic acid (Mollin *et al.*, 1962; Waters, 1963). It therefore appeared that B$_{12}$ was directly involved in the further metabolism of the serum folate compound, which has been shown to be the coenzyme methyl-tetrahydrofolate in normal subjects (Herbert *et al.*, 1962), and in patients with pernicious anemia (Jaenicke and Waters, unpublished observations).

These observations suggested the "methyl folate trap" hypothesis as a possible explanation for the interrelationship of B$_{12}$ and folate in the pathogenesis of megaloblastic anemia (Herbert and Zalusky, 1962; Waters and Mollin, 1963; Buchanan, 1964). This is based on two reactions (Fig. 5); the methylation of deoxyuridylic to thymidylic acid which requires a folate coenzyme (for reviews see Beck, (1962) and O'Brien, (1962)), but is independent of B$_{12}$ (Wahba and Friedkin, 1961; Greenberg *et al.*, 1961); and the methylation of homocysteine to methionine which requires both methyl folate (Hatch *et al.*, 1961; Larrabee and Buchanan,

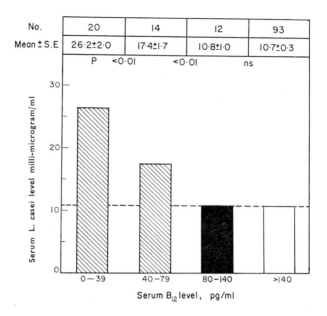

FIG. 4. Correlation of the serum B_{12} and serum folate (*L. casei*) concentrations of 46 patients with B_{12} deficiency and minimal anemia; 34 of these patients had mild pernicious anemia (hemoglobin $> 10g/$ 100 ml) (cross-hatched columns), and 12 had latent pernicious anemia (closed column). For comparison the results in normal subjects are included (open column). The height of each column indicates the mean serum folate (*L. casei*) level for the corresponding serum B_{12} range. From Waters (1963).

1961; Jaenicke, 1961; Sakami and Ukstins, 1961) and methyl-B_{12} (see Table 1, Reaction 5). In the second of these reactions methyl folate transfers its methyl group to homocysteine via methyl-B_{12}, and is converted to tetrahydrofolate (FH_4), which is essential for thymidylate methyl synthesis (McDougall and Blakley, 1961). Thus, B_{12} deficiency would block the reconversion of methyl folate to FH_4, resulting in a "metabolic trap" for methyl folate (reflected in high serum folate levels), and a fall in the level of FH_4, which would lead to defective DNA synthesis and megaloblastic anemia. Low levels of FH_4 in B_{12} deficiency would also explain the increased urinary excretion of formimino-glutamic acid (FIGlu) after histidine loading in many patients with pernicious anemia (Jukes, 1962), since FH_4 is required to accept the formimino group of

FIGlu, as shown in Fig. 6. The administration of B$_{12}$ allows methyl folate to be converted to FH$_4$, which can then accept the formimino group of FIGlu. This explains the observed reversion of FIGlu excretion to normal in such patients after B$_{12}$ therapy (Kohn *et al.*, 1961; Mollin *et al.*, 1962; Zalusky and Herbert, 1961; Knowles and Prankerd, 1962).

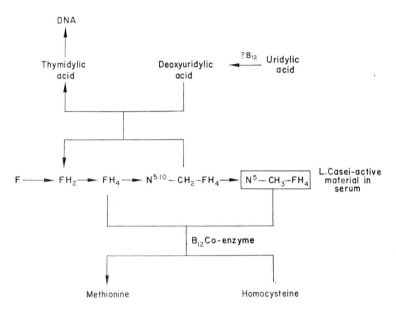

FIG. 5. The "methyl folate trap" hypothesis to explain the possible metabolic interrelationships of B$_{12}$ and folate in the pathogenesis of megaloblastic anemia. B$_{12}$ deficiency may have an indirect limiting effect on DNA synthesis by blocking the reconversion of methyl folate (^{5}N—CH$_3$—FH$_4$) to tetrahydrofolate (FH$_4$), the concentration of which is rate-limiting for the methylation of deoxyuridylic to thymidylic acid. From Waters (1963).

While this hypothesis provides a direct explanation for the development of megaloblastic anemia in patients with B$_{12}$ or folate deficiency, unfortunately it does not appear to explain the hematological relapses that may occur when patients with pernicious anemia are treated with large doses of folic acid, which should bypass the methyl folate trap. This suggests that B$_{12}$ may affect DNA synthesis in other ways. In this respect it has been shown that B$_{12}$ acts as a co-factor in the reduction of ribonucleotides to deoxyribonucleotides in some bacterial systems, and Beck (1962, 1964) has suggested that this is the main cause of impaired DNA synthesis in B_{12} deficiency. However, this reaction has not been demonstrated in mammalian systems and is not present in all bacteria (for a review see Buchanan (1964)). If B_{12} does control this reaction in man, it may only be an important limiting factor in DNA synthesis when the stores of B_{12} are completely exhausted (Waters, 1963), as occurs when patients with pernicious anemia relapse during folic acid therapy (Will *et al.*, 1959).

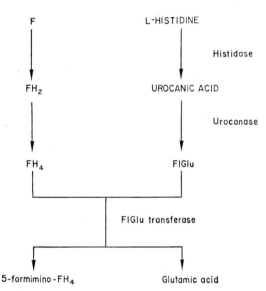

Fig. 6. The mammalian pathway of histidine metabolism. F, folic acid (pteroylglutamic acid); FH_2, dihydrofolic acid; FH_4, tetrahydrofolic acid; FIGlu, formimino-glutamic acid.

Neurological lesions in B_{12} deficiency

Whatever the role of B_{12} in DNA synthesis, failure of DNA synthesis is unlikely to be responsible for the development of nervous system lesions in severe B_{12} deficiency, since DNA turnover is low in cells not undergoing mitosis, such as the neurones of the central nervous system. On the other hand, the RNA content of these cells is high and intensive protein synthesis is necessary to maintain the integrity of the neuronal axons (Bodian, 1947).

It has been suggested by Nieweg *et al.* (1954) that B$_{12}$ may be required for RNA synthesis, thus accounting for the development of nervous lesions in severe B$_{12}$ deficiency. However, there is little evidence for this, and it has recently been suggested that severe B$_{12}$ deficiency may lead to subacute combined degeneration of the cord (SACD) by exposing the central nervous system to toxic damage, possibly due to a disturbance of endogenous cyanide metabolism (Smith, 1961; Wokes and Smith, 1962; Wilson and Langman, 1966). It has also been suggested that the accumulation of methylmalonic acid in severe B$_{12}$ deficiency (see p. 33) may exert a toxic effect on the central nervous system (Cox and White, 1962), but there is no definite evidence to support this (Brozovic *et al.*, 1967).

PHYSIOLOGICAL ASPECTS

Nutritional requirement

It is well established that only microorganisms can synthesize B$_{12}$. With the exception of the small amounts of B$_{12}$ present in the root-nodule microorganisms of legumes (Evans and Kliewer, 1964), plants do not contain B$_{12}$, so that herbivorous animals derive their B$_{12}$ from bacterial synthesis in the rumen and subsequent absorption in the small intestine. Carnivorous animals and man depend on the vitamin stored in animal protein for their requirements.

The normal adult requirement for B$_{12}$ in the form of food is unknown, but therapeutic trials in patients with pernicious anemia show that 1 mcg of cyanocobalamin daily by injection is required (Rickes *et al.*, 1948; West and Reisner, 1949; Darby *et al.*, 1958), and whole-body turnover studies of tracer doses of radioactive B$_{12}$ suggest a similar figure (Heinrich, 1964; Heyssel *et al.*, 1966; Reizenstein *et al.*, 1966). However, much smaller amounts will probably prevent the onset of anemia and other symptoms of B$_{12}$ deficiency (Mollin, 1962a; Herbert, 1966). The additional requirements imposed by growth, pregnancy, and increased metabolism are unknown.

The B$_{12}$ content of different foods has been summarized by McCance and Widdowson (1960), and the U.S. Department of Agriculture (1961). The principal dietary source of B$_{12}$ is animal protein (Table 2). Unlike folate, B$_{12}$ is relatively stable, but severe heating of food, especially in an alkaline medium, leads to definite but variable loss of B$_{12}$ (Heyssel *et al.*, 1966). Calculated from figures based on microbiological assay (McCance and Widdowson, 1960), the average British diet contains 5–6 mcg of B_{12} (Waters, 1963), and similar figures have been reported for American diets (Estren *et al.*, 1958; Chung *et al.*, 1961). Although we cannot assume that all of the B_{12} in food is available, at least 50% of amounts up to 3 mcg are absorbed (Heyssel *et al.*, 1966). Based on these figures, the amount of B_{12} absorbed is therefore in excess of the estimated minimal adult daily requirement.

TABLE 2. DIETARY SOURCES OF VITAMIN B_{12}[a]

	mcg/100 g
Rich sources:	
Beef liver	50–130
Beef kidney	20–50
Beef heart	25
Herring, sardines	10
Other sources:	
Chicken liver	8
Leg of lamb	8
Beef	2–8
Veal	2
Pork	0.1–5
Tinned salmon	2
White fish	1
Milk	1.4 (per pint)
Cheese	1.4–3.6
Eggs	1.2 (per yolk)
No B_{12}:	
Vegetables, fruit and nuts	

[a] Based on data from McCance and Widdowson (1960) and Lester Smith (1965).
Note: Cooking losses are variable, but severe heating in a strongly alkaline medium tends to destroy the vitamin.

It can therefore be seen that provided B_{12} absorption is normal, there is a good safety margin in the dietary intake of B_{12} over requirement, and deficiency from dietary causes is therefore very rare. However, dietary deficiency of B_{12} does occur after many years in strict vegetarians (e.g. Vegans), who take no animal protein in their diet (Wokes *et al.*, 1955; Harrison *et al.*, 1956; Smith, 1962; Wokes and Smith, 1962; Hines, 1966; Winawer *et al.*, 1967), and has been reported in India in breast-fed babies of B$_{12}$ deficient mothers (Jadhav *et al.*, 1962). Even under these conditions the deficiency is rarely as severe as that seen in patients with defective absorption of B$_{12}$. In fact, if an adult suffers from severe megaloblastic anemia due to B$_{12}$ deficiency, defective absorption of B$_{12}$ is always found to be present.

Intestinal absorption

The classical experiments of Castle and co-workers showed that B$_{12}$ absorption is a unique and complex process, depending on the adequate secretion of gastric intrinsic factor (for reviews see Castle (1953, 1966)). The introduction of cyanocobalamin labeled with radioisotopes of cobalt (Chaiet *et al.*, 1950; Lester Smith *et al.*, 1952; Bradley *et al.*, 1954) greatly facilitated the study of B$_{12}$ absorption.

It is now established that there are two mechanisms of B$_{12}$ absorption: one is mediated by intrinsic factor, which is operative in the presence of the small amounts of B$_{12}$ in the diet; the other, probably passive diffusion, only occurs in the presence of excessive and unphysiological amounts of B$_{12}$.

(*a*) *The intrinsic factor mechanism.* Intrinsic factor, which has been the subject of many reviews (Castle, 1953; Ellenbogen and Highley, 1963; Glass, 1963, 1965; Herbert and Castle, 1964), has not yet been isolated in pure form. The available evidence suggests that it is a mucoprotein with a molecular weight of the order of 50,000, or a multiple of this. Recent studies suggest that in man intrinsic factor is secreted by the acid-secreting parietal cells of the gastric fundus (Hoedemaeker *et al.*, 1964, 1966). Normally the amount of intrinsic factor secreted is far in excess of that needed for B$_{12}$ absorption, only 1–2% of the total output being required under physiological conditions to promote normal B$_{12}$ absorption (Abels and Schilling, 1964; Ardeman and Chanarin, 1965). The absorption of B$_{12}$ by fasting normal subjects is therefore usually not improved by histamine or carbachol stimulation. However, the amount of B$_{12}$ that can be absorbed from a single oral dose by the intrinsic factor mechanism is limited (Glass *et al.*, 1954a; Swendseid *et al.*, 1954b; Baker and Mollin, 1955). Thus, normal subjects absorb from 50–90% of an oral dose of 1 mcg of B$_{12}$, 25–30% of 10 mcg., but only 5% of 50 mcg (Mollin, 1959a). Within the limits of B$_{12}$ absorption there is a linear relationship between the amount of intrinsic factor and the amount of B$_{12}$ absorbed (Baker and Mollin, 1955; Schilling and Schloesser, 1957). Furthermore, there is a subsequent "refractory period" during which absorption is depressed (Abels *et al.*, 1959).

In man, B_{12} is absorbed in the ileum (Booth and Mollin, 1959), and observations on patients subjected to intestinal resection show that removal of 4–6 feet or more of ileum impairs the absorption of B_{12} (Booth *et al.*, 1964). The restricted site of absorption and the strict limitation of the amount of B_{12} absorbed at any one time suggest that absorption of this vitamin is an active process mediated by special receptors.

The physiological absorption of B_{12} is a sequential process, the formation of the B_{12}–IF complex being the first stage (Cooper and Castle, 1960). The second phase, which is calcium dependent and does not require energy (Herbert, 1959a; Gräsbeck *et al.*, 1959), involves adsorption of the B_{12}–IF complex onto special intestinal receptors (Strauss *et al.*, 1960; Sullivan *et al.*, 1963; Boass and Wilson, 1964; Ukyo and Cooper, 1965; Cooper, 1967). A new approach by Donaldson *et al.* (1967), using hamster intestinal brush borders and microvillous membranes, has confirmed these previous observations, as to the site and nature of adsorption of the B_{12}–IF complex. However, the third phase of B_{12} absorption, which involves transport of B_{12} into the cell, and the ultimate fate of intrinsic factor is still uncertain (for reviews see Wilson (1964) and Glass (1965)). Recent studies in man have shown that, when B_{12} enters the portal circulation, it is bound to a protein, probably Transcobalamin II, which is not the same as intrinsic factor, but nevertheless may be derived from it (Hall and Finkler, 1965; Cooper, 1967; Cooper and White, 1968; Lindstrand, 1965—unpublished observations). The time course of events after an oral dose of radio-active-B_{12} shows that the vitamin is taken up by the intestinal mucosa and held there for at least 2–3 hr before it appears in the peripheral blood where it reaches peak levels after 8–12 hr (Fig. 7) (Booth and Mollin, 1956, Doscherholmen and Hagen, 1956). The same pattern of absorption has been demonstrated in the portal vein (Doscherholmen and Hagen, 1959; Cooper and White, 1968). Although most of the radioactive-B_{12} is transferred to the blood during the first 24 hr after a labeled test dose, the remainder is slowly released over several days; the ileal mucosa thus acting as a temporary storage for absorbed B_{12} (Doscherholmen *et al.*, 1960). Once released, radioactive-B_{12} accumulates rapidly in the liver, and by 5–6 days 60–70% of the absorbed radioactivity is in the liver (Glass *et al.*, 1954b; 1955; Doscherholmen *et al.*, 1960).

Other cobalamins, such as hydroxocobalamin, co-enzyme B_{12} (adenosyl-B_{12}) and methyl B_{12} are also absorbed, but the precise nature of the chemical form in which B$_{12}$ is finally absorbed is uncertain (Latner *et al.*, 1961; Chosy *et al.*, 1962a; Uchino *et al.*, 1962; Glass and Castro-Curel, 1964; Heinrich and Gabbe, 1964; Herbert and Sullivan, 1964).

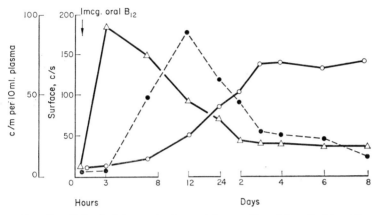

FIG. 7. Abdominal (△— △), plasma (● – – – ●) and hepatic (○— ○) radioactivity in a control subject given an oral dose of 1 mcg of ^{56}Co-B$_{12}$. From Booth and Mollin (1956).

(b) *Passive diffusion mechanism.* This mechanism is less important clinically and only becomes operative in the presence of larger amounts of B$_{12}$ than are usually present in the diet (Ross *et al.*, 1954; Doscherholmen and Hagen, 1957). It is possible that both absorption mechanisms may operate simultaneously, if the diet contains excessive amounts of B$_{12}$.

Excretion

Some B$_{12}$ is re-excreted into the alimentary tract, mainly in the bile, and under normal conditions most of this is reabsorbed giving rise to an entero hepatic circulation of B$_{12}$ (Gräsbeck *et al.*, 1958; Willigan *et al.*, 1958; Reizenstein, 1959). This is a significant drain on the B$_{12}$ stores of patients who are unable to absorb B$_{12}$, and an important economy measure for patients taking a B$_{12}$ deficient diet (Herbert, 1965).

The urinary loss of B$_{12}$ under physiological conditions is very small (Booth and Mollin, 1956; Mollin *et al.*, 1956; Gräsbeck *et al.*, 1958). On the other hand, large parenteral doses of cyanocobalamin are rapidly excreted in the urine, and from a therapeutic point of view this is very uneconomical. The amount excreted increases almost exponentially with the dose, and up to 90 % of 1000 mcg is excreted (see Fig. 16). Once excreted by the renal glomeruli, B_{12} does not appear to be reabsorbed, and it has been possible to use the urinary excretion of radioactive-B_{12} to measure renal glomerular filtration rate in patients previously given large injections of B_{12} to saturate the tissue and plasma B_{12} binding sites (Miller *et al.*, 1957b; Rath *et al.*, 1957; Watkin *et al.*, 1961; Nelp *et al.*, 1964; Brecken-ridge and Metcalfe-Gibson, 1965; Jeremy and McIver, 1966; Malamos *et al.*, 1966). This also has practical application in the assessment of B_{12} absorption using the Schilling test (p. 39). About one-third of any absorbed radioactive-B_{12} is "flushed" into the urine by an injection of 1000 mcg of "cold" B_{12}, given at the same time as the oral test dose of radioactive-B_{12} or up to 2 hr later (Callender and Evans, 1955).

VITAMIN B_{12} DEFICIENCY

Clinical syndromes

In man, B_{12} deficiency, like folate deficiency causes megaloblastic anemia. The clinical syndromes associated with B_{12} deficiency are sum-marized in Table 3. As shown previously, dietary deficiency of B_{12} is rare, and malabsorption is the main cause of deficiency of this vitamin. This may be due either to inadequate secretion of intrinsic factor by the stomach or to impaired intestinal absorption of the B_{12}–I.F. complex. Defective absorption of B_{12} develops long before the serum B_{12} concentration falls to subnormal levels, and the deficiency is often present for years before the development of overt megaloblastic anemia. In fact, although B_{12} deficiency may occur in a wide variety of conditions, severe megaloblastic anemia only occurs in pernicious anemia, chronic tropical sprue and in some patients with total or partial gastrectomy, or anatomical lesions of the small intestine.

The syndromes associated with B_{12} malabsorption will be discussed only briefly, and the reader is referred for further details to the reviews by Mollin (1959b; 1960) and Herbert (1959b). Malabsorption of B_{12} due to lack of intrinsic factor occurs in Addisonian pernicious anemia, and after total or partial gastrectomy. Following partial gastrectomy the secretion of intrinsic factor is impaired, due partly to gastric resection, and partly to atrophy of the gastric remnant, and leads to malabsorption of B_{12} in most patients after this operation (Badenoch *et al.*, 1955a; Deller *et al.*, 1962; Mollin, 1962c; Mollin and Hines, 1964; Adams and Cartwright, 1963;

Turnbull, 1967). The secretion of intrinsic factor is also impaired in patients with atrophic gastritis (Ardeman and Chanarin, 1966), leading to malabsorption of B$_{12}$ which may be associated with subnormal serum B$_{12}$ levels and histamine-fast achlorhydria, as in some patients with early non-anemic pernicious anemia (Mollin *et al.*, 1957; Siurala and Nyberg, 1957; Callender *et al.*, 1960; Glass *et al.*, 1960; Siurala *et al.*, 1960; Whiteside *et al.*, 1964). In such patients, screening the serum for autoantibodies to intrinsic factor and gastric parietal cells may help in the differential, diagnosis from early pernicious anemia (Schwartz, 1958, 1960; Taylor, 1959; Jeffries *et al.*, 1962; Ardeman and Chanarin, 1963; Coghill *et al.*,

TABLE 3. CLINICAL SYNDROMES ASSOCIATED WITH B$_{12}$ DEFICIENCY

1. *Inadequate intake:*
   Strict vegetarians (e.g. Vegans)
   Breast-fed infants of B$_{12}$ deficient mothers

2. *Defective absorption of B$_{12}$:*
   A: *Gastric lesions:*
      1. Addisonian pernicious anemia
      2. Total gastrectomy
      3. Partial gastrectomy
      4. Atrophic gastritis

   B: *Intestinal malabsorption:*
      1. *Anatomical lesions of small intestine:*
         (a) resections
         (b) blind loops, strictures, fistulae and diverticula (associated with abnormal bacterial flora)
         (c) mixed lesions
      2. *Generalized lesions of small intestine:*
         (a) coeliac disease and idiopathic steatorrhoea
         (b) tropical sprue
         (c) Crohn's disease
         (d) infiltrations
      3. Fish tapeworm (Diphyllobothrium latum) infestations
      4. Inherited specific B$_{12}$ malabsorption associated with proteinuria (Imerslund syndrome)
      5. Drugs (e.g. PAS)

   C: Inherited deficiency of intrinsic factor ("Juvenile" pernicious anemia)

B

1965; Doniach *et al.*, 1965; Wangel and Schiller, 1966; Wangel *et al.*, 1968a,b).

In infants and young children, B_{12}-deficient megaloblastic anemia due to inadequate secretion of intrinsic factor is rare, and when this occurs it differs from adult pernicious anemia in that achlorhydria and gastric atrophy are usually absent and antibodies to gastric parietal cells and intrinsic factor cannot be demonstrated. The cause of this defect is still uncertain, but there is some evidence that juvenile pernicious anemia is related to classical Addisonian pernicious anemia (Mollin *et al.*, 1955; Waters and Murphy, 1963). In slightly older children with multiple auto-immune disease, a condition analagous to adult pernicious anemia may occur (Doniach *et al.*, 1965; McIntyre *et al.*, 1965). However, these children differ from adults having pernicious anemia in that, although intrinsic factor antibodies are present in the serum, gastric parietal cell antibodies are absent.

Defective intestinal absorption of B_{12} may be associated with generalized lesions of the small intestine (e.g. idiopathic steatorrhoea, coeliae disease and tropical sprue), with ileal resection or operations which by-pass the B_{12} absorbing site, or with lesions producing stagnation associated with an abnormal bacterial flora (e.g. blind loops, strictures, fistulae and single or multiple diverticula). These conditions will be discussed more fully when we consider the clinical interpretation of radioactive B_{12} absorption tests. Intestinal malabsorption of B_{12} may also be associated with pancreatic steatorrhoea (Perman *et al.*, 1960; Veeger *et al.*, 1962), with certain drugs, such as para-amino salicylic acid (Heinivaara and Palva 1965) and with fish tapeworm infestation (von Bonsdorff, 1956). Rare causes of B_{12} malabsorption include intestinal lymphangectasia (Mistilis *et al.*, 1965), and the inherited selective intestinal malabsorption of B_{12} associated with proteinuria (Imerslund, 1959; Gräsbeck *et al.*, 1960).

Hematological and clinical features

In contrast to the characteristic megaloblastic anemia of severe B_{12} deficiency, the earliest symptoms of deficiency are often vague and non-specific—anorexia, lassitude and irritability. Even at this stage, however, definite hematological changes are usually present. These changes may be overlooked, especially if the hemoglobin concentration is within the normal range, but careful examination of the stained blood films will reveal increased anisocytosis, with some macrocytosis and occasional hyper-segmented neutrophils. In the bone marrow, a proportion of the developing polychromatic erythroblasts will show early megaloblastic change ("intermediate megaloblasts"), and there will be occasional giant metamyelocytes. As the deficiency progresses, these changes become more obvious until the patient presents with overt megaloblastic anemia.

Through its role in DNA synthesis, vitamin B$_{12}$ deficiency also affects other rapidly proliferating tissues. It may produce widespread epithelial changes involving the skin and hair, the buccal and vaginal mucosa, and the alimentary tract. It may also affect the reproductive system leading to sterility.

The skin may be atrophic and show abnormal pigmentation or vitiligo (Wintrobe, 1961; Imerslund, 1959; Baker *et al.*, 1963). The authors have seen a patient with pernicious anemia who presented as a result of an exacerbation of dermatitis which subsided following B$_{12}$ therapy. The hair tends to be dry and brittle, and some patients may even present with alopecia (Booth and Mollin, unpublished observations). Premature greying is said to be more common in patients with pernicious anemia.

Atrophic glossitis is often a presenting symptom in B$_{12}$ (and folate) deficiency. The occurrence of megaloblastic changes in the cells of the buccal mucosa is well recognized (Boen, 1957; Farrant, 1958, 1960; Boddington, 1959; Jacobs, 1960), and similar changes occur in the vaginal mucosa (see below). Dysphagia due to a post-cricoid web has also been reported in patients with pernicious anemia (Jacobs and Kilpatrick, 1964; Procopis and Vincent, 1966). The relationship of gastric atrophy to B$_{12}$ deficiency is a controversial point (Mollin, 1959b), but there is evidence to suggest that classical adult pernicious anemia is due to the combined inheritance of gastric atrophy and impaired secretion of intrinsic factor (Mollin *et al.*, 1955; Waters and Murphy, 1963).

Severe B$_{12}$ deficiency *per se* may have a local effect on the intestinal mucosa (Foroozan and Trier, 1967), and thus impair the absorption of B$_{12}$, which improves after B$_{12}$ therapy (Schloesser and Schilling, 1963; Haurani *et al.*, 1964; Brody *et al.*, 1966; Matthews, 1967; Mollin and Waters, 1968). Another possibility is that B$_{12}$ deficiency may cause deficiency of the β-binder (Transcobalamin II) and thereby impair the uptake of B$_{12}$ from the intestinal cell (Lawrence, 1966). However, these two possibilities are not necessarily exclusive, especially if the β-binder is derived from intrinsic factor, which may enter the intestinal cell with B$_{12}$ (Cooper, 1967; Cooper and White, 1968). Reversible impairment of B$_{12}$ absorption also occurs in patients with severe folate deficiency due to acute tropical sprue (O'Brien and England, 1966), and in some patients with megaloblastic anemia associated with anticonvulsant therapy (Lees, 1961; Reynolds *et al.*, 1965).

Perhaps the most striking clinical changes are produced in the nervous system, where both psychiatric and neurological complications may develop. The psychiatric changes vary from mild irritability and lassitude to frank psychosis, the latter having been referred to as "megaloblastic madness" (Holmes, 1956; Smith, 1960; Strachan and Henderson, 1965; Edwin *et al.*, 1965; Hunter *et al.*, 1967; Smith and Oliver, 1967). The neurological complications range from vague parasthesiae to fully developed subacute combined degeneration of the cord (Ungley, 1949; Victor and Lear, 1956; Wilson and Langman, 1966). Optic neuropathy has also been reported as a less common, but important neurological complication of B_{12} deficiency, which may present before the onset of megaloblastic anemia (Cohen, 1936; Turner, 1940; Benham, 1951; Hamilton *et al.*, 1959; Enoksson and Norden, 1960; Freeman and Heaton, 1961; Matthews, 1961; Bjorkenheim, 1966). However, many workers believe that B_{12} deficiency alone cannot explain the optic neuropathy, and that an additional factor such as smoking, as in tobacco amblyopia, may be involved (Heaton *et al.*, 1958; Smith, 1961; Freeman and Heaton, 1961; Foulds *et al.*, 1969). In fact, as discussed previously (p. 14) the pathogenesis of the whole range of neurological lesions in B_{12} deficiency is obscure.

Severe B_{12} deficiency may produce sterility in some patients, which can be corrected by B_{12} therapy (Adams, 1958; Sharp and Witts, 1962; Jackson *et al.*, 1967; Mollin and Waters, unpublished observations). It has been suggested that the seminal B_{12} level is reduced in the majority of infertile men with abnormal sperm (Watson, 1962). A common complication is the megaloblastic change produced in the vaginal epithelium of women with B_{12} deficiency (Boddington and Spriggs, 1959). In some patients the vaginal cytology may be so bizarre as to simulate malignancy (Lloyd and Garry, 1963).

In view of its widespread effects and insidious onset, the early diagnosis of B_{12} deficiency is therefore a matter of great clinical importance, and the methods now available for studying B_{12} metabolism make diagnosis possible at a very early stage. For this reason, the first step in diagnosis is to suspect that the deficiency may be present, either because the patient has overt megaloblastic anemia or, in the absence of anemia, because the stained blood film shows the characteristic early megaloblastic changes mentioned previously. Even in the absence of these early changes, B_{12} deficiency should always be suspected if a patient suffers from any condition known to be associated with this deficiency (see Table 3).

Diagnosis of B$_{12}$ deficiency

The hematological diagnosis of megaloblastic anemia is usually the first step in the diagnosis of B$_{12}$ (or folate) deficiency. Until recently, the differential diagnosis of the underlying deficiency was based on the procedure of therapeutic trial, which is obviously limited to those patients who present at a late stage of the deficiency with overt megaloblastic anemia. However, recent laboratory methods have made it possible to diagnose B$_{12}$ and folate deficiency at an early stage before the onset of symptoms or anemia. The diagnosis of folate deficiency is discussed by Dr. Chanarin in Chapter 2, and we propose in this section to deal with the laboratory methods for the diagnosis of B$_{12}$ deficiency.

(1) *Therapeutic trial.* The availability of synthetic folic acid and B$_{12}$ made it possible to rationalize the procedure of therapeutic trials which developed from the classical studies of reticulocyte responses by Minot and Castle (1935). The usual therapeutic dose of folic acid (5–15 mg) will produce a hematological response in pernicious anemia, and although the blood picture may become normal, the patient may subsequently relapse or develop neurological complications. On the other hand, some patients with folate-deficient megaloblastic anemia may respond to the usual therapeutic dose of B$_{12}$ (100–1000 mcg), but the response is always incomplete (Mollin and Ross, 1957; Zalusky *et al.*, 1962). However, by adjusting the dose of B$_{12}$ and folic acid, it has been possible to avoid nonspecific hematological responses to large doses of the vitamin which is not causing the deficiency. Thus, patients with Addisonian pernicious anemia will respond to as little as 1 mcg of B$_{12}$ daily by injection, but not to small "physiological" doses of folic acid (50–200 mcg daily); on the other hand, patients with megaloblastic anemia attributed to folate deficiency fail to respond to these small doses of B$_{12}$, but have an optimal response to small doses of folic acid (Fig. 8) (Marshall and Jandl, 1960; Chosy *et al.*, 1962b; Hansen and Weinfeld, 1962; Herbert, 1963; Thirkettle *et al.*, 1964; Waters, 1966).

Correlation with the results of other methods for assessing B$_{12}$ and folate deficiency indicates that a specific response to treatment with small doses of B$_{12}$ or folic acid provides evidence of the underlying deficiency. However, therapeutic trials are time-consuming, and can only be carried out on selected anemic patients who are not suffering from other conditions likely to interfere with a full hematological response, such as infection, renal disease or deficiency of other hematinics (e.g. iron). Furthermore, it provides no direct measure of the degree of deficiency.

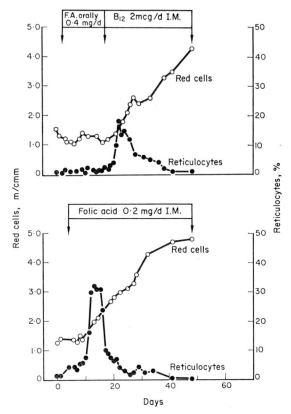

FIG. 8. Therapeutic trials using small doses of B_{12} and/or folic acid in two patients with megaloblastic anemia—one with pernicious anemia (upper response), the other with severe folate deficiency associated with idiopathic steatorrhoea (lower response).

(2) *Assay of B_{12} in serum*

(a) *Microbiological assay.* The development of a sensitive micro-biological assay for B_{12} using *Euglena gracilis* (Ross, 1950, 1952; Mollin and Ross, 1952, 1954, 1957; Lear *et al.*, 1954) or *Lactobacillus leichmanii* (Rosenthal and Sarett, 1952; Girdwood, 1954) made it possible to diagnose B_{12} deficiency directly by measuring the serum B_{12} concentration. Subsequent experience with these assays led to improvements in technique. An enriched assay medium and the use of a different "strain" of *Euglena gracilis* (z strain) led to a faster and more sensitive assay (Hutner *et al.*,

1956), and more recently Anderson (1964) has shown that the addition of a trace of serum of low B_{12} content to the standards will improve the reproducibility of the assay. In the *L. leichmanii* assay it was shown that the presence of cyanide increased the liberation of B_{12} from protein during the extraction of serum for assay, and this modification has improved the diagnostic value of the assay (Boger *et al.*, 1955; Spray, 1955; Killander, 1957; Girdwood, 1960; Matthews, 1962).

Patients with Addisonian pernicious anemia were found to have subnormal serum (see reviews: Mollin and Ross, 1957; Spray and Witts,

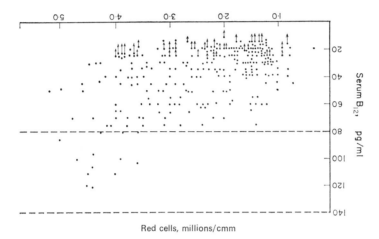

FIG. 9. The serum B_{12} concentrations of patients with Addisonian pernicious anemia plotted against the red cell count. The B_{12} concentrations of all the patients were subnormal (i.e. less than 140 pg/ml) and 96% had levels less than 80 pg/ml, which included all of the anemic patients with red cell counts less than 3.5 million/cmm. Modified from Fig. 8, Mollin (1959b).

1958) and tissue B_{12} levels (Girdwood, 1952; Ross and Mollin, 1957; Nelson and Doctor, 1958; Anderson, 1965), which established the presence of B_{12} deficiency in this condition. A more detailed analysis of the serum B_{12} levels in pernicious anemia is shown in Fig. 9, where the serum B_{12} level is plotted against the red cell count. While all of the anemic patients had B_{12} levels less than 80 pg/ml many of the non-anemic patients also had levels in this range. These latter patients often presented with neurological lesions (Fig. 10, Group 2). However, some patients were detected at an early non-anemic and asymptomatic stage of pernicious anemia as a result of careful examination of the blood film during routine clinical screening. The serum B_{12} levels of these patients, although subnormal, were often above the level found in overt pernicious anemia (Fig. 10, Group 1). Similar results were found in patients whose only symptom was glossitis (Fig. 10, Group 3). The serum B_{12} level is thus a sensitive index of B_{12} deficiency, and becomes subnormal long before the patient presents with overt megaloblastic anemia (Mollin, 1959b; Witts, 1960; Callender and Spray, 1962).

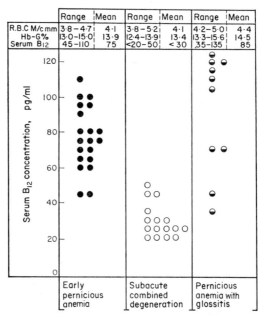

	Range	Mean	Range	Mean	Range	Mean
R.B.C M/c mm	3·8 – 4·7	4·1	3·8 – 5·2	4·1	4·2 – 5·0	4·4
Hb–G%	13·0–15·0	13·9	12·4–13·9	13·4	13·3–15·6	14·5
Serum B12	45–110	75	<20–50	< 30	35–135	85

FIG. 10. The serum B_{12} concentrations in (1) a group of patients with early pernicious anemia who were not anemic and not complaining of symptoms of B_{12} deficiency, (2) a group of patients with subacute combined degeneration of the cord without anemia, and (3) a group of non-anemic patients with pernicious anemia whose only symptom was glossitis. From Mollin (1959b).

Serum B_{12} concentrations similar in distribution to those seen in pernicious anemia are found in patients with megaloblastic anemia associated with (1) total or partial gastrectomy, although folate deficiency is occasionally the main cause following partial gastrectomy (Mollin and Ross, 1954; Badenoch *et al.*, 1955a; Mollin, 1962a; Deller and Witts, 1962; Waters,

1963; Deller *et al.*, 1964; Mollin and Hines, 1964; Gough *et al.*, 1965; Hines *et al.*, 1967); (2) anatomical lesions of the small intestine (Mollin and Ross, 1954; 1957; Meynell *et al.*, 1957; Booth and Mollin, 1960; (3) fish tapeworm (*Diphyllobothrium latum*) infestation (von Bonsdorff, 1956; Nyberg and Ostling, 1956; Gräsbeck *et al.*, 1962); and (4) some patients with chronic tropical sprue (Mollin, 1962a; Booth and Mollin, 1964).

Serum B$_{12}$ levels below the normal range, but usually above the range found in pernicious anemia, occur in atrophic gastritis (Callender *et al.*, 1960; Glass *et al.*, 1960; Siurala *et al.*, 1960; Whiteside *et al.*, 1964), idiopathic steatorrhoea (Mollin and Ross, 1954; Meynell *et al.*, 1957; Spray and Witts, 1958), and during pregnancy (Heinrich, 1954; Mollin and Ross, 1954; Lowenstein *et al.*, 1955, 1966; Boger *et al.*, 1957; Spray and Witts, 1958; Ball and Giles, 1964; Chanarin *et al.*, 1965; Giles, 1966). The levels may be subnormal even in non-anemic patients with these conditions, and although megaloblastic anemia is common (except in atrophic gastritis), this is due to folate deficiency, and not to B$_{12}$ deficiency.

Subnormal serum B$_{12}$ levels also occur in another group of patients, viz., those who present with *severe* megaloblastic anemia due to folate deficiency (Mollin and Ross, 1954, 1957; Mollin *et al.*, 1962; Johnson *et al.*, 1962; Waters, 1963). Although subnormal, these levels are usually higher than in pernicious anemia of comparable severity (Mollin and Ross, 1957), and their precise significance as an index of B$_{12}$ deficiency is uncertain. Most of the patients in this group either fail to respond, or respond slowly and incompletely to treatment with B$_{12}$, but have an optimal response to folic acid, even in small doses (Fig. 11). In many cases, the serum B$_{12}$ level increases rapidly to within the normal range on treatment with folic acid alone (Mollin and Ross, 1957; Mollin *et al.*, 1962; Johnson *et al.*, 1962; Waters, 1963), whereas in pure B$_{12}$ deficiency the serum B$_{12}$ level remains unchanged or falls when folic acid is given (Mollin and Ross, 1953; Lear and Castle, 1956; Will *et al.*, 1959). The explanation for this is uncertain. In some cases it may be due partly to improvement in B$_{12}$ absorption following folic acid therapy, which has been reported in acute tropical sprue (O'Brien and England, 1966). However, this does not appear to be the full explanation, for in many cases no significant change in B$_{12}$ absorption is found. Furthermore, recent observations on the B$_{12}$ content of liver biopsy specimens (Anderson, 1965), and on the urinary excretion of methylmalonic acid (Brozovic *et al.*, 1967) in such patients (see p. 33) suggest that these low serum B$_{12}$ levels do not necessarily reflect the tissue

B*

B_{12} stores. It is possible that in severe folate deficiency the low levels of methyl-folate in serum and liver (Waters, 1963) impair the formation of methyl-B_{12} (Lindstrand *et al.*, 1967), which is the main serum B_{12} component (see p. 5), leaving most of the B_{12} in the form of adenosyl-B_{12}

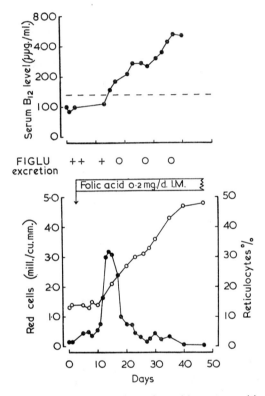

FIG. 11. Therapeutic response of a patient with severe nutritional megaloblastic anemia due to folate deficiency to 200 mcg of folic acid daily by injection. The red cell count is indicated by the open circles, and the reticulocyte count by the closed circles. The effect of this treatment on the serum B_{12} concentration and the urinary excretion of formimino-glutamic acid (FIGlu) after histidine loading is also shown. From Waters (1963).

which is the main liver B_{12} component (see p. 5). Treatment with folic acid might then facilitate the conversion of adenosyl-B_{12} in the liver to methyl-B_{12}, leading to a rise in the serum B_{12} level.

To summarize, the serum B_{12} assay is an extremely reliable method for diagnosing B_{12} deficiency. In fact, the assay is perhaps the single most useful test in the differential diagnosis of megaloblastic anemia, in that it serves not only to diagnose B_{12} deficiency, but also allows a diagnosis of folate deficiency to be made with reasonable certainty in many cases. Thus, if a patient with megaloblastic anemia has a normal serum B_{12} level, he is by exclusion suffering from folate deficiency. A firm diagnosis of folate deficiency can also be made if the serum B_{12} level is subnormal providing (1) the level is above that found in pernicious anemia of similar severity, and (2) the patient responds to treatment with physiological doses of folic acid. A rise in the subnormal serum B_{12} level after folic acid therapy will confirm the diagnosis of folate deficiency.

(b) *Radioisotope assay.** A radioisotope method has been introduced as a possible alternative to microbiological assay. In principle, a known amount of radioactive-B_{12} is added to serum. The B_{12} already present in the serum will dilute the added radioactive-B_{12}, and the aim of the assay is to determine this dilution factor, from which the amount of B_{12} serum can be calculated. As pointed out previously, most of the B_{12} in serum is protein-bound (p. 7), and the first stage is to "free" the bound B_{12} giving rise to a homogenous mixture of "cold" and radioactive-B_{12}. A source of B_{12} binder is added to "biopsy" a representative sample of this mixture. The "bound" B_{12} is then separated from the "free" B_{12} by various methods such as dialysis (Barakat and Ekins, 1961), ultrafiltration (Friedner et al., 1969), gel filtration (Mantzos et al., 1967), adsorption of the "free" B_{12} onto protein coated charcoal (Lau et al., 1965), precipitation of the binder (Rothenberg, 1961), or removal of the binder by ion-exchangers (Frenkel et al., 1966; Roos, 1970). The radioactivity of the "free" and/or "bound" fractions is measured. By comparison with cyanocobalamin standards, treated in the same way as the test serum, the dilution factor can be estimated and the B_{12} concentration of the test serum calculated.

Over 20 methods have been described. Some use human serum, either from normal subjects (Barakat and Ekins, 1961, 1963; Grossowicz et al., 1962; Ekins and Sgherzi, 1965; Frenkel et al., 1966; Mantzos et al., 1967; Matthews et al., 1967; Roos, 1970), or from patients with chronic myeloid leukemia (Rothenberg, 1968); others use intrinsic factor as the B_{12} binding agent (Rothenberg, 1961, 1963; Lau et al., 1935; Herbert et al., 1966;

---

*The authors wish to acknowledge the valuable help of Dr. P. Newmark in the preparation of this section.

Raven *et al.*, 1966, 1969; Friedner, 1969; Rubini, 1970). In addition, human saliva (Carmel and Coltman, 1969), purified hog pylorus protein (Puntula *et al.*, 1969), and chicken serum (Green *et al.*, 1969) have also been suggested as suitable B_{12} binding proteins for radioisotope assays.

Most of these methods show a general overall correlation with standard microbiological methods, but in the most critical assessment of the method so far published, the results obtained by radioisotope assay have been generally higher than those by microbiological assay (Raven *et al.*, 1969), a finding which has been confirmed in this laboratory (Green, Musso and Newmark, unpublished observations). In addition there is evidence that in certain conditions, particularly after partial gastrectomy, there can be a marked discrepancy between microbiological and radioisotope assays (Raven *et al.*, 1969).

The radioisotope method thus provides the first rapid (in hours instead of days) B_{12} assay, a feature which has obvious clinical advantages, and also avoids the interference by antibiotics which may be a pitfall in microbiological techniques. There is, however, still considerable room for improvement and standardization of radioisotope methods. One might, for example, improve reproducibility and precision by increasing the homogeneity of the B_{12}-binding agent used and by paying more attention to the conditions under which the "biopsy" takes place. In addition the speed of the assay might be increased even further by making use of tubes coated with B_{12}-binding agent in order to simplify the separation of "free" from "bound" B_{12} (Rubini, 1970). However, it remains to be seen whether radioisotope methods will replace the familiar and reliable microbiological methods.

(3) *Assay of B_{12} in red cells*. Microbiological (Sobotka *et al.*, 1960; Biggs *et al.*, 1964) and radioisotope dilution methods (Kelly and Herbert 1967) have also been used to measure red cell B_{12} concentrations. However, this investigation is less helpful than the serum B_{12} level in diagnosing B_{12} deficiency, because there is a considerable overlap in the red cell B_{12} levels of patients with megaloblastic anemia due to B_{12} or folate deficiency. A similar overlap is also found in the red cell folate levels of such patients (Hansen and Weinfeld, 1962; Cooper and Lowenstein, 1964; Hoffbrand *et al.*, 1966).

(4) *Urinary methylmalonic acid excretion*. Adenosyl-B_{12} is required as a coenzyme in the conversion of methylmalonyl-CoA to succinyl-CoA (see Table 1, Reaction 2), the last step in the propionate-succinate meta-

bolic pathway (Fig. 12), and methylmalonic acid may accumulate in B$_{12}$-dependent bacteria and in animals rendered B$_{12}$ deficient (Arnstein and Simkin, 1959; Marston *et al.*, 1961; Arnstein and White, 1962). This reaction was first demonstrated in man by Cox and White (1962), who showed that patients with pernicious anemia excreted an abnormal metabolite in their urine, which was identified as methylmalonic acid (MMA). Other workers using a variety of different methods have confirmed and extended these observations (Barness *et al.*, 1963a; Giorgio and Plaut, 1965; Kahn *et al.*, 1965; Bashir *et al.*, 1966; Holmberg *et al.*, 1966; Vivacqua *et al.*, 1966; Brozovic *et al.*, 1967).

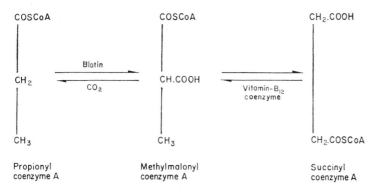

FIG. 12. Metabolic pathway for the conversion of propionyl CoA to succinyl CoA via methylmalonyl CoA, showing the site of action of coenzyme B$_{12}$. From Brozovic *et al.* (1967).

The recent observations of Brozovic *et al.* (1967) show that there is a correlation between urinary MMA excretion and the serum B$_{12}$ level in uncomplicated B$_{12}$ deficiency (Fig. 13). However, when subnormal serum B$_{12}$ levels were associated with iron or folate deficiency, MMA excretion was often normal, and if increased, tended to be lower than in patients with pernicious anemia who had similar serum B$_{12}$ levels. In particular, it was of interest that MMA excretion was invariably normal in patients with severe folate deficiency who also had subnormal serum B$_{12}$ levels. As mentioned previously (p. 29), these patients respond completely to treatment with small "physiological" doses of folic acid, and on this treatment alone the serum B$_{12}$ level returns to normal. These observations suggest that in these patients the tissue B$_{12}$ stores are not critically depleted, thus confirming the findings of Anderson (1965), that the liver B_{12} levels of such patients are higher than in patients with primary B_{12} deficiency who have comparable serum B_{12} levels.

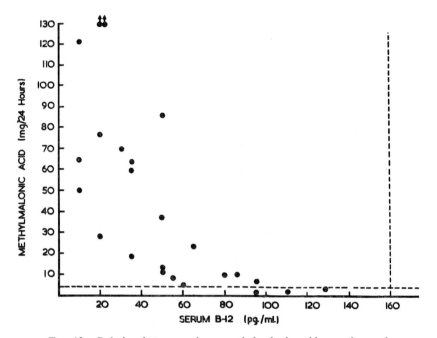

FIG. 13. Relation between urinary methylmalonic acid excretion and the serum B_{12} concentration in patients with uncomplicated B_{12} deficiency. The horizontal broken line indicates the upper limit of normal MMA excretion, and the vertical broken line the lower limit of the normal serum B_{12} concentration. All of the patients with increased MMA excretion had serum B_{12} levels less than 100 pg/ml, and most had levels less than 80 pg/ml, which are the levels found in overt pernicious anemia (see Fig. 9).
Modified from Fig. 2, Brozovic *et al.* (1967).

It has been shown by Gompertz *et al.*, (1967), that the urinary MMA excretion may be increased in patients with B_{12} deficiency by giving a loading dose of valine, and to a lesser extent by loading with isoleucine and sodium propionate, which are all metabolized through MMA. Thymine has also been shown to produce a ten-fold increase in MMA excretion in a patient with pernicious anemia (Lord, 1968—personal communication), and similar results have been produced in B_{12}-deficient rats

(Barness *et al.*, 1963b; Williams, 1968). These observations suggest the possibility of a loading test for B$_{12}$ deficiency similar to the histidine loading (FIGlu excretion) test for folate deficiency.

The measurement of urinary MMA has had limited clinical application, because the methods are in general too complicated. However, semi-quantitative results can be obtained with colorimetric (Giorgio and Plaut, 1965) and thin-layer chromatographic methods (Bashir *et al.*,1966), and this may bring the measurement of urinary MMA within the scope of the routine diagnostic laboratory.

MEASUREMENT OF B$_{12}$ ABSORPTION

Measurement of B$_{12}$ absorption in patients with megaloblastic anemia helps to define the underlying clinical syndrome. The introduction of radioactive-B$_{12}$ has greatly facilitated the measurement of B$_{12}$ absorption and brought it within the scope of clinical medicine.

(1) *Radioactive-B$_{12}$*

(a) *Cobalt isotopes of B$_{12}$.* These isotopes are compared in Table 4. The biological half-life of B$_{12}$ is approximately one year (Schloesser *et al.*, 1958), so it is important that the radiation dose delivered by the labeling isotope should be small. ^{60}Co delivers a relatively high radiation dose to the liver, and is therefore undesirable for radioactive-B$_{12}$ tracer studies in man. On the other hand, the radiation dose due to the other three Co-isotopes is low, and of these ^{57}Co and ^{58}Co are readily available for

TABLE 4. RADIOACTIVE ISOTOPES OF COBALT

Isotope	Half-life	Comparative liver dose	Counting efficiency		
			Geiger-Müller counter	Well-type scintillation counter	Whole-body counter
^{60}Co	5.27 years	28	Good	Good	Good
^{56}Co	77.3 days	4	Good	Good	Good
^{58}Co	71 days	2	Good	Good	Good
^{57}Co	267 days	1	Poor	Very good	Poor

labeling B_{12} for routine clinical studies. ^{58}Co can be counted efficiently in all types of counters and is therefore the most suitable label for general use. ^{57}Co is unsuitable for use with Geiger-Müller counters, but ideally suited for well-type scintillation counters (Rosenblum, 1960, 1962a).

(b) *Stability of radioactive-B_{12}.* Great care must be taken in the handling and storage of radioactive-B_{12}. Mollin and Baker (1955) first drew attention to errors that might arise from the instability of aqueous solutions of radioactive-B_{12}, and the need for care in the handling of such solutions has been emphasized by subsequent workers (Lester Smith, 1959; Rosenblum, 1962b). Radiation-induced decomposition can be satisfactorily reduced, even at high specific activities, by the addition of 0.9% benzyl alcohol (Bayly and Evans, 1966). Furthermore, as B_{12} is photosensitive, it should be protected from light during storage, and it is also essential to avoid bacterial contamination.

(c) *Availability of radioactive-B_{12}.* Radioactive-B_{12} is available commercially either freeze-dried or in aqueous solution containing benzyl alcohol. The radiochemical purity of labeled B_{12} is determined for each batch by reverse isotope dilution and electrophoretic analysis, and this information is usually provided with each consignment. However, if unexpected results are obtained with a particular consignment, the radiochemical purity should be checked. Microbiological assay with *Euglena gracilis* or *Lactobacillus leichmanii* will demonstrate gross discrepancies in the B_{12} content of the solution.

(2) Procedure

The measurement of B_{12} absorption is essentially a two-stage procedure. The test is first carried out by giving the patient a small oral dose of radioactive B_{12} alone. If the patient fails to absorb B_{12} normally, the test must then be repeated with the addition of intrinsic factor.

(a) *Oral dose.* Single doses of between 0.5 and 2.0 mcg of radioactive-B_{12} have been used for the oral test dose. We have found a dose of 1 mcg labeled with 0.5–1 mcc of ^{58}Co or ^{57}Co to be most convenient. These are conveniently available as single doses in ampoules or in gelatin capsules. ^{57}Co is the most suitable label if urinary and plasma radioactivity are to be measured by scintillation counting. ^{58}Co-B_{12} is preferable if whole-body radioactivity is to be measured.

(b) *Intrinsic factor.* Ideally, normal human gastric juice should be used as a source of intrinsic factor, but in practice it is often more convenient to use commercially available B_{12}-free hog intrinsic factor concentrate (HIFC). The dose of HIFC should be large enough to produce maximal possible absorption from the particular dose of B_{12} used. This is the dose usually recommended by the manufacturer, and single doses in gelatin capsules may be obtained. It is advisable to obtain enough of the same batch of HIFC for many tests, so as to ensure strict comparibility of results.

(3) *Methods*

The absorption of B_{12} can be assessed by one of the following methods:

> Fecal excretion method
>
> Hepatic uptake method
>
> Whole-body radioactivity method
>
> Urinary excretion method (Schilling test)
>
> Plasma radioactivity method

The first three methods enable the amount of B_{12} absorbed to be measured, whereas the last two provide only indirect evidence of absorption, but are nevertheless most useful for clinical purposes. It is essential that these tests should be carried out on a fasting subject. In practice the patient fasts from 10 p.m. and the dose of radioactive-B_{12} is given at 8 a.m. the following morning. No food or fluids are allowed for 2 hr after the dose. A light breakfast may then be taken.

Technical details of the above methods have been described in full by Doscherholmen (1965) and Mollin and Waters (1968a, 1970), and we shall confine the present account to discussion of the principles of these methods and the significance of the results obtained in different clinical syndromes.

(a) *Fecal excretion method.* (Heinle *et al.*, 1952). The test dose of 1 mcg (0.5–1.0 mcc) radioactive-vitamin B_{12} is given by mouth and the amount excreted in the feces is measured. The difference between the amount excreted and the amount given is considered to be the amount absorbed. Patients with pernicious anemia absorb less than 30% of the test dose, and usually less than 20%; normal subjects absorb more than 50% of the dose (Mollin *et al.*, 1957).

The advantage of this method is that the amount of vitamin B_{12} absorbed can be measured directly. The disadvantage is that stools may have to be collected for periods of up to six or seven days. Furthermore, if the collection is incomplete, it appears as if the patient had absorbed vitamin B_{12}, an error that may lead to mis-diagnosis. It is doubtful if the method should be used for diagnostic purposes unless the results are checked by the hepatic uptake method or by concurrent measurement of plasma radioactivity (see below).

"Snatch" methods have been suggested as a means for overcoming the need for a complete stool collection. In the method described by Ganatra *et al.* (1965), a labeled unabsorbable marker (^{51}Cr-labeled chromic oxide) is administered orally with ^{58}Co-B_{12}. The ratio of the two isotopes in the test dose is compared with the ratio of these two isotopes in a random stool sample. Any change in the ratio is assumed to be due to absorption of B_{12}, and from this the amount of B_{12} absorbed can be calculated. So far this method has not proved satisfactory in our hands (Brozovic and Mollin, 1965, unpublished data).

(b) *Hepatic uptake method* (Glass *et al.*, 1954a, 1954b). A dose of radioactive-B_{12} is given by mouth, and after all the unabsorbed radioactivity has been excreted the radioactivity that accumulates in the liver can be detected by surface scintillation counting. The amount of B_{12} absorbed can be calculated by comparing the hepatic radioactivity after the oral dose with the increase in radioactivity produced by a subsequent injection of a known amount of radioactive-B_{12}. A disadvantage of this method is that it requires two successive periods of at least one week each before results are available. During this time the patient's condition may change and thereby affect the results. However, this disadvantage has been largely overcome by using a double isotope technique (Weisberg and Glass, 1966). In a single procedure, the hepatic uptake of an oral dose of ^{60}Co-B_{12} can be compared with that of a simultaneous intravenous dose of ^{57}Co-B_{12} by correcting for the different counting characteristics of the two cobalt isotopes. Using this modification, results can often be obtained as early as 48 hr after the test dose.

The main disadvantage of the method is that an injection of radioactive-B_{12} is required to enable the amount of B_{12} absorbed to be calculated. However, the test can be used on a qualitative basis without the injection, and serves as a valuable check on the results of the fecal excretion method. The great advantage of the hepatic uptake method lies in the fact that it is not dependent on the collection of excreta.

(c) *Whole-body radioactivity method.* This method, in contrast to the fecal excretion method, measures the radioactivity retained in the body after an oral test dose, thereby giving a direct measure of the amount of radioactivity absorbed. It thus obviates the need for a fecal collection, and all the uncertainties associated with this.

An initial measurement on the patient is essential before any radio-activity is given ("patient" background). A test dose of ^{58}Co-B$_{12}$ (1 mcg/1 mcc) is given by mouth, and a second measurement taken; this value, less the patient's background, corresponds to 100% retention of the dose. About a week later, when all the unabsorbed radioactivity has been excreted, the patient's radioactivity is again measured. The retained activity can now be calculated as a percentage of the administered dose. All measurements are referred to a standard to allow for instrumental variation and physical decay.

Where whole-body counters are available this is undoubtedly the best method for measuring B$_{12}$ absorption (International Atomic Energy Agency, 1966). Clinical application of the counter described by Warner and Oliver (1966) has been reported by Callender *et al.* (1966).

(d) *Urinary excretion method of Schilling* (1953). In this method 1 or 2 mcg of radioactive-B$_{12}$ is given by mouth and an injection of 1000 mcg of non-radioactive-B$_{12}$ is given at the same time or soon after. This injection flushes out about one-third of the absorbed radioactive-B$_{12}$ into the urine (Callender and Evans, 1955). A *repeat test* can be carried out three days after the first test, provided that a second injection of 1000 mcg of non-radioactive-B$_{12}$ is given to the patient 24 hr after the first test dose to flush out any residual radioactive-B$_{12}$ that can be mobilized (Ellenbogen *et al.*, 1955). The results of the Schilling test in pernicious anemia and other conditions are discussed on p. 41, where we consider the clinical interpretation of radioactive-B$_{12}$ absorption tests.

The Schilling test requires collection of urine for only 24 hr, and an error due to incomplete collection will not mask malabsorption of vitamin B$_{12}$. Its main disadvantages are that the patient has to be treated with large doses of vitamin B$_{12}$, and the results may be inaccurate in serious renal disease (Miller *et al.*, 1957b; Rath *et al.*, 1957). It is the method of choice in the patient who is already being treated with B$_{12}$.

(d') *Modifications of the Schilling test.* A modified test has been introduced by Ellenbogen *et al.*, (1955), who used an oral dose of 2 mcg of radioactive-B$_{12}$ and collected urine for 48 hr. Two flushing injections were given—one at the beginning of the test and the other 24 hr later. The results of the 48-hr test are statistically more reproducible than those of the standard 24-hr test. The longer test is therefore valuable for comparative studies, especially for the assessment of the potency of different intrinsic factor preparations.

A double-isotope modification of Schilling's original test has been described which combines the two stages of the test into a single diagnostic procedure (Katz *et al.*, 1963; Bell *et al.*, 1965; Bayly *et al.*, 1969). This depends on the widely different scintillation spectra of ^{57}Co and ^{58}Co, which make it possible to measure these isotopes separately in a mixture of the two, by scintillation spectrometry. The two isotopes of B_{12} are given to the patient simultaneously, one free and the other previously bound to intrinsic factor. Normal subjects excrete equal amounts of the two isotopes in the urine after a flushing dose of unlabeled B_{12}, whereas patients with pernicious anemia excrete significantly more of the bound isotope than of the isotope which was free when administered. Patients with intestinal malabsorption of B_{12} excrete equal, but subnormal amounts of the two isotopes.

(e) *Plasma radioactivity method* (Booth and Mollin, 1956; Doscher-holmen and Hagen, 1956; Doscherholmen, 1962; Woodliff and Armstrong, 1966; Forshaw and Harwood, 1966; Harwood and Forshaw, 1967). In this method the radioactivity of plasma is measured at intervals after the oral dose. In normal subjects, there is an increase in plasma radioactivity 3 hr after the dose which rises to a peak at 8–12 hr. There is little or no alteration in the plasma radioactivity of patients with pernicious anemia unless the dose is given with intrinsic factor (Fig. 14).

The amount of absorbed vitamin B_{12} present in the plasma of even normal subjects after physiological doses of vitamin B_{12} is small, peak levels being only about 10 pg/ml (Booth and Mollin, 1956). The amount of radioactivity in the serum is therefore small, and initially ^{56}Co-vitamin B_{12} of high specific activity was used for this test. However, the changes in plasma radioactivity after a standard test dose (1.0 mcg ^{58}Co or ^{57}Co-vitamin B_{12}, specific activity 0.5–1.0 mcc) can easily be measured with modern equipment (Doscherholmen, 1962).

The method is simple, does not depend on the collection of excreta and allows a result to be obtained within 8–12 hr of giving the oral dose. The test is particularly helpful in bedridden or incontinent patients, or when tests have to be carried out on patients at a distance. In the latter case, a sample of serum can be sent to a central laboratory with suitable radio-isotope counting equipment.

The plasma radioactivity method does not measure the amount of B_{12} absorbed, but if used in conjunction with fecal excretion or whole-body methods, it provides a quick assessment of B_{12} absorption while waiting for the result of the actual amount absorbed.

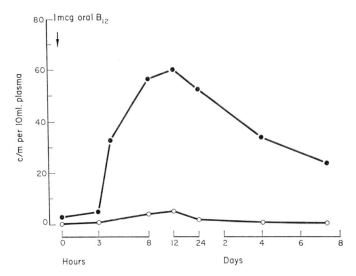

FIG. 14. Plasma radioactivity after an oral dose of 1 mcg. ^{56}Co-B_{12} given to a patient with pernicious anemia, with (●—●) and without (○—○) the addition of intrinsic actor. From Booth and Mollin, (1956).

(4) *Clinical interpretation of radioactive-B_{12} absorption tests*

As mentioned previously, B_{12} malabsorption develops long before the onset of B_{12} deficiency, and the deficiency is often present for years before such patients develop megaloblastic anemia. In fact, absorption tests with radioactive-B_{12} may provide the first evidence for impaired gastric or intestinal function. The diagnostic application of radioactive-B_{12} absorption tests is summarized in Table 5. These tests have their most useful application in the diagnosis of pernicious anemia, but they are also useful for demonstrating intestinal malabsorption of B_{12} even in the absence of other evidence of the intestinal malabsorption syndrome.

In the diagnosis of pernicious anemia, the Schilling test is probably most widely used in clinical medicine, and we propose to discuss the diagnostic

TABLE 5. DIAGNOSTIC APPLICATION OF RADIOACTIVE B_{12} ABSORPTION TESTS[a]

Method	Nutritional megaloblastic anemia	Pernicious anemia	Total gastrectomy	Partial gastrectomy	Loop syndrome	Idiopathic steatorrhoea	Tropical sprue
Dose alone	normal	subnormal	subnormal	subnormal	subnormal	50% of patients subnormal	subnormal
Dose with I.F.	normal	improvement	improvement	improvement	no improvement	no improvement	no improvement
Dose after antibiotics	normal	—	—	—	improvement if the ileum is intact	no improvement	improvement in many

[a] From Mollin (1962b).

interpretation of results obtained with this method. Normal subjects and healthy hospital controls given an oral dose of 1 mcg of radioactive-B$_{12}$ excrete 10% or more of the administered radioactivity in 24 hr, whereas patients with pernicious anemia excrete less than 5% and usually less than 3% of the dose. Patients with atrophic gastritis or the intestinal malabsorption syndrome may have results in the pernicious anemia range, but border-line results between 5 and 10% are also found. If a patient excretes 5% or less of the administered radioactivity in 24 hr, the test should be repeated with the addition of intrinsic factor to the dose of radioactive-B$_{12}$.

The significance of results falling between 3 and 5% is sometimes very difficult to interpret. As pointed out above, these levels may be found in some patients with pernicious anemia, but are more common in the intestinal malabsorption syndrome, and in patients with atrophic gastritis who may have no evidence of B$_{12}$ deficiency. In assessing the significance of such results the use of parasympathetic stimulants like carbachol or histamine may be valuable (Baker and Mollin, 1955; Ardeman *et al.*, 1964).

The maximum urinary excretion in patients with pernicious anemia following a 1 mcg test dose of B$_{12}$ with intrinsic factor is usually 10–15%, but results between 6 and 20% may be found. In practice, we take an increase in excretion of 3% of a 1 mcg dose as being significant in a patient whose initial absorption was in the pernicious anemia range. Very rarely the actual increase may be as little as 2 or 3%, and in these patients interpretation of the results is very difficult. This poor improvement may be due to technical errors (Mollin and Waters, 1968a, 1968b), but is often related to differences in the patients themselves. Sometimes a cause can be found for this. For example, the patient may have previously received hog intrinsic factor and become resistant to this material (Schwartz *et al.*, 1958; Lowenstein *et al.*, 1961; Ramsey and Herbert, 1965; Gullberg *et al.*, 1966), or the patient's gastric juice and intestinal secretions may contain an antibody to the B$_{12}$-IF complex which inhibits the intestinal absorption of B$_{12}$ (Schade *et al.*, 1966, 1967; Cooper and Yates, 1967). On the other hand, there may be unexpected bacterial contamination associated with single or multiple jejunal diverticula, or with an afferent blind loop following partial gastrectomy (Mollin and Hines, 1964; Tabaqchali *et al.*, 1966).

Defective intestinal absorption of B$_{12}$ occurs in all patients with B$_{12}$-deficient megaloblastic anemia associated with anatomical lesions of the small intestine (Table 6). Malabsorption may be present in the absence of anemia in such patients, and this is certainly the case if the ileum has been

resected or by-passed, (Booth and Mollin, 1959; Booth *et al.*, 1964), or
if there is heavy bacterial contamination due to stagnation associated with
blind loops, strictures, fistulae, or diverticula (Badenoch, *et al.*, 1955b;
Halsted *et al.*, 1956; Mollin *et al.*, 1957; Scudamore *et al.*, 1958; Cooke
et al., 1963; Donaldson, 1964, 1965; Mollin and Hines, 1964; Paulk and
Farrar, 1964; Barrett and Holt, 1966; Tabaqchali *et al.*, 1966; Tabaqchali
and Booth, 1967). Malabsorption of B_{12} is almost invariably found in
patients with acute or chronic tropical sprue (Booth and Mollin, 1964;
O'Brien and England, 1964, 1966).

TABLE 6. ABSORPTION OF ^{58}CO-B_{12} BY PATIENTS WITH MEGALOBLASTIC ANEMIA DUE
TO MALABSORPTION SYNDROME[a]

Condition	Number of patients studied (1)	Number (percentage) of patients with results in P.A. range (2)	Percentage of dose[b] absorbed by patients in (2)	
			Range (3)	Mean (4)
Anatomical lesions of small intestine	44	44 (100%)	0–27	8
Idiopathic steatorrhoea	55	32 (58%)	0–28	12
Tropical sprue	8	7 (89%)	0–19	9

[a] From: Mollin (1962c).
[b] Oral test dose: 1 mcg ^{58}Co-B_{12}. Normal subjects absorb more than 50% of this
dose, and patients with pernicious anemia absorb less than 30%.

On the other hand, malabsorption of B_{12} occurs in only 50–60% of
patients with idiopathic steatorrhoea (Table 6; and Mollin *et al.*, 1959).
In pancreatic steatorrhoea, the incidence of malabsorption of B_{12} appears
to be directly related to the severity of the lesion. If this is severe enough
to cause changes in the pH of the lower intestinal contents, there is defective absorption of B_{12} which may be improved by the administration of
bicarbonate and pancreatin or secretin (Perman *et al.*, 1960; Veeger *et al.*,
1962; Glass, 1965).

Administration of intrinsic factor does not improve B_{12} absorption in
patients with intestinal lesions. However, there may be an improvement
in absorption after specific treatment, and this may be of diagnostic value.
Thus, the absorption of B_{12} may return to normal in patients with idiopathic steatorrhoea treated with a gluten-free diet (Mollin *et al.*, 1957).

Treatment with broad-spectrum antibiotics will improve absorption in patients with anatomical lesions of the small intestine associated with heavy bacterial contamination, providing the absorptive surface of the ileum is intact or has not been by-passed (see previous references, p. 44). Treatment with folic acid will improve the absorption of B$_{12}$ in acute tropical sprue (O'Briens and England, 1966), but may be ineffective in patients with chronic tropical sprue (Booth and Mollin, 1964). In these latter patients absorption is usually improved, albeit slowly, by treatment with antibiotics, which will also improve the absorption in acute tropical sprue (French *et al.*, 1956; Sheehy and Perez-Santiago, 1961; Booth and Mollin, 1964; Klipstein, 1964a,b; Klipstein *et al.*, 1966; O'Brien and England, 1966).

VITAMIN-B$_{12}$ THERAPY

In a recent review Castle (1966) has traced the improvements in the treatment of pernicious anemia from the liver meals of Minot and Murphy (1926), through the various liver fractions for oral and parenteral use, to the isolation of crystalline cyanocobalamin in 1948.

Parenteral cyanocobalamin and hydroxocobalamin

Today, pernicious anemia and other B$_{12}$ deficiency syndromes are most commonly treated by intramuscular injections of cyanocobalamin. However, the body is very uneconomical in its handling of large parenteral doses of cyanocobalamin (CN-B$_{12}$). Less than 10% of a parenteral dose of 20 mcg of CN-B$_{12}$ is excreted in the urine, but approximately 50% of a dose of 100 mcg, and 90% of a dose of 1000 mcg is excreted (Fig. 15). Hydroxocobalamin (OH-B$_{12}$), on the other hand, is better retained in the body than CN-B$_{12}$ (Fig. 15), owing to its strong binding to proteins (Bauriedel *et al.*, 1956; Skeggs *et al.*, 1960; Meyer *et al.*, 1963; Hertz *et al.*, 1964). Thus after a large parenteral dose, OH-B$_{12}$ is retained longer at the site of the injection, produces a more sustained rise in the serum B$_{12}$ level, and results in a smaller short-term urinary loss than an equivalent dose of CN-B$_{12}$ (Glass *et al.*, 1961a,b; Glass and Lee, 1966a,b; Killander and Schilling, 1961; Heinrich and Gabbe, 1962; Shearman *et al.*, 1965). Moreover, since OH-B$_{12}$ appears to have the same hemopoietic effects as CN-B$_{12}$ (Lichtman *et al.*, 1949; Schilling *et al.*, 1951; Ungley, 1951), a case can be made out for the use of OH-B$_{12}$ in preference to CN-B$_{12}$ in the treatment of pernicious anemia (Bourne *et al.*, 1964; Withey and Kilpatrick, 1964; Adams and Kennedy, 1965; Chalmers and Shinton,

1965). Thus, OH-B$_{12}$ has the theoretical advantage that it will probably replenish the tissue stores of B$_{12}$ more rapidly than an equivalent dose of CN-B$_{12}$, and when used in large doses has the advantage of prolonging the intervals between maintenance injections. Furthermore, OH-B$_{12}$ may have an advantage over CN-B$_{12}$ in treating the neurological complications of B$_{12}$ deficiency. However, the evidence for this is still tentative and is

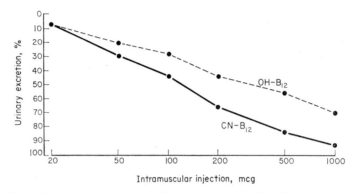

FIG. 15. Comparison of the urinary excretion of radioactivity (as a percentage of the injected dose) in normal subjects after intramuscular injections of 20–1000 mcg of ^{60}Co-labeled-cyanocobalamin (CN-B$_{12}$) and ^{60}Co-labeled-hydroxocobalamin (OH-B$_{12}$) respectively. Each point represents the mean value for 10 subjects. Modified from Fig. 3, Heinrich (1964).

related to the fact that OH-B$_{12}$ is readily converted to CN-B$_{12}$ in the presence of cyanide, which may cause neurological damage in B$_{12}$ deficiency (Smith, 1961; Wokes and Smith, 1961; Wilson and Langman, 1966), and in tobacco amblyopia (Heaton *et al.*, 1958; Wokes, 1958; Smith, 1961; Smith and Duckett, 1965; Lindstrand *et al.*, 1966; Wilson and Matthews, 1966; Chisholm *et al.*, 1967; Foulds *et al.*, 1968, 1969, 1970).

Coenzyme B$_{12}$

Like hydroxocobalamin, coenzyme B$_{12}$ is better retained in the body after parenteral administration than an equivalent dose of cyanocobalamin (Heinrich and Gabbe, 1964; Herbert and Sullivan, 1964; Uchino *et al.*, 1964). Preliminary therapeutic trials in patients with uncomplicated pernicious anemia suggest that in very small doses (0.1 mcg) coenzyme B$_{12}$ may be more potent than cyanocobalamin (Herbert and Sullivan, 1964;

Sullivan and Herbert, 1965). However, further studies are necessary to define the place of coenzyme B_{12} in the treatment of B_{12} deficiency syndromes. Furthermore, coenzyme B_{12} is very unstable, and is rapidly converted to hydroxocobalamin on exposure to light and oxygen. This could make it difficult to provide large quantities of coenzyme B_{12} for therapeutic purposes.

Dosage

A significant, though suboptimal, hematological response can be initiated in a patient with pernicious anemia with as little as 0.1 mcg of cyanocobalamin daily by injection (Sullivan and Herbert, 1965). However, to achieve a complete hematological remission a dose of the order of 1 mcg daily is required. This dose of B_{12} will not produce a hematological response in a patient with folate-deficient megaloblastic anemia, and is the basis of the procedure of therapeutic trial discussed previously.

In routine clinical practice larger doses of B_{12} are used, the therapeutic regime depending largely on the individual physician. The initial treatment should aim at restoring the depleted tissue reserves of B_{12} and thereafter enough B_{12} should be given to maintain the serum B_{12} level within the normal range. In the case of CN-B_{12} we have found it convenient in uncomplicated pernicious anemia to initiate therapy with weekly injections of 100–200 mcg of cyanocobalamin until the blood count is normal, and thereafter to continue monthly injections for life. If OH-B_{12} is used, it will lead to better replacement of the depleted body stores during initial therapy, and thereafter an injection of 1000 mcg of OH-B_{12} every two months will provide adequate maintenance therapy (Glass *et al.*, 1963; Chalmers and Shinton, 1965; also see Adams, 1962; Adams and Kennedy, 1965; Herbert *et al.*, 1963). Ideally, patients should be seen at least every six months for routine blood counts and clinical examination.

It is usually believed that larger doses of B_{12} are necessary in patients with neurological complications, but there is no definite evidence for this belief. However, as mentioned above, it is possible that OH-B_{12} may have an advantage over CN-B_{12} in patients with the neurological complications of B_{12} deficiency, and is recommended as the treatment of choice in tobacco amblyopia and Leber's hereditary optic atrophy (Chisholm *et al.*, 1967; Foulds *et al.*, 1968, 1970).

Other B_{12} preparations

Other preparations which have been advocated from time to time will be considered briefly. Some of these may be used under special circumstances, but in general they are less satisfactory and often more expensive than parenteral B_{12}.

Oral Cyanocobalamin in relatively large daily doses of 500 mcg or more will allow enough B_{12} to be absorbed by the "passive diffusion" mechanism to produce a hematological response in some patients with pernicious anemia (Meyer *et al.*, 1960; Ungley, 1951; Ross *et al.*, 1954; Chalmers and Shinton, 1958). There is so much variation in response from one patient to another that this is unsatisfactory for routine B_{12} therapy. Perhaps a reasonable exception, on physiological grounds, is the strict vegetarian with nutritional B_{12} deficiency. Such patients could be given 5–10 mcg of cyanocobalamin daily by mouth.

Oral B_{12} and intrinsic factor concentrate. This combined preparation should provide the most natural form of therapy for patients with B_{12} deficiency due to inadequate secretion of intrinsic factor. However, patients with pernicious anemia may become refractory to this therapy, owing to the production of antibody to some fraction of the heterologous intrinsic factor concentrate, which impairs the absorption of B_{12} (Schwartz *et al.*, 1958). Until intrinsic factor is available in pure form for further clinical trials, this form of therapy should be discontinued.

Liver extracts for injection or oral use are only effective in proportion to their B_{12} content and should be abandoned in favour of parenteral cyanocobalamin or hydroxocobalamin.

Various depot preparations have been made to minimize the urinary loss of $CN-B_{12}$ and thereby facilitate the replacement of tissue stores and reduce the interval between maintenance injections (Thompson and Hecht, 1959; Glass *et al.*, 1961a; Schwartz *et al.*, 1962; Bastrup-Madsen *et al.*, 1966; Tudhope *et al.*, 1967). Clinical experience with these preparations is limited, and further studies are needed to determine whether the therapeutic benefits claimed for them warrant their general application.

Oral B_{12}-peptide complexes have been claimed to be effective in pernicious anemia from time to time, but " such claims are not supported by controlled studies, have been refuted by many competent investigators, and should be regarded as completely invalid " (Herbert, 1965).

Other preparations. It has also been shown that cyanocobalamin can be administered by nasal insufflation (Israels and Shubert, 1954), aerosol inhalation (Shinton and Singh, 1967), and *per rectum* (Ross *et al.*, 1954; Ungley, 1955), presumably as a result of mucosal diffusion. These methods are mentioned out of interest, without intending to imply any practical therapeutic application.

REFERENCES

(a) BOOKS, REVIEWS AND MONOGRAPHS

ADAMS, J. F. (1962). Considerations governing the maintenance therapy of patients with pernicious anaemia. In: *Vitamin B_{12} und Intrinsic Factor. Second Europ. Symp.*, Hamburg, 1961, p. 628. Enke, Stuttgart.

BOGER, W. P., WRIGHT, L. D. and BAYNE, G. M. (1957). Serum vitamin B_{12} concentrations of pregnant women and newborn infants. In: *Vitamin B_{12} und Intrinsic Factor. First Europ. Symp.*, Hamburg, 1956, p. 443. Enke, Stuttgart.

CHOSY, J. J., KILLANDER, A. and SCHILLING, R. F. (1962a). Studies on hydroxocobalamin. Estimates of absorption from the gut and binding to serum and liver. In: *Vitamin B_{12} und Intrinsic Factor. Second Europ. Symp.*, Hamburg, 1961, p. 668. Enke, Stuttgart.

COATES, M. E. and KON, S. K. (1957). Biological and microbiological activities of purine and benzimidazole analogues of vitamin B$_{12}$. In: *Vitamin B$_{12}$ und Intrinsic Factor. First Europ. Symp., Hamburg*, 1956, p. 72. Enke, Stuttgart.

DOSCHERHOLMEN, A. (1962). Scintillation spectrometry of Co^{57}-vitamin B$_{12}$ in the, diagnosis of pernicious anaemia. In: *Vitamin B$_{12}$ und Intrinsic Factor. Second Europ. Symp., Hamburg*, 1961, p. 345. Enke, Stuttgart.

DOSCHERHOLMEN, A. (1965). *Studies in the metabolism of vitamin B$_{12}$*. University of Minnesota Press, Minneapolis, pp. 271.

EKINS, R. P. and SGHERZI, A. M. (1965). The microassay of vitamin B$_{12}$ in human plasma by the saturation assay technique. In: *Radiochemical methods of analysis*, Vol. II, p. 239. I.A.E.A., Vienna.

FOSTER, M. A. (1966). Vitamin B$_{12}$ and folic acid in the synthesis of methionine by human liver. In: *B-Vitamine: Klinische und physiologisch-chemische probleme. Symposion veranstaltet von der I Medizinischen Klinik der Freien Universitat Berlin*, 1965. (Eds. VON KRESS, H. F. & BLUM, K-U). Schattauer, Stuttgart. p. 103.

HEINRICH, H. C. (1964). Metabolic basis of the diagnosis and therapy of vitamin B$_{12}$ deficiency. In: *Seminars in Haematology*, vol. **1**, 199. Grune and Stratton, New York.

HERBERT, V. (1959b). *The megaloblastic anaemias*. Grune and Stratton, New York.

HERBERT, V. (1965). Drugs effective in megaloblastic anemias: vitamin B$_{12}$ and folic acid. In: *The pharmacological basis of therapeutics*. 3 Ed. GOODMAN, L. S. and GILMAN, A. (Eds.), p. 1410. Collier-MacMillan, London.

HERBERT, V. (1966). Nutritional requirements for vitamin B$_{12}$ and folic acid. *Proc. Plenary Sessions XI Congr. Int. Soc. Haemat., Sydney*, 1966, p. 109. Government Printer, Sydney.

HUENNEKENS, F. M. (1966). Biochemical functions and interrelationships of folic acid and vitamin B$_{12}$. In: *Progress in Haematology*, BROWN, E. B. and MOORE, C. V. (Eds.), vol. **5**, p. 83. Grune & Stratton, N.Y.

IMERSLUND, O. (1959). Idiopathic chronic megaloblastic anaemia in children. *Acta paediat., Suppl.* **119**. Oslo Univ. Press, Oslo.

INTERNATIONAL ATOMIC ENERGY AGENCY (1966). *Clinical uses of whole body counting*. I.A.E.A., Vienna, pp. 291.

JAENICKE, L. (1961). Mechanism of action of tetrahydrofolate cofactors in one-carbon transfer. Ciba Found. Study Group vol., **11**, p. 38. Churchill, London.

LESTER SMITH, E. (1962). Report of round table discussion on nomenclature. In: *Vitamin B$_{12}$ und Intrinsic Factor, Second Europ. Symp., Hamburg*, 1961, p. 764. Enke, Stuttgart.

LESTER SMITH, E. (1965). *Vitamin B$_{12}$*. 3 ed. Methuen, London, pp. 180.

MANSON, L. A. (1962). Vitamin B$_{12}$ and deoxyribose synthesis. In: *Vitamin B$_{12}$ und Intrinsic Factor. Second Europ. Symp., Hamburg*, 1961, p. 191. Enke, Stuttgart.

MOLLIN, D. L. (1959b). The megaloblastic anaemias. *Lectures on the Scientific Basis of Medicine*, 1957–1958, vol. **7**, p. 94. Athlone Press, London.

MOLLIN, D. L. (1962b). The use of radioisotopes in the study of vitamin B$_{12}$ and folic acid deficiencies. In: *Radioisotopes in Tropical Medicine*, p. 29. I.A.E.A., Vienna.

MOLLIN, D. L. and BAKER, S. J. (1955). The absorption and excretion of vitamin B$_{12}$ in man. *Biochem. Soc. Symp. No.* 13, p. 52. Cambridge Univ. Press.

MOLLIN, D. L. and ROSS, G. I. M. (1957). The pathophysiology of vitamin B$_{12}$ deficiency in the megaloblastic anaemias. In: *Vitamin B$_{12}$ und Intrinsic Factor. First Europ. Symp., Hamburg*, 1956, p. 413. Enke, Stuttgart.

MOLLIN, D. L. and WATERS, A. H. (1968a). *The study of vitamin B$_{12}$ absorption using labelled cobalamins*. Medical Monograph 6. U.K.A.E.A., R.C.C., Amersham, England.

MOLLIN, D. L. and WATERS, A. H. (1970). Vitamin B$_{12}$ and folic acid absorption and metabolism. In: *Radioisotopes in medical diagnosis*. VETTER, H. and BELCHER, E. H. (Eds.). Butterworth, London (In press).

MOLLIN, D. L., BOOTH, C. C. and CHANARIN, I. (1959). The pathogenesis of deficiency of vitamin B_{12} and folic acid in idiopathic steatorrhoea. In: *Proc. Wld. Congr. Gastroenterology*, Washington, D.C. 1958, p. 483. Williams and Wilkins, Baltimore.

MOLLIN, D. L., WATERS, A. H. and HARRISS, E. (1962). Clinical aspects of the metabolic interrelationships between folic acid and vitamin B_{12}. In: *Vitamin B_{12} und Intrinsic Factor. Second Europ. Symp., Hamburg*, 1961, p. 737. Enke, Stuttgart.

McCANCE, R. A. and WIDDOWSON, E. M. (1960). *The composition of Foods*. M.R.C. Special Report Series No. 297. H.M.S.O., London.

NEWMAN, G. E., O'BRIEN, J. R. P., SPRAY, G. H. and WITTS, L. J. (1962a). Distribution of vitamin B_{12} in rat liver cell fractions. In: *Vitamin B_{12} und Intrinsic Factor. Second Europ. Symp., Hamburg*, 1961. p. 424. Enke, Stuttgart.

ROSENBLUM, C. (1962a). Radioactive vitamin B_{12} and its application in biochemical research. In: *Vitamin B_{12} und Intrinsic Factor. Second Europ. Symp., Hamburg*, 1961, p. 306. Enke, Stuttgart.

ROSENBLUM, C. (1962b). Stability of radioactive vitamin B_{12}. In: *Vitamin B_{12} und Intrinsic Factor. Second Europ. Symp., Hamburg*, 1961, p. 294. Enke, Stuttgart.

ROSS, G. I. M. and MOLLIN, D. L. (1957). Vitamin B_{12} in tissues in pernicious anaemia and other conditions. In: *Vitamin B_{12} und Intrinsic Factor. First Europ. Symp., Hamburg*, 1956, p. 437. Enke, Stuttgart.

SCHILLING, R. F. and SCHLOESSER, L. L. (1957). Intrinsic factor studies. V. Some aspects of the quantitative relationship between vitamin B_{12}, intrinsic factor, binding, and the absorption of vitamin B_{12}. In: *Vitamin B_{12} und Intrinsic Factor. First Europ. Symp., Hamburg*, 1956, p. 194. Enke, Stuttgart.

UNITED STATES DEPARTMENT OF AGRICULTURE (1961). *Vitamin B_{12}. Home Economics Research Report No.* 13, pp. 15.

WATERS, A. H. (1966). Haematological responses in vitamin B_{12} and folate deficiencies In: *Proc. Symp. on Folic Acid*, 25th *April* 1966. Glaxo Laboratories, Greenford, Middlesex, England. p. 86.

WINTROBE, M. M. (1951). *Clinical Hematology*. 3 ed., p. 96. Kimpton, London.

WINTROBE, M. M. (1961). *Clinical Hematology*. 5 ed., p. 473. Kimpton, London.

WOKES, F. and SMITH, A. D. M. (1962). Vitamin B_{12} and vegetarians. In: *Vitamin B_{12} und Intrinsic Factor. Second Europ. Symp., Hamburg*, 1961, p. 602. Enke, Stuttgart.

(b) ORIGINAL PAPERS

ABELES, R. H. and LEE, H. A., JR. (1961). Intramolecular oxidation-reduction requiring cobamide coenzyme. *J. biol. Chem.*, **236:** 2347.

ABELS, J. and SCHILLING, R. F. (1964). Protection of intrinsic factor by vitamin B_{12}. *J. lab. clin. Med.*, **64:** 375.

ABELS, J., VEGTER, J. J. M., WOLDRING, M. G., JANS, J. H. and NIEWEG, H. O. (1959). The physiologic mechanism of vitamin B_{12} absorption. *Acta med. Scand.*, **165:** 105.

ADAMS, J. F. (1958). Pregnancy and Addisonian pernicious anaemia. *Scot. med. J.*, **3:** 21.

ADAMS, J. F. and CARTWRIGHT, E. J. (1963). The reliability and reproducibility of the Schilling test in primary malabsorption disease and after partial gastrectomy. *Gut*, **4:** 32.

ADAMS, J. F. and KENNEDY, E. H. (1965). Hydroxocobalamin: excretion and retention after parenteral doses in anaemic and non-anaemic subjects with reference to the treatment of vitamin B_{12} deficiency states. *J. lab. clin. Med.*, **65:** 450.

ANDERSON, B. B. (1964). Investigations into the Euglena method for the assay of vitamin B_{12} in serum. *J. clin. Path.*, **17:** 14.

ANDERSON, B. B. (1965). Investigations into the Euglena method of assay of vitamin B$_{12}$: the results obtained in human serum and liver using an improved method of assay. Ph.D. Thesis, University of London, pp. 224.

ARDEMAN, S. and CHANARIN, I (1963). A method for the assay of human gastric intrinsic factor and for the detection and titration of antibodies against intrinsic factor. *Lancet*, ii: 1350.

ARDEMAN, S. and CHANARIN, I. (1965). Assay of gastric intrinsic factor in the diagnosis of Addisonian pernicious anaemia. *Brit. J. Haemat.*, 11: 305.

ARDEMAN, S. and CHANARIN, I. (1966). Intrinsic factor secretion in gastric atrophy. *Gut*, 7: 99.

ARDEMAN, S., CHANARIN, I. and DOYLE, J. C. (1964). Studies on secretion of gastric intrinsic factor in man. *Brit. med. J.* ii: 600.

ARNSTEIN, H. R. V. (1964). The metabolic functions of folic acid and vitamin B$_{12}$. *Series Haematologica*, 3: 38.

ARNSTEIN, H. R. V. and SIMKIN, J. L. (1959). Vitamin B$_{12}$ and biosynthesis in rat liver. *Nature (Lond.)*, 183: 523.

ARNSTEIN, H. R. V. and WHITE, A. M. (1962). The function of vitamin B$_{12}$ in the metabolism of propionate by the protozoan *Ochromonas malhamensis*. *Biochem, J.*, 83: 264.

BADENOCH, J., EVANS, J. R., RICHARDS, W. C. D. and WITTS, L. J. (1955a). Megaloblastic anaemia following partial gastrectomy and gastroenterostomy. *Brit. J. Haemat.*, 1: 339.

BADENOCH, J., BEDFORD, P. D. and EVANS, J. R. (1955b). Massive diverticulosis of the small intestine with steatorrhoea and megaloblastic anaemia. *Quart. J. Med.*, 24: 321.

BAKER, H., HERBERT, V., FRANK, O., PASHER, I., HUTNER, S. H., WASSERMAN, L. R. and SOBOTKA, H. (1959). A microbiologic method for detecting folic acid deficiency in man. *Clin. Chem.*, 5: 275.

BAKER, S. J. and MOLLIN, D. L. (1955). The relationship between intrinsic factor and the intestinal absorption of vitamin B$_{12}$. *Brit. J. Haemat.*, 1: 46.

BAKER, S. J., IGNATIUS, M., JOHNSON, S. and VAISH, S. K. (1963). Hyperpigmentation of skin. A sign of vitamin B$_{12}$ deficiency. *Brit. med. J.*, i: 1713.

BALL, E. W. and GILES, C. (1964). Folic acid and vitamin B$_{12}$ levels in pregnancy and their relation to megaloblastic anaemia. *J. clin. Path.*, 17: 165.

BARAKAT, R. M. and EKINS, R. P. (1961). Assay of vitamin B$_{12}$ in blood. A simple method. *Lancet*, ii: 25.

BARAKAT, R. M. and EKINS, R. P. (1963). An isotopic method for the determination of vitamin B$_{12}$ levels in blood. *Blood*, 21: 70.

BARKER, H. A., WEISSBACH, H. and SMYTH, R. D. (1958). Coenzyme containing pseudovitamin B$_{12}$. *Proc. Nat. Acad. Sci.*, 44: 1093.

BARNESS, L. A., YOUNG, D., MELLMAN, W. J., KAHN, S. B. and WILLIAMS, W. J. (1963a). Methylmalonate excretion in a patient with pernicious anaemia. *New Engl. J. Med.*, 268: 144.

BARNESS, L. A., FLAKS, J., YOUNG, D., TEDESCO, T. and NOCHO, R. (1963b). Sources of urinary methylmalonate-thymine metabolism. *Fed. Proc.*, 22: 259.

BARRETT, C. R. JR. and HOLT, P. R. (1966). Postgastrectomy blind loop syndrome, megaloblastic anaemia secondary to malabsorption of folic acid. *Amer. J. Med.*, 41: 629

BASHIR, H. V., HINTERBERGER, H. and JONES, B. P. (1966). Methylmalonic acid excretion in vitamin B$_{12}$ deficiency. *Brit. J. Haemat.*, 12: 704.

BASTRUP-MADSEN, P., NØRREGAARD, S., SCHWARTZ, M., HANSEN, T. and MEULENGRACHT, E. (1966). Serum vitamin B$_{12}$ during maintenance therapy in pernicious anaemia with a depot preparation of vitamin B$_{12}$. *Lancet*, i: 739.

BAURIEDEL, W. R., PICKEN, J. C., JR. and UDERKOFLER, L. A. (1956). Reactions of cyanocobalamin and aquocobalamin with proteins. *Proc. Soc. exp. Biol., N.Y.,* **91**: 377.

BAYLY, R. J. and EVANS, E. A. (1966). Stability and storage of compounds labelled with radioisotopes. *J. labeled Compounds* **2**: 1.

BAYLY, R. J., BELL, T. K. and WATERS, A. H. (1969). A dual isotope modification of the Schilling test. *Proc. Society Nuclear Med. Zurich,* Sept. 1969 (to be published).

BECK, W. S. (1962). The metabolic functions of vitamin B_{12}. *New Eng. J. Med.,* **266**: 708.

BECK, W. S. (1964). The metabolic basis of megaloblastic erythropoiesis. *Medicine,* **43**: 715.

BECK, W. S., GOULIAN, M., LARSSON, A. and REICHARD, P. (1966). Hydrogen donor specificity of cobamide-dependent ribonucleotide reductase and allosteric regulation of substrate specificity. *J. biol. Chem.,* **241**: 2177.

BELL, T. K., BRIDGES, J. M. and NELSON, M. G. (1965). Simultaneous free and bound radioactive vitamin B_{12} urinary excretion test. *J. clin. Path.,* **18**: 611.

BENHAM, G. H. H. (1951). The visual field defects in subacute combined degeneration of the spinal cord. *J. Neurol. Neurosurg. Psychiat.,* **14**: 40.

BERK, L., CASTLE, W. B., WELCH, A. D., HEINLE, R. W., ANKER, R. and EPSTEIN, M. (1948). Observations on etiologic relationship of achylia gastrica to pernicious anemia. X. Activity of vitamin B_{12} as food (extrinsic) factor. *New Engl. J. Med.,* **239**: 911.

BIGGS, J. C., MASON, S. L. A. and SPRAY, G. H. (1964). Vitamin B_{12} activity in red cells. *Brit. J. Haemat.,* **10**: 36.

BJORKENHEIM, B. (1966). Optic neuropathy caused by vitamin B_{12} deficiency in carriers of the fish tapeworm, *Diphyllobothrium latum. Lancet,* **i**: 688.

BLAKLEY, R. L. and BARKER, H. A. (1964). Cobamide stimulation of the reduction of ribotides to deoxyribotides in *Lactobacillus leichmanii. Biochim. Biophys. Res. Comm.,* **16**: 391.

BLAKLEY, R. L., GHAMBEER, R. K., NIXON, P. F. and VITOLS, E. (1965). The cobamide dependent ribonucleoside triphosphate reductase of *Lactobacilli. Biochim. Biophys. Res. Comm.,* **20**: 439.

BOASS, A. and WILSON, R. H. (1964). Intestinal absorption of intrinsic factor and B_{12} intrinsic factor complex. *Amer. J. Physiol.,* **207**: 27.

BODDINGTON, M. M. (1959). Changes in buccal cells in the anaemias. *J. clin. Path.,* **12**: 222.

BODDINGTON, M. M. and SPRIGGS, A. I. (1959). The epithelial cells in megaloblastic anaemias. *J. clin. Path.,* **12**: 228.

BODIAN, D. (1947). Nucleic acid in nerve cell regeneration. *Symp. Soc. exp. Biol.,* **i**: 163.

BOEN, S. T. (1957). Changes in the nuclei of squamous epithelial cells in pernicious anaemia. *Acta med. Scand.,* **159**: 425.

BOGER, W. P., WRIGHT, L. D., STRICKLAND, S. C., GYLFE, J. S. and CIMINERA, J. L. (1955). Vitamin B_{12}: correlation of serum concentration and age. *Proc. Soc. exp. Biol., N.Y.,* **89**: 375.

BOOTH, C. C. and MOLLIN, D. L. (1956). Plasma tissue and urinary radioactivity after oral administration of ^{56}Co-labelled vitamin B_{12}. *Brit. J. Haemat.,* **2**: 223.

BOOTH, C. C. and MOLLIN, D. L. (1959). The site of absorption of vitamin B_{12} in man. *Lancet,* **i**: 18.

BOOTH, C. C. and MOLLIN, D. L. (1960). The blind loop syndrome. *Proc. Roy. Soc. Med.,* **53**: 658.

BOOTH, C. C. and MOLLIN, D. L. (1964). Chronic tropical sprue in London. *Amer. J. dig. Dis.,* **9**: 770.

BOOTH, C. C., MACINTYRE, I. and MOLLIN, D. L. (1964). Nutritional problems associated with extensive lesions of the distal small intestine in man. *Quart. J. Med.*, **33**: 401.

BOURNE, M. S., BOTTOMLEY, A. C. and ISRAELS, M. C. G. (1964). Hydroxocobalamin for pernicious anaemia. *Lancet*, **ii**: 173.

BRADLEY, J. E., LESTER SMITH, E., BAKER, S. J. and MOLLIN, D. L. (1954). The use of the radioactive isotope of cobalt Co^{58} for the preparation of labelled vitamin B$_{12}$. *Lancet*, **ii**: 476.

BRECKENRIDGE, A. and METCALFE-GIBSON, A. (1965). Methods of measuring glomerular filtration rate. A comparison of inulin, vitamin B$_{12}$ and creatinine clearances. *Lancet*, **ii**: 265.

BRODY, E. A., ESTREN, S. and WASSERMAN, L. R. (1960). The kinetics of intravenously injected radioactive vitamin B$_{12}$: Studies on normal subjects and patients with chronic myelocytic leukaemia and pernicious anaemia. *Blood*, **15**: 646.

BRODY, E. A., ESTREN, S. and HERBERT, V. (1966). Coexistent pernicious anemia and malabsorption in four patients: including one whose malabsorption disappeared with vitamin B$_{12}$ therapy. *Ann. int. Med.*, **64**: 1246.

BROZOVIC, M., HOFFBRAND, A. V., DIMITRIADOU, A. and MOLLIN, D. L. (1967). The excretion of methylmalonic acid and succinic acid in vitamin B$_{12}$ and folate deficiency. *Brit. J. Haemat.*, **13**: 1021.

BUCHANAN, J. M. (1964). The function of vitamin B$_{12}$ and folic acid coenzymes in mammalian cells. *Medicine*, **43**: 697.

BUCHANAN, N. M., ELFORD, H. L., LOUGHLIN, R. E., MCDOUGALL, B. M. and ROSENTHAL, S. (1964). The role of vitamin B$_{12}$ in methyl transfer to homocysteine. *Ann. N.Y. Acad. Sci.*, **112**: 756.

CAHN, A. and VON MERING, J. (1886). Die Sauren des gesunden und kranken Magens. *Deutsch. Arch. Klin. Med.*, **39**: 233.

CALLENDER, S. T. and EVANS, J. R. (1955). The urinary excretion of labelled vitamin B$_{12}$. *Clin. Sci.*, **14**: 295.

CALLENDER, S. T. and SPRAY, G. H. (1962). Latent pernicious anaemia. *Brit. J. Haemat.*, **8**: 230.

CALLENDER, S. T., RETIEF, F. P. and WITTS, L. J. (1960). The augmented histamine test with special reference to achlorhydria. *Gut*, **1**: 326.

CALLENDER, S. T., WITTS, L. J., WARNER, G. T. and OLIVER, R. (1966). The use of a simple whole-body counter for haematological investigations. *Brit. J. Haemat.*, **12**: 276.

CARMEL, R. and COLTMAN, A., Jr. (1969). Radioassay for serum vitamin B$_{12}$ with the use of saliva as the vitamin B$_{12}$ binder. *J. Lab. clin. Med.*, **74**: 967.

CASTLE, W. B. (1929). Observations on etiologic relationship of achylia gastrica to pernicious anemia. I. The effect of administration to patients with pernicious anemia of the contents of the normal human stomach recovered after the ingestion of beef muscle. *Amer. J. med. Sci.*, **178**: 748.

CASTLE, W. B. (1953). Development of knowledge concerning the gastric intrinsic factor and its relation to pernicious anaemia. *New Eng. J. Med.*, **249**: 603.

CASTLE, W. B. (1966). Treatment of pernicious anaemia: historical aspects. *Clin. Pharmacol. Therapeutics*, **7**: 147.

CASTLE, W. B. and TOWNSEND, W. C. (1929). Observations on etiologic relationship of achylia gastrica to pernicious anemia. II. The effect of the administration to patients with pernicious anemia of beef muscle after incubation with normal human gastric juice. *Amer. J. med. Sci.*, **178**: 764.

CASTLE, W. B., TOWNSEND, W. C. and HEATH, C. W. (1930). Observations on etiologic relationship of achylia gastrica to pernicious anemia. III. The nature of the reaction between normal human gastric juice and beef muscle leading to clinical improvement and increased blood formation similar to the effect of liver feeding. *Amer. J. med. Sci.* **180**: 305.

C

CHAIET, L., ROSENBLUM, C. and WOODBURY, T. (1950). Biosynthesis of radioactive vitamin B_{12} containing cobalt-60. *Science*, **111**: 360.

CHALMERS, J. N. M. and SHINTON, N. K. (1958). Absorption of orally administered vitamin B_{12} in pernicious anaemia. *Lancet*, **ii**: 1298.

CHALMERS, J. N. M. and SHINTON, N. K. (1965). Comparison of hydroxocobalamin and cyanocobalamin in the treatment of pernicious anaemia. *Lancet*, **ii**: 1305.

CHANARIN, I., ROTHMAN, D. and BERRY, V. (1965). Iron deficiency and its relation to folic acid status in pregnancy. Results of a clinical trial. *Brit. med. J.*, **i**: 480.

CHISHOLM, I. A., BRONTE-STEWART, J. and FOULDS, W. S. (1967). Hydroxocobalamin versus cyanocobalamin in the treatment of tobacco amblyopia. *Lancet*, **ii**: 450.

CHOSY, J. J., CLATANOFF, D. V. and SCHILLING, R. F. (1962b). Responses to small doses of folic acid in pernicious anaemia. *Amer. J. clin. Nutr.*, **104**: 349.

CHUNG, A. S. M., PEARSON, W. M., DARBY, W. J., MILLER, O. N. and GOLDSMITH, G. A. (1961). Folic acid, vitamin B_6, pantothenic acid and vitamin B_{12} in human dietaries. *Amer. J. clin. Nutr.*, **9**: 573.

COHEN, H. (1936). Optic atrophy as the presenting sign in pernicious anaemia. *Lancet* **ii**: 1202.

COOKE, W. T., COX, E. V., FONE, D. J., MEYNELL, M. J. and GADDIE, R. (1963). Clinical and metabolic significance of jejunal diverticula. *Gut*, **4**: 115.

COOPER, B. A., (1967). Disparity between biological and immunological characteristics of apparent IF-B_{12} in human ileum during B_{12} absorption *in vivo*. *J. clin. Invest.*, **46**: 1047.

COOPER, B. A. and CASTLE, W. B., (1960). Sequential mechanisms in the enhanced absorption of vitamin B_{12} by intrinsic factor in the rat. *J. clin. Invest.*, **39**: 199.

COOPER, B. A. and LOWENSTEIN, L. (1964) Relative folate deficiency of erythrocytes in pernicious anemia and its correction with cyanocobalamin. *Blood*, **24**: 502.

COOPER, B. A. and WHITE, J. J. (1968). Absence of intrinsic factor from human portal plasma during $^{57}Co\ B_{12}$ absorption in man. *Brit. J. Haemat.*, **14**: 73.

COOPER, B. A. and YATES, T. (1967). Antibody to intrinsic factor—vitamin B_{12} complex in pernicious anaemia. *Brit. J. Haemat.*, **13**: 687.

COGHILL, N. F., DONIACH, D., ROITT, I. M., MOLLIN, D. L. and WILLIAMS, A. W. (1965). Autoantibodies in simple atrophic gastritis. *Gut*, **6**: 48.

COX, E. V. and WHITE, A. M. (1962). Methylmalonic acid excretion: an index of vitamin B_{12} deficiency. *Lancet*, **ii**: 853.

DARBY, W. J., BRIDGEFORTH, E. B., LeBROCQUY, J., CLARK, S. L., JR., DE OLIVIERA, J. D., KEVANY, J., McGANITY, W. J. and PEREZ, C. (1958). Vitamin B_{12} requirement of adult man. *Amer. J. Med.*, **25**: 726.

DAVIDSON, J. N., LESLIE, I. and WHITE, J. C. (1951). The nucleic-acid content of the cell. *Lancet*, **i**: 1287.

DELLER, D. J. and WITTS, L. J. (1962). Changes in the blood after partial gastrectomy with special reference to vitamin B_{12}. I. Serum vitamin B_{12}, haemoglobin, serum iron and bone marrow. *Quart. J. Med.*, **31**: 71.

DELLER, D. J., RICHARDS, W. C. D. and WITTS, L. J. (1962). Changes in the blood after partial gastrectomy with special reference to vitamin B_{12}. II. The cause of the fall in serum vitamin B_{12}. *Quart. J. Med.*, **31**: 89.

DELLER, D. J., IBBOTSON, R. N. and CROMPTON, B. (1964). Metabolic effects of partial gastrectomy with special reference to calcium and folic acid. Part II. The contribution of folic acid deficiency to the anaemia. *Gut*, **5**: 225.

DONALDSON, R. M., JR. (1964). Normal bacterial population of the intestine and their relation to intestinal function. *New Engl. J. Med.*, **270**: 938.

DONALDSON, R. M., JR. (1965). Malabsorption in the blind loop syndrome. *Gastroenterology*, **48**: 388.

DONALDSON, R. M., JR., MACKENZIE, I. L. and TRIER, J. S. (1967). Intrinsic factor-mediated attachment of vitamin B$_{12}$ to brush borders and microvillous membranes of hamster intestine. *J. clin. Invest.*, **46**: 1215.

DONIACH, D., RIOTT, I. M. and TAYLOR, K. B. (1965). Autoimmunity in pernicious anaemia and thyroiditis: a family study. *Ann. N.Y. Acad. Sci.*, **124**: 605.

DOSCHERHOLMEN, A. and HAGEN, P. S. (1956). Radioactive vitamin B$_{12}$ absorption studies: results of direct measurement of radioactivity in the blood. *J. clin. Invest.*, **35**: 699.

DOSCHERHOLMEN, A. and HAGEN, P. S. (1957). A dual mechanism of vitamin B$_{12}$ plasma absorption. *J. clin. Invest.*, **36**: 1551.

DOSCHERHOLMEN, A. and HAGEN, P. S. (1959). Delay of absorption of radiolabelled cyanocobalamin in the intestinal wall in the presence of intrinsic factor. *J. lab. clin. Med.*, **54**: 434.

DOSCHERHOLMEN, A., FINLEY, P. R. and HAGEN, P. S. (1960). Distribution of radio-activity in man after the oral ingestion of small test doses of radiolabelled cyanoco-balamin. *J. Lab. clin. med.*, **56**: 547.

DOWNING, M. and SCHWEIGERT, B. S. (1956). Role of vitamin B$_{12}$ in nucleic acid meta-bolism. IV. Metabolism of C^{14} labelled thymidine by *Lactobacillus leichmanii*. *J. biol. Chem.*, **220**: 521.

DUBNOFF, J. W. (1950). The effect of B$_{12}$ concentrates on the reduction of S–S groups. *Arch. Biochem.*, **27**: 466.

EDWIN, E., HOLTEN, K., NORUM, K. R., SCHRUMPF, A. and SKAUG, O. E. (1965). Vitamin B$_{12}$ hypovitaminosis in mental diseases. *Acta med. Scand.*, **177**: 689.

ELLENBOGEN, L. and HIGHLEY, D. R. (1963). Intrinsic factor. *Vitamins and Hormones*, **21**: 1.

ELLENBOGEN, L., WILLIAMS, W. L., RABINER, S. F. and LICHTMAN, H. C. (1955). An improved urinary excretion test as an assay for intrinsic factor. *Proc. Soc. exp. Biol. (N.Y.)*, **89**: 357.

ENOKSSON, P. and NORDEN, A. (1960). Vitamin B$_{12}$ deficiency affecting the optic nerve. *Acta med. Scand.*, **167**: 199.

ESTREN, S., BRODY, E. A. and WASSERMAN, L. R. (1958). The metabolism of vitamin B$_{12}$ in pernicious and other megaloblastic anemias. *Adv. int. Med.*, **9**: 11.

EVANS, H. J. and KLIEWER, M. (1964). Vitamin B$_{12}$ compounds in relation to the requirements of cobalt for higher plants and nitrogen-fixing organisms. *Ann. N.Y. Acad. Sci.*, **112**: 735.

FARRANT, P. C. (1958). Nuclear changes in oral epithelium in pernicious anaemia. *Lancet*, **i**: 830.

FARRANT, P. C. (1960). Nuclear changes in squamous cells from buccal mucosa in pernicious anaemia. *Brit. med. J.*, **i**: 1694.

FENWICK, S. (1870). On atrophy of the stomach. *Lancet*, **ii**: 78.

FINKLER, A. E. and HALL, C. A. (1966). Specific cyanocobalamin transport in human cell culture. *Fed. Proc.*, **25**: 430.

FINKLER, A. E. and HALL, C. A. (1967). Nature of the relationship between vitamin B$_{12}$ binding and cell uptake. *Arch. Biochem. Biophys.*, **120**: 79.

FINKLER, A. F., GREEN, P. D. and Hall, C. A. (1970). Immunological properties of human vitamin B$_{12}$ binders. *Biochim. Biophys. Acta*, **200**: 151.

FINKLER, A. E., HALL, C. A. and LANDAU, J. V. (1965). Uptake of HeLa cells of normal and abnormal B$_{12}$ binding proteins. *Fed. Proc.*, **24**: 679.

FLOYD, K. W. and WHITEHEAD, R. W. (1960). Role of vitamin B$_{12}$ in thymidine syn-thesis. *Biochem. Biophys. Res. Comm.*, **3**: 220.

FOROOZAN, P. and TRIER, J. S. (1967). Mucosa of the small intestine in pernicious anemia. *New Eng. J. Med.*, **277**: 553.

FORSHAW, J. and HARWOOD, L. (1966). Measurement of intestinal absorption of ^{57}Co vitamin B_{12} by serum counting. *J. clin. Path.*, **19**: 606.

FOULDS, W. S., CANT, J. S., CHISHOLM, I. A., BRONTE-STEWART, J. and WILSON, J. (1968). Hydroxocobalamin in the treatment of Leber's hereditary optic atrophy. *Lancet*, **i**: 896.

FOULDS, W. S., CHISHOLM, I. A., BRONTE-STEWART, J. and WILSON, T. M. (1969). Vitamin B_{12} absorption in tobacco amblyopia. *Brit. J. Opthal.*, **53**: 393.

FOULDS, W. S., FREEMAN, A. G., PHILLIPS, C. I. and WILSON, J. (1970). Cyanocobalamin: a case for withdrawal. *Lancet*, **i**: 35.

FREEMAN, A. G. and HEATON, J. M. (1961). The aetiology of retrobulbar neuritis in Addisonian pernicious anaemia. *Lancet*, **i**: 908.

FRENCH, J. M., GADDIE, R., and SMITH, N. M. (1956). Tropical sprue: a study of seven cases and their response to chemotherapy. *Quart. J. Med.*, **25**: 333.

FRENKEL, E. P., KELLER, S. and McCALL, M.S. (1966). Radioisotopic assay of serum vitamin B_{12} with the use of DEAE cellulose. *J. lab. clin. Med.*, **68**: 510.

FRIEDKIN, M. and WOOD, H. (1956). Conversion of uracil deoxyriboside to thymidine of deoxyribosenucleic acid. *J. biol. Chem.*, **220**: 645.

FRIEDNER, S., JOSEPHSON, B. and LEVIN, K. (1969). Vitamin B_{12} determination by means of radioisotope dilution and ultrafiltration. *Clin. Chim. Acta*, **24**: 171.

GANATRA, R. D., SUNDARAM, K., DESAI, K. B. and GAITONDE, B. B. (1965). Determination of absorption of vitamin B_{12} by a double isotope tracer technique. *J. nucl. Med.*, **6**: 459.

GILES, C. (1966). An account of 335 cases of megaloblastic anaemia of pregnancy and the puerperium. *J. clin. Path.*, **19**: 1.

GIORGIO, A. J. and PLAUT, G. W. E. (1965). A method for the colorimetric determination of urinary methylmalonic acid in pernicious anemia. *J. lab. clin. Med.*, **66**: 667.

GIRDWOOD, R. H. (1952). The occurrence of growth factors for *Lactobacillus leichmanii*, *Streptococcus faecalis* and *Leuconostoc citrovorum* in the tissues of pernicious anaemia patients and controls. *Biochem. J.*, **52**: 58.

GIRDWOOD, R. H. (1954). Rapid estimation of the serum vitamin B_{12} level by a microbiological method. *Brit. med. J.*, **ii**: 954.

GIRDWOOD, R. H. (1960). Microbiological methods of assay in clinical medicine with particular reference to the investigation of deficiency of vitamin B_{12} and folic acid. *Scot. med. J.*, **5**: 10.

GLASS, G. B. J. (1963). Gastric intrinsic factor and its function in the metabolism of vitamin B_{12}. *Physiol. Rev.*, **43**: 529.

GLASS, G. B. J. (1965). Intrinsic factor: properties and physiology. Series Haematologica, **3**: 61.

GLASS, G. B. J. and CASTRO-CUREL, Z. (1964). Activity of coenzyme B_{12} on guinea pig intestinal mucosa homogenates. *Ann. N. Y. Acad. Sci.*, **112**: 904.

GLASS, G. B. J. and LEE, D. H. (1966a). Hydroxocobalamin 4. Biological half-life of hydroxocobalamin in the human liver. *Blood*, **27**: 234.

GLASS, G. B. J. and LEE, D. H. (1966b). Hydroxocobalamin 5. Prolonged maintenance of high vitamin B_{12} blood levels following a short course of hydroxocobalamin injections. *Blood*, **27**: 227.

GLASS, G. B. J., BOYD, L. J. and STEPHANSON, L. (1954a). Intestinal absorption of vitamin B_{12} in man. *Science*, **120**: 74.

GLASS, G. B. J., BOYD, L. J., GELLIN, G. A. and STEPHANSON, L. (1954b). Uptake of radioactive vitamin B_{12} by the liver in humans: test of measurement of intestinal absorption of vitamin B_{12} and intrinsic factor activity. *Arch. Biochem.*, **51**: 251.

GLASS, G. B. J., BOYD, L. J. and GELLIN, G. A. (1955). Surface scintillation measurements in humans of the uptake of parenterally administered radioactive vitamin B_{12}. *Blood*, **10**: 95.

GLASS, G. B. J., SPEER, F. D., NIEBURGS, H. E., ISHIMORI, A., JONES, E. L., BAKER, H., SCHWARTZ, S. A. and SMITH, R. (1960). Gastric atrophy, atrophic gastritis and gastric secretory failure. *Gastroenterology*, **39**: 429.

GLASS, G. B. J., SKEGGS, H. R., LEE, D. H., JONES, E. L. and HARDY, W. W. (1961a). Hydroxocobalamin. I. Blood levels and urinary excretion of vitamin B$_{12}$ in man after a single parenteral dose of aqueous hydroxocobalamin, aqueous cyanocobalamin and cyanocobalamin zinctannate complex. *Blood*, **18**: 511.

GLASS, G. B. J., LEE, D. H. and HARDY, W. W. (1961b). Hydroxocobalamin. II. Absorption from the site of injection and uptake by the liver and calf muscle in man. *Blood*, **18**: 522.

GLASS, G. B. J., LEE, D. H., SKEGGS, H. R. and STANLEY, J. L. (1963). Hydroxocobalamin. III. Long acting effects of massive parenteral doses on vitamin B$_{12}$ blood levels in man. *J. Amer. med. Ass.*, **183**: 425.

GLAZER, H. S., MUELLER, J. F., JARROLD, R., SAKURAI, K., WILL, J. J. and VILTER, R.W. (1954). The effect of vitamin B$_{12}$ and folic acid on nucleic acid composition of the bone marrow of patients with megaloblastic anaemia. *J. lab. clin. Med.*, **43**: 905.

GOMPERTZ, D., JONES, J. H. and KNOWLES, J. P. (1967). Metabolic precursors of methylmalonic acid in vitamin B$_{12}$ deficiency. *Clin. Chim. Acta*, **18**: 197.

GOTTLIEB, C. W., RETIEF, F. P., PRATT, P. W. and HERBERT, V. (1966). Correlation of B$_{12}$ binding proteins with disorders of B$_{12}$ metabolism: relation to hypo- and hyperleucocyte states and leucocyte turnover. *J. clin. Invest.*, **45**: 1016.

GOUGH, K. R., THIRKETTLE, J. L. and READ, A. E. (1965). Folic acid deficiency in patients after gastric resection. *Quart. J. Med.*, **34**: 1.

GRÄSBECK, R., NYBERG, W. and REIZENSTEIN, P. G., (1958). Biliary and fecal vitamin B$_{12}$ excretion in man. An isotope study. *Proc. Soc. exp. Biol., N.Y.*, **97**: 780.

GRÄSBECK, R., KANTERO, I. and SIURALA, M. (1959). Influence of calcium ions on vitamin B$_{12}$ absorption in steatorrhoea and pernicious anaemia. *Lancet*, **i**: 234.

GRÄSBECK, R., GORDON, R., KANTERO, I. and KUHLBACK, B. (1960). Selective vitamin B$_{12}$ malabsorption and proteinuria in young people: a syndrome. *Acta med. Scand.*, **167**: 289.

GRÄSBECK, R., NYBERG, W., SAARNI, M. and VON BONSDORFF, B., (1962). Lognormal distribution of serum vitamin B$_{12}$ levels and dependence of blood values on the B$_{12}$ level in a large population heavily infected with *Diphyllobothrium latum*. *J. lab. clin. Med.*, **59**: 419.

GREEN, R., MUSSO, A. M. and NEWMARK, P. A. (1969). Assay of serum vitamin B$_{12}$ levels by saturation analysis (Abstract). *Clin. Sci.*, **37**: 571.

GREENBERG, D. M., NATH, R. and HUMPHREY, G. K. (1961). Purification and properties of thymidylate synthetase from calf thymus. *J. biol. Chem.*, **236**: 2271.

GROSSOWICZ, N., HOCHMAN, A., ARONOVITCH, J., IZAK, G. and RACHMILEWITZ, M. (1957). Malignant growth in the liver and serum vitamin B$_{12}$ levels. *Lancet*, **i**: 1116.

GROSSOWICZ, N., SULITZEANU, D. and MERZBACH, D. (1962). Isotopic determination of vitamin B$_{12}$ binding capacity and concentration. *Proc. Soc. exp. Biol., N.Y.*, **109**: 604.

GUEST, J. R., HELLEINER, C. W., CROSS, M. J. and WOODS, D. D. (1960). Cobalamin and the synthesis of methionine by ultrasonic extracts of *Escherichia coli*. *Biochem. J.*, **76**: 396.

GULLBERG, R., KISTNER, S., BOTTIGER, L. E. and EVALDSSON, U. (1966). Precipitating serum antibodies to intrinsic factor in pernicious anaemia. *Acta med. Scand.*, **180**: 87.

GURNANI, S., MISTRY, S. P. and JOHNSON, B. C. (1960). Functions of vitamin B$_{12}$ in methylmalonate metabolism. 1. Effect of a cofactor form of B$_{12}$ on the activity of methylmalonyl-CoA isomerase. *Biochim. Biophys. Acta, Amst.*, **38**: 187.

HALL, C. A. (1961). The plasma disappearance of radioactive vitamin B$_{12}$ in myeloproliferative diseases and other blood disorders. *Blood*, **18**: 717.

HALL, C. A. and FINKLER, A. E. (1962). *In vitro* plasma vitamin B_{12} binding in B_{12} deficient and non-deficient subjects. *J. lab. clin. Med.*, **60**: 765.

HALL, C. A. and FINKLER, A. E., (1963). A second vitamin B_{12} binding substance in human plasma. *Biochim. Biophys. Acta*, **78**: 233.

HALL, C. A. and FINKLER, A. E. (1965). The dynamics of transcobalamin II. A vitamin B_{12} binding substance in plasma. *J. lab. clin. Med.*, **65**: 459.

HALL, C. A. and FINKLER, A. E. (1966). Measurement of the amounts of the individual vitamin B_{12} proteins in plasma. I. Studies of normal plasma. II. Abnormalities in leukemia and pernicious anemia. *Blood*, **27**: 611, 618.

HALSTED, J. A., LEWIS, P. M. and GASSTER, M. (1956). Absorption of radioactive vitamin B_{12} in syndrome of megaloblastic anemia associated with intestinal stricture or anastomosis. *Amer. J. Med.*, **20**: 42.

HAMILTON, H. E., ELLIS, P. P. and SHEETS, R. F. (1959). Visual impairment due to optic neuropathy in pernicious anaemia: Report of a case and review of the literature. *Blood*, **14**: 378.

HANSEN, H. A. and WEINFELD, A. (1962). Metabolic effects and diagnostic value of small doses of folic acid and B_{12} in megaloblastic anemias. *Acta med. Scand.*, **172**: 427.

HARRISON, R. J., BOOTH, C. C. and MOLLIN, D. L. (1956). Vitamin B_{12} deficiency due to defective diet. *Lancet*, **i**: 727.

HARWOOD, L. and FORSHAW, J. (1967). Vitamin B_{12} absorption studies: effect of parenteral non-radioactive vitamin B_{12} on serum level of ^{57}Co vitamin B_{12}. *J. clin. Path.*, **20**: 687.

HATCH, F. T., LARRABEE, A. R., CATHOU, R. E. and BUCHANAN, J. M. (1961). Enzymatic synthesis of the methyl group of methionine. I. Identification of the enzymes and co-factors involved in the system isolated from *Escherichia coli*. *J. biol. Chem.*, **236**: 1095.

HAURANI, F. I., SHERWOOD, W. and GOLDSTEIN, F. (1964). Intestinal malabsorption of vitamin B_{12} in pernicious anemia. *Metabolism*, **13**: 1342.

HEATON, J. M., McCORMICK, A. J. A. and FREEMAN, A. G. (1958). Tobacco amblyopia: a clinical manifestation of vitamin B_{12} deficiency. *Lancet*, **ii**: 286.

HEINIVAARA, O. and PALVA, I. P. (1965). Malabsorption and deficiency of vitamin B_{12} caused by treatment with para-amino-salicylic acid. *Acta med. Scand.*, **177**: 337.

HEINLE, R. W., WELCH, A. D., SCHARF, V., MEACHAM, G. C. and PRUSOFF, W. H. (1952). Studies of excretion (and absorption) of Co^{60} labelled vitamin B_{12} in pernicious anemia. *Trans. Ass. Amer. Phycns.*, **65**: 214.

HEINRICH, H. C. (1954). Die biochemischen Grundlagen der Diagnostik und Therapie der vitamin B_{12} Mangelzustande (B_{12}-Hypo-und Avitaminosen) des Menschen und der Haustiere. II. Untersuchungen zum Vitamin B_{12}-stoffwechsel des Menschen wahrend der Graviditat und Lactation. *Klin. Wschr.*, **32**, 205.

HEINRICH H. C. and GABBE, E. E. (1962). Intravitale Retention und Exkretion des Aquacobamids einer für die Therapie geeigneten naturlichen vitamin B_{12}-depot Form. *Klin. Wschr.*, **39**: 689.

HEINRICH, H. C. and GABBE, E. E. (1964). Metabolism of the vitamin B_{12} coenzyme in rats and man. *Ann. N.Y. Acad. Sci.*, **112**: 871.

HELLER, P., EPSTEIN, R. CUNNINGHAM, B. HENDERSON, W. and YAKULIS, V. (1964). Vitamin B_{12} binding capacity of serum in B_{12} deficiency. *Proc. Soc. exp. Biol., N.Y.*, **115**: 342.

HERBERT, V. (1959a). Mechanism of intrinsic factor action in everted sacs of rat small intestine. *J. clin. Invest.*, **38**: 102.

HERBERT, V. (1961). The assay and nature of folic acid activity in human serum. *J. clin. Invest*, **40**: 81.

HERBERT, V. (1963). Current concepts in therapy. Megaloblastic anemia. *New Engl. J. Med.*, **268**, 201.

HERBERT, V. and CASTLE, W. B. (1964). Intrinsic factor. *New Engl. J. Med.*, **270**: 1181.

HERBERT, V. and SULLIVAN, L. W. (1964). Activity of coenzyme B$_{12}$ in man. *Ann. N.Y Acad. Sci.*, **112**: 855.

HERBERT, V. and ZALUSKY, R. (1962). Interrelationships of vitamin B$_{12}$ and folic acid metabolism: folic acid clearance studies. *J. clin. Invest.*, **41**: 1263.

HERBERT, V., LARRABEE, A. R. and BUCHANAN, J. M. (1962). Studies on the identification of a folate compound of human serum. *J. clin. Invest.*, **41**: 1134.

HERBERT, V., ZALUSKY, R. and SKEGGS, H. R. (1963). Retention of injected hydroxocobalamin versus cyanocobalamin versus liver extract-bound cobalamin. *Amer. J. clin. Nutr.*, **12**: 145.

HERBERT, V., STREIFF, R. R. and SULLIVAN, L. W. (1964). Notes on vitamin B$_{12}$ absorption; autoimmunity and childhood pernicious anemia; relation of intrinsic factor to blood group substance. *Medicine*, **43**: 679.

HERBERT, V., GOTTLIEB, C. and LAU, K.-S. (1966). Hemoglobin-coated charcoal assay for serum vitamin B$_{12}$. *Blood*, **28**: 130.

HERTZ, H., KRISTENSEN, H. P. O. and HOFF-JORGENSEN, E. (1964). Studies on vitamin B$_{12}$ retention. Comparison of retention following intramuscular injection of cyanocobalamin and hydroxocobalamin. *Scand. J. Haemat.*, **1**: 5.

HEYSSEL, R. M., BOZIAN, R. C., DARBY, W. J. and BELL, M. C. (1966). Vitamin B$_{12}$ turnover in man. The assimilation of vitamin B$_{12}$ from natural foodstuff by man and estimates of minimal daily dietary requirements. *Amer. J. clin. Nutr.*, **18**: 176.

HINES, J. D. (1966). Megaloblastic anaemia in an adult vegan. *Amer. J. clin. Nutr.*, **19**: 260.

HINES, J. D., HOFFBRAND, A. V. and MOLLIN, D. L. (1967). The hematologic complications following partial gastrectomy. A study of 292 patients. *Amer. J. Med.*, **43**: 555.

HODGKIN, D. C., PICKWORTH, J., ROBERTSON, J. H., TRUEBLOOD, K. N., PROSEN, R. J., WHITE, J. G., BONNETT, R., CANNON, J. R., JOHNSON, A. W., SUTHERLAND, I., TODD, SIR ALEXANDER and LESTER SMITH, E. (1955). The crystal structure of the hexacarboxylic acid derived from B$_{12}$ and the molecular structure of the vitamin. *Nature, Lond.*, **176**: 325.

HOEDEMAEKER, P. J., ABELS, J., WACHTERS, J. J., ARENDS, A. and NIEWEG, H. O. (1964). Investigations about the site of production of Castle's gastric intrinsic factor. *Lab. Invest.*, **13**: 1394.

HOEDEMAEKER, P. J., ABELS, J., WACHTERS, J. J., ARENDS, A. and NIEWEG, H. O. (1966). Further investigations about the site of production of Castle's intrinsic factor. *Lab. Invest.*, **15**: 1163.

HOFFBRAND, A. V., NEWCOMBE, B. F. A. and MOLLIN, D. L. (1966). Method of assay of red cell folate activity and the value of the assay as a test for folate deficiency. *J. clin. Path.*, **19**: 17.

HOLMBERG, C. G., JONEMAR, B., NORDEN, A., STAHLBERG, K.-G. and TRYDING, N. (1966). Methylmalonic acid, excretion and serum vitamin B$_{12}$. *Scand. J. Haemat*, **3**: 399.

HOLMES, J. MacD. (1956). Cerebral manifestations of vitamin B$_{12}$ deficiency. *Brit. med. J.*, **ii**: 1394.

HOM, B. L. (1967). Plasma turnover of [57]Cobalt-vitamin B$_{12}$ bound to transcobalamin I and II. *Scand. J. Haemat.*, **4**: 321.

HOM, B., OLESEN, H. and LOUS, P. (1966). Fractionation of vitamin B$_{12}$ binders in human serum. *J. lab. clin. Med.*, **68**: 958.

HUNTER, R., JONES, M., JONES, T. G. and MATTHEWS, D. M. (1967). Serum B$_{12}$ and folate concentrations in mental patients. *Brit. J. Psychiat.*, **113**: 1291.

HUTNER, S. H., BACH, M. K. and ROSS, G. I. M. (1956). A sugar containing basal medium for vitamin B_{12} assay with Euglena; application to body fluids. *J. Protozool.*, 3: 101.

ISRAËLS, M. C. G. and SHUBERT, S. (1954). The treatment of pernicious anaemia by insufflation of vitamin B_{12}. *Lancet*, i: 341.

JACKSON, I. M. D., DOIG, W. B. and MACDONALD, G. (1967). Pernicious anaemia as a cause of infertility. *Lancet*, ii: 1159.

JACOBS, A. (1960). The buccal mucosa in anaemia. *J. clin. Path.*, 13: 463.

JACOBS, A. and KILPATRICK, G. S. (1964). The Paterson-Kelly syndrome. *Brit. med. J.*, ii: 79.

JADHAV, M., WEBB, J. K. G., VAISHNAVA, S. and BAKER, S. J. (1962). Vitamin B_{12} deficiency in Indian infants. A clinical syndrome. *Lancet*, ii: 903

JEFFRIES, G. H., HOSKINS, D. W. and SLEISENGER, M. H. (1962). Antibody to intrinsic factor in serum from patients with pernicious anemia. *J. clin. Invest.*, 41: 1106.

JEREMY, D. and McIVER, M. (1966). Inulin, ^{57}Co-labelled vitamin B_{12} and endogenous creatinine clearances in the measurement of glomerular filtration rate in man. *Aust. Ann. Med.*, 15: 346.

JOHANSON, A. H. (1929). Achylia in pernicious anaemia after liver treatment. *J. Amer. med. Ass.*, 92: 1928.

JOHNSON, S., SWAMINATHAN, S. P. and BAKER, S. J. (1962). Changes in serum vitamin B_{12} levels in patients with megaloblastic anaemia treated with folic acid. *J. clin. Path.*, 15: 274.

JONES, P. N., MILLS, E. H. and CAPPS, R. B. (1957). The effect of liver disease on serum vitamin B_{12} concentrations. *J. lab. clin. Med.*, 49: 910.

JUKES, T. H. (1962). Some nutritional and biochemical functions of folic acid. In: *Proceedings of the Conference on Intestinal Malabsorption and allied Hematologic Problems, Puerto Rico, 1962. Amer. J. dig. Dis.*, 7: 987.

KACZKA, E. A., WOLF, D. E., KUEHL, F. A., Jr. and FOLKERS, K. (1950). Vitamin B_{12}: Reactions of cyanocobalamin and related compounds. *Science*, 112: 354.

KAHN, S. B., WILLIAMS, W. J., BARNESS, L. A., YOUNG, D., SHAFER, B., VIVACQUA, R. J. and BEAUPRE, E. M. (1965). Methylmalonic acid excretion a sensitive indicator of vitamin B_{12} deficiency in man. *J. lab. clin. Med.*, 66: 75.

KATZ, J. H., DIMASE, J. and DONALDSON, R. M. (1963). Simultaneous administration of gastric juice-bound and free radioactive cyanocobalamin: rapid procedure for differentiating between intrinsic factor deficiency and other causes of vitamin B_{12} malabsorption. *J. lab. clin. Med.*, 61: 266.

KELLY, A. and HERBERT, V. (1967). Coated charcoal assay of erythrocyte vitamin B_{12} levels. *Blood*, 29: 139.

KILLANDER, A. (1957). The assay of vitamin B_{12} in human serum. *Acta Soc. Med. Upsalien*, 62: 39.

KILLANDER, A. and SCHILLING, R. F. (1961). Studies on hydroxocobalamin. I. Excretion and retention of massive doses in control subjects. *J. lab. clin. Med.*, 57: 553.

KISLIUK, R. L. and WOODS, D. D. (1960). Interrelationships between folic acid and cobalamin in the synthesis of methionine by extracts of *Escherichia coli*. *Biochem. J.*, 75: 467.

KLIPSTEIN, F. A., (1964a). Tropical sprue in New York City. *Gastroenterology*, 47: 457.

KLIPSTEIN, F. A. (1964b). Antibiotic therapy in tropical sprue: the role of dietary folic acid in the hematologic remission associated with oral antibiotic therapy. *Ann. int. Med.*, 61: 721.

KLIPSTEIN, F. A., SCHENK, E. A. and SAMLOFF, I. M. (1966). Folate repletion associated with oral tetracycline therapy in tropical sprue. *Gastroenterology*, 51: 317.

KNOWLES, J. P. and PRANKERD, T. A. J. (1962). Abnormal folic acid metabolism in vitamin B$_{12}$ deficiency. *Clin. Sci.*, **22**: 233.

KOHN, J., MOLLIN, D. L. and ROSENBACH, L. M. (1961). Conventional voltage electrophoresis for formiminoglutamic acid determination in folic acid deficiency. *J. clin. Path.*, **14**: 345.

LARRABEE, A. R. and BUCHANAN, J. M. (1961). A new intermediate of methionine biosynthesis. *Fed. Proc.*, **20**: 9.

LATNER, A. L., RAINE, L. ROSS, G. I. M. and UNGLEY, C. C. (1952). A preparative paper-electrophoresis technique and its application to vitamin B$_{12}$ binding in serum. *Biochem. J.*, **52**: xxxiii.

LATNER, A. L., HODSON, A. W. and SMITH, P. A. (1961). Intestinal absorption of coenzyme B$_{12}$ in the normal and fluoroacetate poisoned rat. *Lancet*, **ii**: 230.

LAU, K.-S., GOTTLIEB, C., WASSERMAN, L. R. and HERBERT, V. (1965). Measurement of serum vitamin B$_{12}$ level using radioisotope dilution and coated charcoal. *Blood*, **26**: 202.

LAWRENCE, C. (1966). B$_{12}$ binding protein deficiency in pernicious anaemia. *Blood*, **27**: 389.

LEAR, A. A. and CASTLE, W. B. (1956). Supplemental folic acid therapy in pernicious anemia: The effect on erythropoiesis and serum vitamin B$_{12}$ concentrations in selected cases. *J. lab. clin. Med.*, **47**: 88.

LEAR, A. A., HARRIS, J. W., CASTLE, W. B. and FLEMING, E. M. (1954). The serum vitamin B$_{12}$ concentration in pernicious anaemia. *J. lab. clin. Med.*, **44**: 715.

LEES, F. (1961). Radioactive vitamin B$_{12}$ absorption in the megaloblastic anaemia caused by anticonvulsant drugs. *Quart. J. Med.*, **30**: 231.

LENGYEL, P., MAZUMDER R. and OCHOA, S. (1960). Metabolism of propionic acid in animal tissues. VI. Mammalian methylmalonyl isomerase and vitamin B$_{12}$ coenzymes. *Proc. Nat. Acad. Sci., U.S.A.*, **45**: 1312.

LENHERT, P. G. and HODGKIN, D. C. (1961). Structure of the 5-6 dimethylbenzimidazolyl-cobamide coenzyme. *Nature, Lond.*, **192**: 937.

LESTER SMITH, E. (1951). Vitamin B$_{12}$. Part I. *Nutr. Abs. Rev.*, **20**: 795.

LESTER SMITH, E. (1959). Instability of radioactive vitamin B$_{12}$. *Lancet*, **i**: 388.

LESTER SMITH, E. and PARKER, L. F. J. (1948). Purification of antipernicious anaemia factor. *Biochem. J.*, **43**: viii.

LESTER SMITH, E., HOCKENHULL, D. J. D. and QUILTER, A. R. J. (1952). Tracer studies with the B$_{12}$ vitamins. 2. Biosynthesis of vitamin B$_{12}$ labelled with ^{60}Co and ^{32}P. *Biochem. J.*, **52**: 387.

LICHTMAN, H., WATSON, J., GINSBERG, V., PIERCE, J. V., STOKSTAD, E. L. R. and JUKES, T. H. (1949). Vitamin B$_{12}$b: Some properties and its therapeutic use. *Proc. Soc. exp. Biol., N.Y.*, **72**: 643.

LINDSTRAND, K. and STAHLBERG, K.-G. (1963). On vitamin B$_{12}$ forms in human plasma. *Acta. med. Scand.*, **174**: 665.

LINDSTRAND, K., WILSON, J. and MATTHEWS, D. M. (1966). Chromatography and microbiological assay of vitamin B$_{12}$ in smokers. *Brit. med. J.*, **2**: 988.

LINDSTRAND, K., ANDERSON, B. B., COWAN, J. D., COATES, M. E. and HOFFBRAND, A. V. (1967). The effect of dietary folate deficiency on the synthesis of methylcobalamin in the chick. *Scand. J. Haemat.*, **4**: 181.

LLOYD, H. E. D. and GARRY, J. (1963). Atypical cells in vaginal smears in pernicious anaemia. *Amer. J. Obstet. Gynec.*, **85**: 408.

LOUGHLIN, R. E., ELFORD, H. L. and BUCHANAN, J. M. (1964). Enzymatic synthesis of the methyl group of methionine. VII. Isolation of a cobalamin-containing transmethylase (5-methyltetrahydro-folate homocysteine) from mammalian liver. *J. biol. Chem.*, **239**: 2888.

C*

LOWENSTEIN, L., PICK, C. and PHILPOTT, N. (1955). Megaloblastic anaemia of pregnancy and the puerperium. *Amer. J. Obstet. Gynec.*, 70: 1309.

LOWENSTEIN, L., COOPER, B. A., BRUNTON, L., GARTHA, S. and KERNER, K. (1961). An immunologic basis for acquired resistance to oral administration of hog intrinsic factor and vitamin B_{12} in pernicous anaemia. *J. clin. Invest.*, 40: 1656.

LOWENSTEIN, L., BRUNTON, L. and HSIEH, Y.-S. (1966). Nutritional anaemia and megalblastosis in pregnancy. *Canad. med. Ass. J.*, 94: 636.

MALAMOS, B., DONTAS, A. S., KOUTRAS, D. A., MARKETOS, S., SFONTOURIS, J. and PAPANICOLAOU, N. (1966). The determination of glomerular filtration rate in clinical practice. *Lancet*, i: 943.

MANSON, L. A. (1960). Vitamin B_{12} and deoxyribose synthesis in *Lactobacillus leichmanii. J. biol. Chem.*, 235, 2955.

MANTZOS, J., GYFTAKI, H. and ALEVIZOU, V. (1967). Isotopic determination of serum vitamin B_{12} level using Sephadex G-25. *Nucl. Med., Vienna*, 6: 311.

MARSHALL, R. A. and JANDL, J. H. (1960). Responses to "physiologic" doses of folic acid in the megaloblastic anemias. *Arch. int. Med.*, 105: 352.

MARSTON, H. R., ALLEN, S. H. and SMITH, R. M. (1961). Primary metabolic defect supervening on B_{12} deficiency in the sheep. *Nature, Lond.*, 190: 1085.

MATTHEWS, D. M. (1961). Retrobulbar neuritis in Addisonian pernicious anaemia. *Lancet*, i: 1289.

MATTHEWS, D. M. (1962). Observations on the estimation of serum vitamin B_{12} using *Lactobacillus leichmanii. Clin. Sci.*, 22: 101.

MATTHEWS, D. M. (1967). Absorption of water-soluble vitamins. *Brit. med. Bull.*, 23: 258.

MATTHEWS, D. M., GUNASEGARAM, R. and LINNELL, J. C. (1967). Results with radio-isotopic assay of serum B_{12} using serum binding agent. *J. clin. Path.*, 20: 683.

MEYER, L. M., SAWITSKY, A., COHEN, B. S., KRIM, M., FADEM, R. and RITZ, N. D. (1950). Oral treatment of pernicious anaemia with vitamin B_{12}. *Bull. N.Y. Acad. Med.*, 26: 263.

MEYER, L. M., CRONKITE, E. P., MILLER, I. F., MULZAC, C. W. and JONES, I. (1962). Co^{60}-vitamin B_{12} binding capacity of human leukocytes. *Blood*, 19: 229.

MEYER, L. M., REIZENSTEIN, P. G., CRONKITE, E. P., MILLER, I. F. and MULZAC, C. W. (1963). Serum binding of vitamin B_{12} analogues: identification of binding groups in the B_{12} molecule. *Brit. J. Haemat.*, 9: 158.

MEYNELL, M. J., COOKE, W. T., COX, E. V. and GADDIE, R. (1957). Serum cyanocobalamin level in chronic intestinal disorders. *Lancet*, i: 901.

MILLER, A., CORBUS, H. F. and SULLIVAN, J. F. (1957a). The plasma disappearance, excretion and tissue distribution of cobalt^{60} labelled vitamin B_{12} in normal subjects and patients with chronic myelogenous leukemia. *J. clin. Invest.*, 36: 18.

MILLER, A., CORBUS, H. F. and SULLIVAN, J. F. (1957b). A modified urinary excretion test for measuring oral Cobalt^{60} labelled vitamin B_{12} absorption and its application in certain disease states. *Blood*, 12: 347.

MINOT, G. R. and CASTLE, W. B. (1935). Interpretation of reticulocyte reactions. Their value in determining the potency of therapeutic materials, especially in pernicious anaemia. *Lancet*, ii: 319.

MINOT, G. R. and MURPHY, W. B. (1926). Treatment of pernicious anaemia by special diet. *J. Amer. med. Ass.*, 87: 470.

MISTILIS, S. P., SKYRING, A. P. and STEPHEN, D. D. (1965). Intestinal lymphangiectasia: mechanism of enteric loss of plasma-protein and fat. *Lancet*, i: 77.

MOLLIN, D. L. (1959a). Radioactive vitamin B_{12} in the study of blood diseases. *Brit. med. Bull.*, 15: 8.

MOLLIN, D. L. (1960). The megaloblastic anemias. *Ann. Rev. Med.*, 11: 333.

MOLLIN, D. L. (1962a). The megaloblastic anaemias and the malabsorption syndrome. *Trans. med. Soc. Lond.*, **78**: 51.

MOLLIN, D. L. (1962c). Vitamin B$_{12}$ metabolism in man using cobalt-58 (^{58}Co) as a tracer. *Proc. R. Soc. Med.*, **55**: 141.

MOLLIN, D. L. and BOOTH, C. C. (1959). The plasma clearance of intravenous doses of radioactive vitamin B$_{12}$. *Haemat. lat.* (*Milan*), **2**: 257.

MOLLIN, D. L. and HINES, J. D. (1964). Observation on the nature and pathogenesis of anaemia following partial gastrectomy. *Proc. R. Soc. Med.*, **57**: 575.

MOLLIN, D. L. and ROSS, G. I. M. (1952). The vitamin B$_{12}$ concentrations of serum and urine of normals and of patients with megaloblastic anaemias and other diseases. *J. clin. Path.*, **5**: 129.

MOLLIN, D. L. and ROSS, G. I. M. (1953). Serum vitamin B$_{12}$ concentrations of patients with megaloblastic anaemia after treatment with vitamin B$_{12}$, folic acid or folinic acid. *Brit. med. J.*, **ii**: 640.

MOLLIN, D. L. and ROSS, G. I. M. (1954). Vitamin B$_{12}$ deficiency in the megaloblastic anaemias. *Proc. R. Soc. Med.*, **47**: 428.

MOLLIN, D. L. and WATERS, A. H. (1968). Nutritional megaloblastic anaemia. In: Symposia of the Swedish Nutrition Foundation, VI: 121.

MOLLIN, D. L. and ROSS, G. I. M. (1955). Serum vitamin B$_{12}$ concentrations in leukaemia and in some other haematological conditions. *Brit. J. Haemat.*, **1**: 155.

MOLLIN, D. L., BAKER, S. J. and DONIACH, I. (1955). Addisonian pernicious anaemia without gastric atrophy in a young man. *Brit. J. Haemat.*, **1**: 278.

MOLLIN, D. L., PITNEY, W. R., BAKER, S. J. and BRADLEY, J. E. (1956). The plasma clearance and urinary excretion of parenterally administered ^{58}Co-B$_{12}$. *Blood*, **11**: 31.

MOLLIN, D. L., BOOTH, C. C. and BAKER, S. J. (1957). The absorption of vitamin B$_{12}$ in control subjects, in Addisonian pernicious anaemia and in the malabsorption syndrome. *Brit. J. Haemat.*, **3**: 412.

MUELLER, J. F. and WILL, J. J. (1955). Interrelationship of folic acid, vitamin B$_{12}$ and ascorbic acid in patients with megaloblastic anaemia. *Amer. J. clin. Nutr.*, **3**: 30.

MUELLER, J. F., GLAZER, H. S. and VILTER, R. W. (1952). Preliminary studies on the purine and pyrimidine bases of human bone marrow as determined by paper chromatography. I. Variations in pernicious anaemia in response to therapy. *J. clin. Invest.* **31**: 651.

MCDOUGALL, B. M. AND BLAKLEY, R. L. (1961). Biosynthesis of thymidylic acid. I. Preliminary studies with extract of *Streptococcus faecalis R*. *J. biol. Chem.*, **236**: 832.

MCINTYRE, O. R., SULLIVAN, L. W., JEFFRIES, G. H. and SILVER, R. H. (1965). Pernicious anemia in childhood. *New Engl. J. Med.*, **272**: 981.

MCINTYRE, P. A., HAHN, R., CONLEY, C. L. and GLASS, B. (1959). Genetic factors in predisposition to pernicious anemia. *Bull. Johns Hopk. Hosp.*, **104**: 309.

NEALE, G., CAUGHEY, D. E., MOLLIN, D. L. and BOOTH, C. C. (1966). Effects of intrahepatic and extrahepatic infection on liver function. *Brit. med. J.*, **i**: 382.

NELP, W. B., WAGNER, H. N. and REBA, R. (1964). Renal excretion of vitamin B$_{12}$ and its use in measurement of glomerular filtration rate in man. *J. lab. clin. Med.*, **63**: 480.

NELSON, R. S. and DOCTOR, V. M. (1958). The vitamin B$_{12}$ content of human liver as determined by bio-assay of needle biopsy material. *Ann. int. Med.*, **49**: 1361.

NEWMAN, G. E., O'BRIEN, J. R. P., SPRAY, G. H., WILLIAMS, D. L. and WITTS, L. J. (1962b). Distribution of vitamin B$_{12}$ in cell fractions of rat brains. *Biochem. biophys. Acta*, **64**: 438.

NIEWEG, H. O., FABER, J. G., DE VRIES, J. A. and KROESE, W. F. S. (1954). The relationship of vitamin B$_{12}$ and folic acid in megaloblastic anaemias. *J. lab. clin. Med.*, **44**: 118.

NYBERG, W. and OSTLING, G. (1956). Low vitamin B$_{12}$ concentrations in serum in fish tapeworm anaemia. *Nature, Lond.*, **178**: 934.

O'BRIEN, J. S. (1962). Role of the folate co-enzymes in cellular division: a review. *Cancer Res.*, **22**: 267.

O'BRIEN, W. and ENGLAND, N. W. J. (1964). Folate deficiency in acute tropical sprue. *Brit. med. J.*, **ii**: 1573.

O'BRIEN, W. and ENGLAND, N. W. J. (1966). Military tropical sprue from South East Asia. *Brit. med. J.*, **ii**: 1157.

O'DELL, B. L., ERICKSON, B. A., NEWBERNE, P. M. and FLYNN, L. M. (1961). State of oxidation of non-protein sulfhydryl compounds in vitamin B_{12} deficiency. *Amer. J. Physiol.*, **200**: 99.

PAULK, E. A., JR. and FARRAR, W. E. (1964). Diverticulosis of the small intestine and megaloblastic anemia. Intestinal microflora and absorption before and after tetracycline administration. *Amer. J. Med.*, **37**: 473.

PEEL, J. L. (1962). Vitamin B_{12} derivatives and CO_2-pyruvate exchange reaction: reappraisal. *J. biol. Chem.*, **237**: PC 263.

PERLMAN, D. (Ed.) (1964). Vitamin B_{12} Coenzymes. *Ann. N.Y. Acad. Sci.*, **112**: 547–921.

PERMAN, G., GULLBERG, R., REIZENSTEIN, P. G., SNELLMAN, B. and ALLGEN, L. G. (1960). A study of absorption patterns in malabsorption syndromes. *Acta med. Scand.*, **168**: 117.

PITNEY, W. R., BEARD, M. F. and VAN LOON, E. J. (1954). Observations on the bound form of vitamin B_{12} in human serum *J. biol. Chem.*, **207**: 143.

PITNEY, W. R., BEARD, M. F. and VAN LOON, E. J. (1955). The vitamin B_{12} content of electrophoretic fractions of liver homogenates. *J. biol. Chem.*, **212**: 117.

PROCOPIS, P. G. and VINCENT, P. C. (1966). A case of dysphagia due to post-cricoid web in a patient with pernicious anaemia without iron deficiency. *Med. J. Aust.*, **2**: 991.

PUNTULA, L., ARO, H. and GRASBECK, R. (1969). Hog mucosal protein in the assay of serum vitamin B_{12} by isotope dilution. *Scand. J. clin. Lab. Invest.*, **24**. Suppl. 110, 122.

RACHMILEWITZ, M., ARONOVITCH, J. and GROSSOWICZ, N. (1956). Serum concentrations of vitamin B_{12} in acute and chronic liver disease. *J. lab. clin. Med.*, **48**: 339.

RACHMILEWITZ, M., STEIN, Y., ARONOVITCH, J. and GROSSWICZ, N. (1958). The clinical significance of serum cyanocobalamin (vitamin B_{12}) in liver disease. *Arch. int. Med.*, **101**: 1118.

RACHMILEWITZ, M., STEIN, Y., STEIN, O., ARONOVITCH, J. and GROSSOWICZ, N. (1959). The storage of vitamin B_{12} in the liver. *Haemat. Lat., Milan*, **2**: 297.

RAMSEY, C. and HERBERT, V. (1965). Dialysis assay for intrinsic factor and its antibody; Demonstration of species specificity of antibodies to human and hog intrinsic factor. *J. lab. clin. Med.*, **65**: 143.

RATH, C. E., McCURDY, P. R. and DUFFY, B. J. (1957). Effect of renal disease on the Schilling test. *New Engl. J. Med.*, **256**: 111.

RAVEN, J. L., ROBSON, M. B., WALKER, P. L. and BARKHAN, P. (1969). Improved method for measuring vitamin B_{12} in serum using intrinsic factor, ^{57}Co B_{12} and coated charcoal. *J. clin. Path.*, **22**: 205.

RAVEN, J. L., WALKER, P. L. and BARKHAN, P. (1966). Comparison of the radioisotope dilution coated charcoal method and a microbiological method (*L. leichmanii*) for measuring vitamin B_{12} in serum. *J. clin. Path.*, **19**: 610.

REGISTER, V. D. (1954). Effect of vitamin B_{12} on liver and blood nonprotein sulfhydryl compounds. *J. biol. Chem.*, **206**: 705.

REICHARD, P. (1962). Enzymatic synthesis of deoxyribonucleotides. 1. Formation of deoxycytidine diphosphate from cytidine diphosphate with enzymes from *Escherichia coli. J. biol. Chem.*, **237**: 3513.

REIZENSTEIN, P. G. (1959). Vitamin B_{12} metabolism. Some studies on the absorption, excretion, enterohepatic circulation, turnover rate, body distribution and tissue-binding of B_{12}. *Acta med. Scand.*, **165** (Suppl.): 347.

REIZENSTEIN, P. G. (1967). Conversion of cyanocobalamin to a physiologically occurring form. *Blood*, 29: 494.

REIZENSTEIN, P. G., EK, G. and MATTHEWS, C. (1966). Vitamin B_{12} kinetics in man. Implications on total-body B_{12} determinations, human requirements and normal and pathological cellular B_{12} uptake. *Phys. Med. Biol.*, **11**: 295.

RETIEF, F., GOTTLIEB, C. and HERBERT, V. (1966). Binding of B_{12} by human serum α- in preference to β-globulin. *Clin. Res.*, **14**: 325.

RETIEF, F. P., GOTTLIEB, C. and HERBERT, V. (1967). Delivery of Co^{57} B_{12} to erythrocytes from α- and β-globulin of normal, B_{12} deficient, and chronic myeloid leukemia serum. *Blood*, 29: 837.

REYNOLDS, E. H., HALLPIKE, J. F., PHILLIPS, B. M. and MATTHEWS, D. M. (1965). Reversible absorptive defects in anticonvulsant megaloblastic anaemia. *J. clin. Path.*, **18**: 593.

RICKES, E. L., BRINK, N. G., KONIUSZY, F. R. WOOD, T. R. and FOLKERS, K. (1948). Crystalline vitamin B_{12}. *Science*, **107**: 396.

RILEY, W. H. (1925). Achlorhydria preceding pernicious anaemia. *J. Amer. med. Ass.*, **85**: 1908.

RITZ, N. D. and MEYER, L. M. (1960). Clearance of intravenously injected radioactive cobalt-labelled vitamin B_{12} in chronic myeloid leukemia and other conditions. *Cancer*, **13**: 1000.

Roos, P. (1970). A simple and rapid amberlite saturation analysis of serum B_{12}. *In*: In vitro procedures with radioisotopes in medicine. *Proc. Symp. Vienna, 1969*, p. 359. I.A.E.A., Vienna.

ROSENBLUM, C. (1960). Radiation comparison of cobalt isotopes. *Amer. J. clin. Nutr.*, **8**: 276.

ROSENBLUM, C. (1965). Stability of cyanocobalamin in living systems. *Series Haematologica*, **3**: 48.

ROSENBLUM, C., REIZENSTEIN, P. G., CRONKITE, E. P. and MERIWETHER, H. T. (1963). Tissue distribution and storage forms of vitamin B_{12} injected and orally administered to the dog. (28011). *Proc. Soc. exp. Biol., N.Y.*, **112**: 262.

ROSENTHAL, H. L. and SARETT, H. P. (1952). The determination of vitamin B_{12} activity in human serum. *J. biol. Chem.*, **199**: 433.

Ross, G. I. M. (1950). Vitamin B_{12} assay in body fluids. *Nature, Lond.*, **166**: 270.

Ross, G. I. M. (1952). Vitamin B_{12} assay in body fluids using *Euglena gracilis*. *J. clin. Path.*, **5**: 250.

Ross, G. I. M., MOLLIN, D. L., Cox, E. V. and UNGLEY, C. C. (1954). Hematologic responses and concentration of vitamin B_{12} in serum and urine following oral administration of vitamin B_{12} without intrinsic factor. *Blood*, **9**: 473.

ROTHENBERG, S. P. (1961). Assay of serum vitamin B_{12} concentration using Co^{57}-B_{12} and intrinsic factor. *Proc. Soc. exp. Biol., N.Y.*, **108**: 45.

ROTHENBERG, S. P. (1963). Radioassay of vitamin B_{12} by quantitating the competition between Co^{57}-B_{12} and unlabelled B_{12} for the binding sites of intrinsic factor. *J. clin. Invest.*, **42**: 1391.

ROTHENBERG, S. P. (1968). A radio-assay for serum B_{12} using unsaturated transcobalamin I as the B_{12} binding protein. *Blood*, **31**: 44.

RUBINI, J. R. (1970). Simplified assay for vitamin B_{12} in plastic tubes coated with intrinsic factor. *In*: In vitro procedures with radioisotopes in medicine. *Proc. Symp. Vienna, 1969*, p. 355. I.A.E.A., Vienna.

SAKAMI, W. and UKSTINS, I. (1961). Enzymatic methylation of homocysteine by a synthetic tetrahydrofolate derivative. *J. biol. Chem.*, **236**: PC 50.

SCHADE, S. G., ABELS, J., SCHILLING, R. F., FEICK, P. and MUCKERHEIDE, M. (1967). Studies on antibody to intrinsic factor. *J. clin. Invest.*, **46**: 615.

SCHADE, S. G., FEICK, P., MUCKERHEIDE, M. and SCHILLING, R. F. (1966). Occurrence in gastric juice of antibody to a complex of intrinsic factor and vitamin B_{12}. *New Engl. J. Med.*, **275**: 528.

SCHILLING, R. F. (1953). Intrinsic factor studies. II. The effect of gastric juice on the urinary excretion of radioactivity after the oral administration of radioactive vitamin B_{12}. *J. lab. clin. Med.*, **42**: 860.

SCHILLING, R. F., HARRIS, J. W. and CASTLE, W. B. (1951). Observations on the etiologic relationship of achylia gastrica to pernicious anemia. XIII. Haemopoietic activity of vitamin B_{12a} (vitamin B_{12b}). *Blood*, **6**: 228.

SCHLOESSER, L. L. and SCHILLING, R. F. (1963). Vitamin B_{12} absorption studies in a vegetarian with megaloblastic anemia. *Amer. J. clin. Nutr.*, **12**: 70.

SCHLOESSER, L. L., DESHPANDE, P. and SCHILLING, R. F. (1958). Biologic turnover rate of cyanocobalamin (vitamin B_{12}) in human liver. *Arch. int. Med.*, **101**: 306.

SCHWARTZ, M. (1958). Intrinsic-factor-inhibiting substance in serum of orally treated patients with pernicious anaemia. *Lancet*, **ii**: 61.

SCHWARTZ, M. (1960). Intrinsic factor antibody in serum from patients with pernicious anaemia. *Lancet*, **ii**: 1263.

SCHWARTZ, M., BASTRUP-MADSEN, P., NØRREGAARD, S. and KRISTENSEN, K. (1962). A vitamin-B_{12} preparation with retarded absorption. *Lancet*, **ii**: 1181.

SCHWARTZ, M., LOUS, P. and MEULENGRACHT, E. (1958). Absorption of vitamin B_{12} in pernicious anaemia. Defective absorption induced by prolonged oral treatment. *Lancet*, **ii**: 1200.

SCUDAMORE, H. H., HAGEDORN, A. B., WOLLAEGER, E. E. and OWEN, C. A., JR. (1958). Diverticulosis of small intestine and macrocytic anemia with report of two cases and studies on absorption of radioactive vitamin B_{12}. *Gastroenterology*, **34**: 66.

SHARP, A. A. and WITTS, L. J. (1962). Seminal vitamin B_{12} and sterility. *Lancet*, **ii**: 779.

SHEARMAN, D. J. C., CALVERT, J. A., ALA, F. A. and GIRDWOOD, R. H. (1965). Renal excretion of hydroxocoblamin in man. *Lancet*, **ii**: 1328.

SHEEHY, T. W. and PEREZ-SANTIAGO, E. (1961). Antibiotic therapy in tropical sprue. *Gastroenterology*, **41**: 208.

SHINTON, N. K. and SINGH, A. K. (1967). Vitamin B_{12} absorption by inhalation. *Brit. J. Haemat.*, **13**: 75.

SIMONS, K. (1964). Vitamin B_{12} binders in human body fluids and blood cells. *Societas Scientiarum Fennica, Commentationes Biologicae* XXVII, Helsinki.

SIURALA, M. and NYBERG, W. (1957). Vitamin B_{12} absorption in atrophic gastritis. *Acta med. Scand.*, **157**: 435.

SIURALA, M., ERAMAA, E. and NYBERG, W. (1960). Pernicious anemia and atrophic gastritis. *Acta med. Scand.*, **166**: 213.

SKEGGS, H. R., HANUS, E. J., MCCAULEY, A. B. and RIZZO, V. J. (1960). Hydroxocobalamin: physiological retention in the dog. *Proc. Soc. exp. Biol., N.Y.*, **105**: 518.

SMITH, A. D. M. (1960). Megaloblastic madness. *Brit. med. J.*, **ii**: 1840.

SMITH, A. D. M. (1961). Retrobulbar neuritis in Addisonian pernicious anaemia. *Lancet*, **i**: 1001.

SMITH, A. D. M. (1962). Veganism: a clinical survey with observations on vitamin B_{12} metabolism. *Brit. med. J.*, **i**: 1655.

SMITH, A. D. M. and DUCKETT, S. (1965). Cyanide, vitamin B_{12}, experimental demyelination and tobacco amblyopia. *Brit. J. exp. Path.*, **46**: 615.

SMITH, A. D. M., DUCKETT, S. and WATERS, A. H. (1963). Neuropathological changes in chronic cyanide intoxication. *Nature, Lond.*, **200**: 179.

SMITH, R. and OLIVER, R. A. M. (1967). Sudden onset of psychosis in association with vitamin-B_{12} deficiency. *Brit. med. J.*, **3**: 34.

SOBOTKA, H., BAKER, H. and ZIFFER, H. (1960). Distribution of vitamin B$_{12}$ between plasma and cells. *Amer. J. clin. Nutr.*, **8**: 283.

SPELL, W. H., JR. and DINNING, J. S. (1959). Requirement for vitamin B$_{12}$ in conversion of ribose to deoxyribose by *Lactobacillus leichmanii*. *J. Amer. chem. Soc.*, **81**: 3804.

SPRAY, G. H. (1955). An improved method for the rapid estimation of vitamin B$_{12}$ in serum. *Clin. Sci.*, **14**: 661.

SPRAY, G. H. and WITTS, L. J. (1958). Results of three years' experience with microbiological assay of vitamin B$_{12}$ in serum. *Brit. med. J.*, **i**: 295.

STADTMAN, E. R., OVERØTH, P., EGGERER, H. and LYNEN, F. (1960). Role of vitamin B$_{12}$ coenzyme and biotin in propionate metabolism. *Fed. Proc.*, **19**: 417.

STAHLBERG, K.-G. (1964). Forms of plasma vitamin B$_{12}$ in health and in pernicious anaemia, chronic myeloid leukaemia and acute hepatitis: A preliminary report. *Scand. J. Haemat.*, **1**, 220.

STAHLBERG, K.-G. (1965). On the occurrence of methylcobalamin in human liver. *Scand. J. Haemat.*, **2**: 80.

STAHLBERG, K.-G. (1967). Studies on methyl-P$_{12}$ in man. *Scand. J. Haemat., Suppl*: 1.

STAHLBERG, K.-G., RADNER, S. and NORDEN, ﾟ. (1967). Liver B$_{12}$ in subjects with and without vitamin B$_{12}$ deficiency. A quanatative and qualitative study. *Scand. J. Haemat.*, **4**: 312.

STERN, J. R. and FRIEDMAN, D. L. (1960). Vitamin B$_{12}$ and methylmalonyl CoA isomerase. *Biochem. biophys. Res. Comm.*, **2**: 82.

STRACHAN, R. W. and HENDERSON, J. G. (1965). Psychiatric syndromes due to avitaminosis B$_{12}$ with normal blood and marrow. *Quart. J. Med.*, **34**: 303.

STRAUSS, E. W., WILSON, T. H. and HOTCHKISS, A. (1960). Factors controlling B$_{12}$ uptake by intestinal sacs *in vitro*. *Amer. J. Physiol.*, **198**: 103.

SULLIVAN, L. W. and HERBERT, V. (1965). Studies on the minimum daily requirement for vitamin B$_{12}$. Haemopoietic responses to 0.1 microgram of cyanocobalamin or coenzyme B$_{12}$ and comparison of their relative potency. *New Engl. J. Med.*, **272**: 340.

SULLIVAN, L. W., HERBERT, V. and CASTLE, W. B. (1963). *In vitro* assay for human intrinsic factor. *J. clin. Invest.*, **42**: 1443.

SWENDSEID, M. E., BETHELL, F. H. and ACKERMANN, W. W. (1954a). The intracellular distribution of vitamin B$_{12}$ and folinic acid in mouse liver. *J. biol. Chem.*, **190**: 791.

SWENDSEID, M. E., GASSTER, M. and HALSTED, J. A. (1954b). Limits of absorption of orally administered vitamin B$_{12}$: effect of intrinsic factor sources. *Proc. Soc. exp. Biol., N.Y.*, **86**: 834.

TABAQCHALI, S. and BOOTH, C. C. (1967). Relationship of the intestinal bacterial flora to absorption. *Brit. med. Bull.*, **23**: 285.

TABAQCHALI, S., OKUBADEJO, O. A., NEALE, G. and BOOTH, C. C. (1966). Influence of abnormal bacterial flora on small intestinal function. *Proc. roy. Soc. Med.*, **59**: 1244.

TAKEYAMA, S., HATCH, F. T. and BUCHANAN, J. M. (1961). Enzymatic synthesis of the methyl group of methionine. II. Involvement of vitamin B$_{12}$. *J. biol. Chem.*, **236**: 1102.

TAYLOR, K. B. (1959). Inhibition of intrinsic factor by pernicious anaemia sera. *Lancet*, **ii**: 106.

THIRKETTLE, J. L., GOUGH, K. R. and READ, A. E. (1964). Diagnostic value of small oral doses of folic acid in megaloblastic anaemia. *Brit. med. J.*, **i**: 1286.

THOMPSON, R. E. and HECHT, R. A. (1959). Studies on a long-acting vitamin B$_{12}$ preparation. *Amer. J. clin. Nutr.*, **7**: 311.

THORELL, B. (1947). Studies on the formation of cellular substances during blood cell production. *Acta med. Scand.*, **129**: Suppl. 200: 104.

TOOHEY, J. I. and BARKER, H. A. (1961). Isolation of coenzyme B$_{12}$ from liver. *J. biol. Chem.*, **236**: 560.

TUDHOPE, G. R., SWAN, H. T. and SPRAY, G. H. (1967). Patient variation in pernicious anaemia, as shown in a clinical trial of cyanocobalamin, hydroxocobalamin and cyanocobalamin-zinc tannate. *Brit. J. Haemat.*, **13**: 216.
TURNBULL, A. L. (1967). Absorption of vitamin B_{12} in patients with anaemia after Polya partial gastrectomy. *Brit. J. Haemat.*, **13**: 752.
TURNER, J. W. A. (1940). Optic atrophy associated with pernicious anaemia. *Brain*, **63**: 225.
UCHINO, H. S., UKYO, S., YAGIRI, Y. and WAKISAKA, G. (1962). Absorption and tissue distribution of 5,6-dimethylbenzimidazolyl cobamide coenzyme. *Vitamins*, **25**: 190.
UCHINO, H. S., UKYO, S., YAGARI, Y., YOSHINO, T. and WAKISAKA, G. (1964). Tissue distribution of coenzyme B_{12} in rats following intravenous administration. *Ann. N. Y. Acad. Sci.*, **112**: 844.
UKYO, S. and COOPER, B. A. (1965). Intrinsic-factor-like activity in extracts of guinea pig intestines. *Amer. J. Physiol.*, **208**: 9.
UNGLEY, C. C. (1949). Subacute combined degeneration of the cord. *Brain.*, **72**: 382.
UNGLEY, C. C. (1951). Vitamin B_{12}. Part 2. A review of the clinical aspects. *Nutr. Abstr. Rev.*, **21**: 1.
UNGLEY, C. C. (1955). The chemotherapeutic action of vitamin B_{12}. *Vitamins Hormones*, **13**: 137.
VEEGER, W., ABELS, J., HELLEMANS, N. and NIEWEG, H. O. (1962). Effect of sodium bicarbonate and pancreatin on the absorption of vitamin B_{12} and fat in pancreatic insufficiency. *New Engl. J. Med.*, **267**: 1341.
VICTOR, M. and LEAR, A. A. (1956). Subacute combined degeneration of the spinal cord. *Amer. J. Med.*, **20**: 896.
VIVACQUA, R. J., MYERSON, R. M., PRESCOTT, D. J. and RABINOWITZ, J. L. (1966). Abnormal propionic-methylmalonic-succinic acid metabolism in vitamin B_{12} deficiency and its possible relationship to the neurologic syndrome of pernicious anemia. *Amer. J. med. Sci.*, **251**: 507.
VON BONSDORFF, B. (1956). *Diphyllobothrium latum* as a cause of pernicious anaemia. *Exp. Parasitol.*, **5**: 207.
WAGNER, F. (1966). Vitamin B_{12} and related compounds. *Ann. Rev. Biochem.*, **35**: 405.
WAHBA, A. J. and FRIEDKIN, M. (1961). Direct spectrophotometric evidence for oxidation of tetrahydrofolate during enzymatic synthesis of thymidylate. *J. biol. Chem.*, **236**: PC 11.
WANGEL, A. G. and SCHILLER, K. F. R. (1966). Diagnostic significance of antibody to intrinsic factor. *Brit. med. J.*, **i**: 1274.
WANGEL, A. G., CALLENDER, S. T., SPRAY, G. H. and WRIGHT, R. (1968a). A family study of pernicious anaemia. I. Autoantibodies, achlorhydria, serum pepsinogen and vitamin B_{12}. *Brit. J. Haemat.*, **14**: 161.
WANGEL, A. G., CALLENDER, S. T., SPRAY, G. H. and WRIGHT, R. (1968b). A family study of pernicious anaemia. II. Intrinsic factor secretion, vitamin B_{12} absorption and genetic aspects of gastric autoimmunity. *Brit. J. Haemat.*, **14**: 183.
WARNER, G. T. and OLIVER, R. A. (1966). A whole-body counter for clinical measurements utilizing the "shadow shield" technique. *Phys. Med. Biol.*, **11**: 83.
WATERS, A. H. (1963). Folic acid metabolism in the megaloblastic anaemias. Ph.D. Thesis, University of London, pp. 215.
WATERS, A. H. and MOLLIN, D. L. (1961). Studies on the folic acid activity of human serum. *J. clin. Path.*, **14**: 335.
WATERS, A. H. and MOLLIN, D. L. (1963). Observations on the metabolism of folic acid in pernicious anaemia. *Brit. J. Haemat.*, **9**: 319.
WATERS, A. H. and MURPHY, M. E. B. (1963). Familial juvenile pernicious anaemia a study of the hereditary basis of pernicious anaemia. *Brit. J. Haemat.*, **9**: 1.

WATKIN, D. M., BARROWS, C. H., JR., CHOW, B. F. and SHOCK, N. W. (1961). Renal clearance of intravenously administered vitamin B$_{12}$. *Proc. Soc. exp. Biol., N.Y.*, **107**: 219.

WATSON, A. A. (1962). Seminal vitamin B$_{12}$ and sterility. *Lancet*, **ii**: 644.

WEISBERG, H. and GLASS, G. B. J. (1966). A rapid quantitative method for measuring intestinal absorption of vitamin B$_{12}$ in man using a double label hepatic uptake test. *J. lab. clin. Med.*, **68**: 163.

WEISSBACH, H. and DICKERMAN, H. (1965). Biochemical role of vitamin B$_{12}$. *Physiol. Rev.*, **45**: 80.

WEISSBACH, H., TOOHEY, J. I. and BARKER, H. A. (1959). Isolation and properties of B$_{12}$ coenzymes containing benzimidazole or dimethylbenzimidazole. *Proc. nat. Acad. Sci. Wash.*, **45**; 521.

WEISSBACH, H., LADD, J. N., VOLCANI, B. E., SMYTH, R. D. and BARKER, H. A. (1960). Structure of adenylcobamide coenzyme: degradation by cyanide, acid and light. *J. biol. Chem.*, **235**: 1462.

WEST, R. and REISNER, E. H., JR. (1949). Treatment of pernicious anaemia with crystalline vitamin B$_{12}$. *Amer. J. Med.*, **6**: 643.

WHIPPLE, G. H., HOOPER, W. C. and ROBSCHEIT, F. S. (1920). Blood regeneration following simple anaemia. IV. Influence of meat, liver and various extractives alone or combined with standard diets. *Amer. J. Physiol.*, **53**: 236.

WHITE, J. C., LESLIE, I. and DAVIDSON, J. N. (1953). Nucleic acids of bone marrow cells, with special reference to pernicious anaemia. *J. Path. Bact.*, **66**: 291.

WHITESIDE, M. G., MOLLIN, D. L., COGHILL, N. F., WILLIAMS, A. W. and ANDERSON, B. (1964). The absorption of radioactive vitamin B$_{12}$ and the secretion of hydrochloric acid in patients with atrophic gastritis. *Gut*, **5**: 385.

WICKRAMASINGHE, S. N., CHALMBERS, D. G. and COOPER, E. H. (1967). Disturbed proliferation of erythropoietic cells in pernicious anaemia. *Nature, Lond.*, **212**: 189.

WILL, J. J., MUELLER, J. F., BRODINE, C., KIELY, C. E., FRIEDMAN, B., HAWKINS, V. R., DUTRA, J. and VILTER, R. W. (1959). Folic acid and vitamin B$_{12}$ in pernicious anaemia. *J. lab. clin. Med.*, **53**: 22.

WILLIAMS, D. L. (1968). The distribution of vitamin B$_{12}$ in animals and the effects of dietary deficiency. D.Phil. Thesis, University of Oxford, p. 116.

WILLIGAN, D. A., CRONKITE, E. P., MEYER, L. M. and NOTO, S. L. (1958). Biliary excretion of Co^{60} labelled vitamin B$_{12}$ in dogs. *Proc. Soc. exp. Biol., N.Y.*, **99**: 81.

WILSON, J. and LANGMAN, M. J. S. (1966). Relation of subacute combined degeneration of the cord to vitamin B$_{12}$ deficiency. *Nature, Lond.*, **212**: 787.

WILSON, J. and MATTHEWS, D. M. (1966). Metabolic inter-relationships between cyanide, thiocyanate and vitamin B$_{12}$ in smokers and non-smokers. *Clin. Sci.*, **31**: 1.

WILSON, T. H. (1964). Membrane transport of vitamin B$_{12}$. *Medicine*, **43**: 669.

WINAWER, S. J., STREIFF, R. R. and ZAMCHECK, N. (1967). Gastric and hematological abnormalities in a vegan with vitamin B$_{12}$ deficiency: effect of oral vitamin B$_{12}$. *Gastroenterology*, **53**: 130.

WINTROBE, M. M. (1939). The antianemic effect of yeast in pernicious anemia. *Amer. J. med. Sci.*, **197**: 286.

WITHEY, J. L. and KILPATRICK, G. S. (1964). Hydroxocobalamin and cyanocobalamin in Addisonian anaemia. *Lancet* **i**: 16.

WITTS, L. J. (1960). The development of pernicious anaemia. *Acta haemat.*, **24**: 1

WOKES, F. (1958). Tobacco amblyopia. *Lancet*, **ii**: 526.

WOKES, F., BADENOCH, J. and SINCLAIR, H. M. (1955). Human dietary deficiency of vitamin B$_{12}$. *Amer. J. clin. Nutr.*, **3**: 375.

WOODLIFF, H. J. and ARMSTRONG, B. K. (1966). Vitamin B$_{12}$ absorption studies: comparison of ^{57}Co and vitamin B$_{12}$ plasma levels, urinary excretion and faecal excretion. *Med. J. Aust.*, **i**: 1023.

ZALUSKY, R. and HERBERT, V. (1961). Failure of formimino-glutamic acid (FIGLU) excretion to distinguish vitamin B_{12} deficiency from nutritional folic acid deficiency. *J. clin. Invest. (Abstr.)*, **40**: 1091.

ZALUSKY, R., HERBERT, V. and CASTLE, W. B. (1962). Cyanocobalamin therapy effect in folic acid deficiency. *Arch. int. Med.*, **109**: 545.

CHAPTER 2

FOLIC ACID AND DERIVATIVES

I. Chanarin

*Department of Haematology,
Norwich Park Hospital and Clinical Research Centre,
Harrow, Middlesex*

HISTORICAL

THE demonstration of a hematopoietic factor active in producing a hematological response in patients with megaloblastic anemia, and different from the anti-pernicious anemia factor present in "refined" liver extracts, was made by Lucy Wills in 1931. Working in Bombay, she found that macrocytic anemia in pregnant women and in non-pregnant patients responded to oral treatment with "crude" liver extracts, or with yeast.

Other workers were also active in isolating a biologically active fraction from yeast. Day *et al.* (1936) had found that both yeast and liver extracts were effective in curing what they termed nutritional cytopenia in monkeys and named the factor vitamin M. Stokstad and Manning (1938) had found that a factor in yeast (Factor U) promoted growth in chicks, and a similar factor derived from liver was described by Hogan and Parrott (1939). Meanwhile Snell and Peterson (1940) had obtained a factor, from both yeast and liver by adsorption and elution from activated charcoal, which was required for the growth of *Lactobacillus casei*. They termed this the "Norit-eluate factor", and subsequently Stokstad (1943) demonstrated the similarity of the factor from both these sources by isolating them in relatively pure form.

A further source of this factor proved to be spinach, and Mitchell *et al.* (1941), using four tons of spinach as their starting material obtained the growth factor in a relatively pure form. Because of the relatively high yield from this source, they suggested the term folic acid (Latin: folium, leaf) for the growth factor. Isolation of the active fractions in a relatively pure state was also achieved by Hutchings *et al.* (1941a), Pfiffner *et al.* (1943), and by Stockstad (1943). Its chemical structure was determined by the study of its degradation products, and final proof of the structure of folic acid and related compounds was obtained by their chemical synthesis (Angier *et al.*, 1946). These aspects are reviewed by Jukes and Stokstad (1948).

BIOCHEMISTRY

Nomenclature

The International Union of Pure and Applied Chemistry and the International Union of Biochemistry have suggested tentative rules for the naming of folic acid and related compounds (Jaenicke *et al.*, 1965). These rules are:

(1) Folic acid and folate are to be used as general terms for any members of the family.

(2) The parent compound is pteroic acid, and the salts and the radical derived from pteroic acid are named pteroates and pteroyl respectively.

(3) The numbering of the atoms in pteroic acid is as shown in Fig. 1. The bridge carbons in the pteridine ring are numbered 4a and 8a.

(4) The term pteroylglutamic acid is used when pteroic acid is conjugated with one molecule of glutamic acid. When more than one molecule of glutamic acid is present linked through the gamma carboxyl groups, the compounds are terms pteroyldiglutamic acid, etc. The term pteroylmonoglutamic acid is not used.

(5) Reduced compounds are indicated by prefixes "dihydro-" and "tetrahydro-" with numerals indicating positions of the hydrogen atoms. A tetrahydro-compound is assumed to be 5,6,7,8-tetrahydro-.

(6) *Abbreviations*:

(a) The generic terms, folate and folic, should not be abbreviated.
(b) Pteroic acid, pteroate or pteroyl is indicated by the symbol Pte; thus $PteGlu_1$, $PteGlu_3$, $PteGlu_y$, etc., the number indicating the number of glutamic acid units.
(c) Reduced derivatives are indicated as follows: $7,8\text{-}H_2PteGlu$, $H_4PteGlu$ but $H_2Folate$ and $H_4folate$ may be used without specifying the number of glutamic acid molecules.

(d) Substituents are indicated as follows and prefixed by the position of substitution:

Formimino	HCNH—
Formyl	HCO—
Hydroxymethyl	$HOCH_2$—
Methyl	CH_3—
Methylene	—CH_2—
Methylidyne	—CH=

(7) Substituents at the 6 position may be associated with optical activity and this may be designated by the symbols $(+)$ $(-)$ or $(\pm)$

Examples:

10-HCO-H_4PteGlu	10-Formyl-5,6,7,8-tetrahydropteroylglutamic acid
5,10-CH_2-H_4PteGlu	5,10-Methylenetetrahydropteroylglutamic acid
$(\pm)$-5,6-H_2PteGlu	racemic 5,6-Dihydropteroylglutamic acid.

Folate compounds from "natural" sources

A number of folate derivatives have been isolated from natural sources. These include pteroylglutamic acid, pteroic acid, pteroyltriglutamic acid, pteroylheptaglutamic acid, 10-formylpteroylglutamic acid, 5-formyl-tetrahydropteroylglutamic acid, and 5-methyltetrahydropteroylglutamic acid. Isolation of many of these compounds is not evidence that they exist naturally in these forms but merely that these forms are more stable chemically than the biologically active forms from which they are derived.

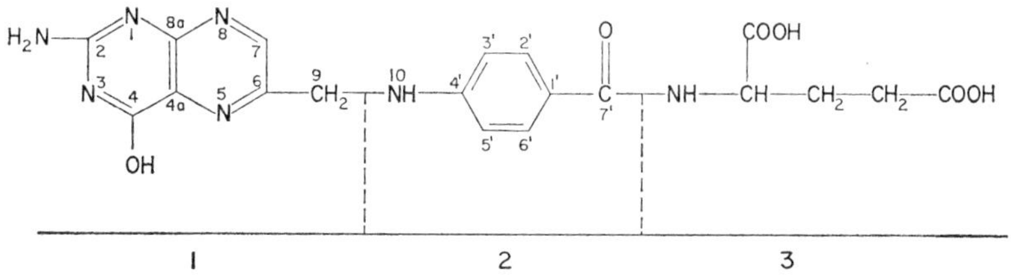

FIG. 1. Pteroylglutamic acid.

The parent compound is pteroylglutamic acid (Fig. 1). It consists of a pteridine or pterin portion (1), *p*-amino-benzoic acid (2) and *l*-glutamic acid (3). The pteridine (1) is a 2-amino-4-hydroxy derivative. The moiety composed of the pteridine and *p*-aminobenzoic acid portions (1 and 2) is

called pteroic acid, and was isolated by Keresztesy *et al.* (1943), from
cultures of *Rhizopus nigricans*.

The identification of *p*-amino-benzoic acid as part of the folic acid
molecule, coupled with the observation by Woods (1940) that *p*-amino-
benzoic acid would nullify the antibacterial effects of the sulfonamides,
suggested to Tschesche (1947) that sulfonamides interfered with the synthesis of folic acid at the stage of combination of either *p*-aminobenzoic
acid or *p*-aminobenzoyl-glutamic acid with the pteridine aldehyde to
produce dihydrofolate. Only those organisms that synthesize folic acid
are sensitive to the antibacterial action of sulfonamides and generally those
microorganisms such as *Lactobacillus casei, Str. faecalis R, Pediococcus
cerevisiae,* and *Tetrahymena geleii* which required the preformed folate
molecule, are insensitive to these drugs (Lampen and Jones, 1947; Nimmo-
Smith *et al.,* 1948). Similarly, the need for preformed folic acid by vertebrates explains why the sulfonamide drugs generally do not affect their
metabolism.

Pteroyltriglutamic acid (Fig. 2) also called "Teropterin" was isolated
from a *corynebacterium* by Hutchings *et al.* (1948a). It contains 3 glutamic
acid residues linked by γ-glutamyl peptide bonds.

F<small>IG</small>. 2.   Pteroyltriglutamic acid.

Pteroylheptaglutamate was isolated from yeast, and was shown by
Pfiffner *et al.* (1946) to contain 7 glutamic acid residues. The folate
compounds containing 3 and 7 glutamic acid residues have been termed
polyglutamates, and also folic acid "conjugates". Although these three
forms of folate were found to be equally active in promoting growth of
chicks and rats on folate free diets, they differ markedly in their activity for
microorganisms (Stokstad, 1954). *Streptococcus faecalis* grows only in
the presence of pteroylglutamic acid. *Lactobacillus casei* grows in the
presence of either pteroylglutamic acid or the triglutamate. Neither
organism is able to utilize the heptaglutamate. Polyglutamates may con-
stitute between 57 to 97% of folate present in a normal diet (Butterworth
et al., 1963).

10-formylpteroylglutamic (Fig. 3) acid was isolated from horse liver by Silverman *et al.* (1954).

5-formyltetrahydropteroylglutamic acid, also called folinic acid, leucovorin, citrovorum factor (Fig. 4) has been obtained from both liver and yeast and was found to be a necessary growth factor for *Pediococcus cerevisiae* (previously termed *Leuconostoc citrovorum*) by Sauberlich and Baumann (1948). It differs from pteroylglutamic acid in that the pyrazine ring of the pteridine moiety is reduced, i.e. there are 4 additional hydrogen atoms at positions 5, 6, 7, and 8, and that there is a formyl group at position 5. It has been obtained in a relatively pure form from horse liver by Keresztesy and Silverman (1951). Polyglutamyl derivatives of the

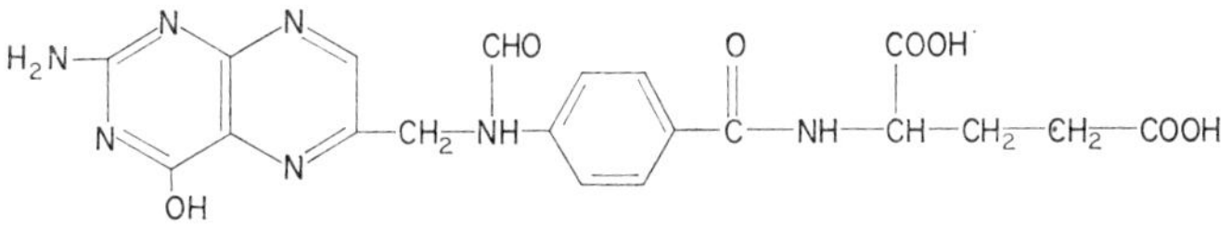

FIG. 3.   10-formylpteroylglutamic acid.

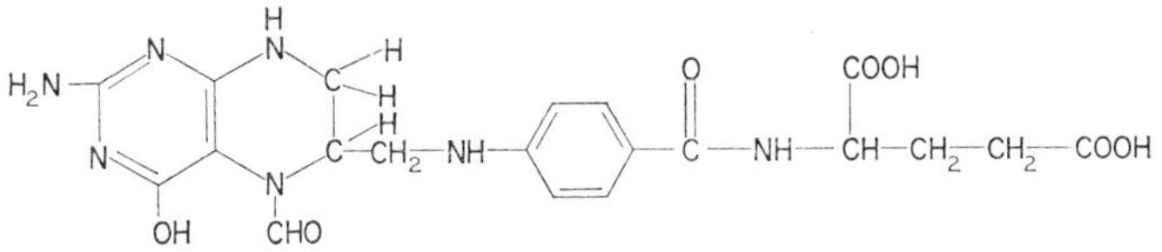

FIG. 4.   5-formyltetrahydropteroylglutamic acid.

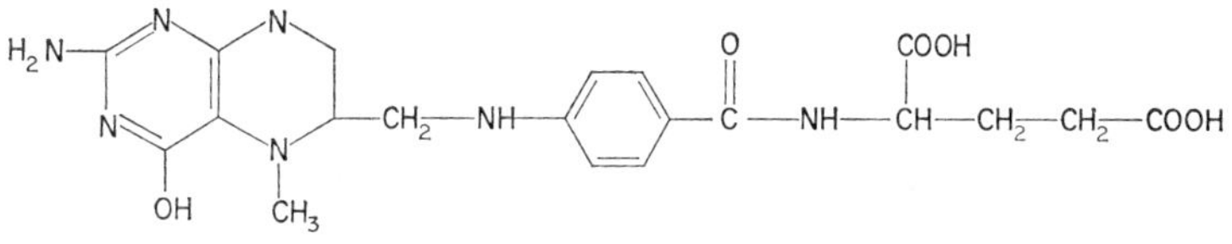

FIG. 5.   5-methyltetrahydropteroylglutamic acid.

reduced forms of folic acid occur in natural materials, since it has been observed that preliminary enzymatic treatment is required in order to obtain maximum growth with *P. cerevisiae* (Sauberlich, 1952). These have been demonstrated in algae, yeast, chick liver, and bacterial cells (Doctor and Couch, 1953; Bánhidi and Ericson, 1953).

5-methyltetrahydropteroylglutamic acid (Fig. 5) was isolated from horse liver by Donaldson and Keresztsey in 1959, and characterized by Larrabee *et al.* (1961). It is the main form of folate in the liver of the horse, in the liver of the mouse (Silverman *et al.*, 1961), and in the liver of man (Chanarin *et al.*, 1966). It is also the major constituent of serum folate (Herbert *et al.*, 1962).

Pteroylglutamic acid. Pteroylglutamic acid may be crystallized from solution as yellow spear-shaped crystals. Its molecular weight is 441.4, and contains 2 molecules of water, which are lost on heating above 140°.

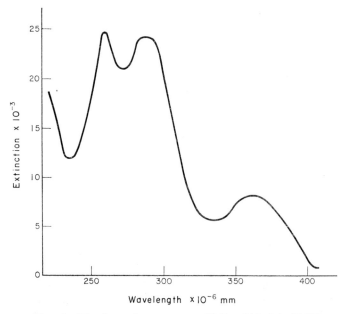

FIG. 6.   The absorption spectrum of folic acid in 0.1N KOH.

The free acid is relatively insoluble in water and in most organic solvents. It is slightly soluble in acetic acid. The disodium salt, however, is very soluble (15 g per l).

The absorption spectrum is shown in Fig. 6. Like most pteridines, pteroylglutamic acid exhibits fluorescence (Kyeda and Rabinowitz, 1963). It is optically active since there is an asymmetric carbon in the glutamic acid moiety.

Reduction of pteroylglutamic acid in the presence of platinum oxide results in the uptake first of one mole of hydrogen, to give H_2folate, and subsequently to give H₄folate (O'Dell *et al.*, 1947). The reduced forms are highly unstable, and can be preserved only under strict anaerobic conditions.

Exposure to concentrated formic acid at 100° results in the formation of 10-formylpteroylglutamic acid (Gordon *et al.*, 1948). Acid or alkaline hydrolysis with heat, exposure to sulfurous acid, or treatment with zinc and dilute acid, produces a split in the molecule at the 9,10 link to yield an aromatic amine, *p*-aminobenzoylglutamic acid, and a free pteridine (Hutchings *et al.*, 1948b). The rapid inactivation of pteroylglutamic acid on exposure to ultraviolet light (Stokstad *et al.*, 1947) is partly effected by cleavage of the molecule in this position.

5-formyltetrahydropteroylglutamic acid (*folinic acid*). This compound is one of the few stable forms among the reduced folate analogues. It may be obtained by catalytic hydrogenation of 10-formylfolate, followed by heat in alkaline solution (Flynn *et al.*, 1951; Roth *et al.*, 1952). In this

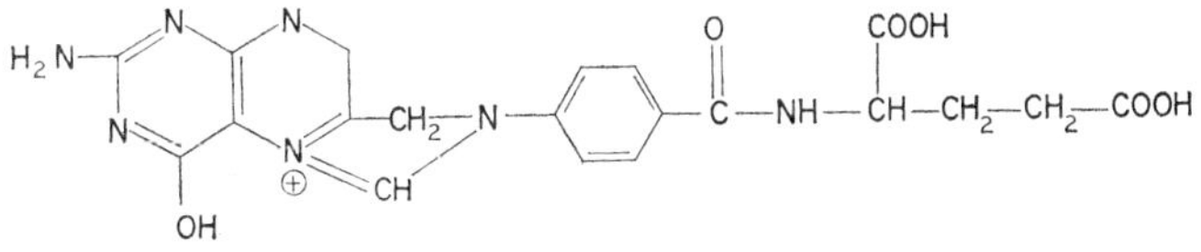

FIG. 7.   5,10-methenyltetrahydropteroylglutamic acid.

reaction 10-formylfolate is first reduced to 10-formylH₄folate, and this in turn is converted to the 5-formyl compound by alkali treatment. Unlike the form derived from horse liver, the synthetic compound is a mixture of diastereoisomers, which can in fact be separated on the basis of the differing solubility of their calcium salts (Cosulich *et al.*, 1952a). This mixture of isomers has only half the microbiological activity for *P. cerevisiae* possessed by the form from natural sources and this resides in the 1(L)-isomer, which has a specific rotation of − 15.1°.

On the addition of acid, 5-formylH₄folate loses a molecule of water, to form 5,10-methenylH₄folate or anhydroleucovorin (Fig. 7). (May *et al.*, 1951; Cosulich *et al.*, 1952b). The absorption spectrum of the 5,10-methenylH₄folate (Fig. 8) shows a peak at 350×10^{-6} mm in acid solution, and this has proved of value in devising quantitative procedures for the assay of various compound concerned with the folate coenzymes (Tabor and Wyngarden, 1958; Chanarin and Bennett, 1962a).

Polyglutamates. Enzymes are present in tissues which convert the poly-glutamate forms of naturally occurring folate compounds to forms active in microbiological assay (Wright and Welch, 1943a). Such enzymes were termed "folic acid conjugases". These enzymes are peptidases (Pfiffner *et al.*, 1946), and that purified from chicken pancreas was shown to be a γ-glutamic acid carboxypeptidase (Kazenko and Laskowski, 1948). Similar enzymes have been prepared from liver (Mims *et al.*, 1944), from kidney (Bird *et al.*, 1946) and Simpson and Schweigert (1949), and more

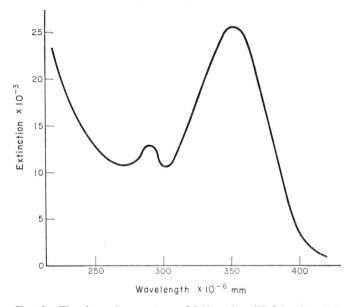

FIG. 8.   The absorption spectrum of 5,10-methenylH$_4$folate in N HCl.

recently Santini *et al.* (1966) have demonstrated these conjugases in the blood in man. Human intestinal juice has been found to be as effective as chick pancreas in making polyglutamates available for microbiological assay (Santini *et al.*, 1962). Although polyglutamates appear to be able to replace the monoglutamates in the nutrition of growing chicks and rats, and are able to produce hematological responses when given orally in large doses to patients with megaloblastic anemia (Wilkinson and Israëls, 1949), there is some doubt as to whether they are as effective in man as is pteroylglutamic acid when used in smaller doses (Bethell *et al.*, 1947).

Hematological responses may be obtained in patients with folic acid deficiency given small doses of pteroylglutamic acid, although the diets of the patients contain relatively large amounts of polyglutamates (Crosby, 1960; Butterworth *et al.*, 1963).

Folic acid reductase

The forms of folate functioning as coenzymes are all tetrahydrofolate derivatives. The conversion of less reduced forms to the tetrahydro-form is the function of the enzyme, folic acid reductase. Reduction of folic acid was demonstrated in man by Sauberlich (1949), in liver slices by Nichol and Welch (1950), in bacteria by Broquist *et al.* (1953), and in cell-free systems in Heisler and Schweigert (1955). The usual substrate is H_2folate, which is the primary product of folate biosynthesis (Brown *et al.*, 1961). H_2folate also arises from H_4folate in the course of thymidylate synthesis (McDougall and Blakley, 1960).

The reduction of folate to dihydrofolate is also catalysed by folic acid reductase, but this reaction takes place more slowly than the subsequent reduction of the dihydro to the tetrahydro form. Triglutamate compounds are equally effective as substrates for dihydrofolate reductase. Food folates are presumably converted to monoglutamates, and thereafter converted to H_4folate by this enzyme.

Two assays have been used to estimate reductase activity. One is based on the decrease of absorption at 350×10^{-6} mm due to loss of hydrogen from the reduced form of nicotinamide-adenine dinucleotide, and the change in the absorption as H_2folate is converted to H_4folate (Osborn and Huennekens, 1958; Blakley and McDougall, 1962; Friedkin *et al.*, 1962).

Another assay method is based on the spontaneous breakdown of the end product of reductase activity, viz. H_4folate, with the release of the diazotizable *p*-aminobenzoylglutamate which is estimated by the Brattan-Marshall reaction (Zakrzewski, 1960).

Folic acid reductase is also the specific site of action of the folic acid antagonists, aminopterin, amethopterin and dichloroamethopterin which bind irreversibly to this enzyme (Werkheiser, 1961; Delmonte and Jukes, 1962). Thus these antagonists prevent the regeneration of H_4folate from H_2folate. H_2folates accumulate as a result of the action of thymidylate synthetase which converts deoxyuridylic acid to thymidylic acid by the transfer of a carbon unit. In the course of this transfer the carbon is reduced to the methyl form, and the two hydrogen atoms for this reduction are obtained from H_4folate which is thereby reduced to H_2folate. The effect of the folate antagonists is to prevent regeneration of H_4folate from H_2folate produced in this way. This in turn results in a general reduction in the supply of H_4folate, and so leads to interference with the function of other folate coenzymes.

Resistance to the action of these folic acid antagonists is due to a marked increase in the folic acid reductase content of the cells (Hakala *et al.*, 1960). The same mechanism is operative in the development of a resistance to methotrexate in leukaemia in man (Bertino *et al.*, 1961).

The folate coenzymes

The biochemical role of folic acid was suggested by:

(a) Nutritional studies with bacteria showing that their folic acid requirement was decreased by purines, pyrimidines such as thymine and by serine (Snell and Mitchell, 1941; Stokes, 1944; Holland and Meinke, 1949). This suggested that folic acid played some function in the biosynthesis of these compounds.

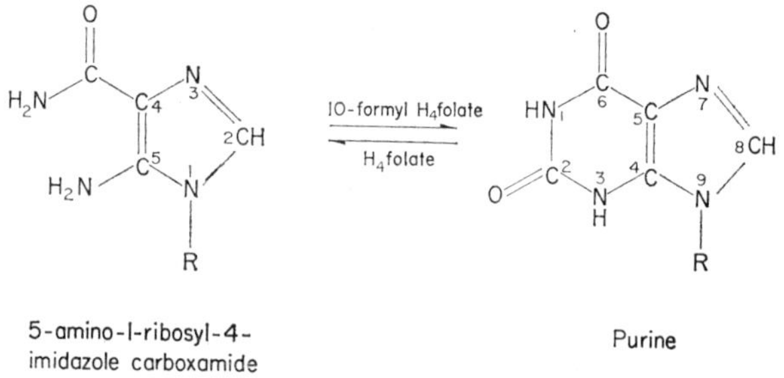

5-amino-l-ribosyl-4-
imidazole carboxamide   Purine

FIG. 9.   Closure of the purine nucleus.

(b) More particularly, Shive *et al.* (1947) found that, when *E. coli* was incubated in the presence of sulfanilamide, a purine precursor, 5-amino-4-imidazolecarboxamide, which lacked the carbon 2 atom of the purine nucleus accumulated. They postulated that the function of *p*-aminobenzoic acid (and hence of folic acid) was to transfer a carbon atom to complete the purine ring (Fig. 9).

(c) The characterization of 5-formylH_4folic acid (folinic acid), indicating that it differed from folic acid in the possession of an additional C unit, was a further stimulus to the view that folate compounds were concerned in the transfer of this single carbon unit.

(d) The use of ^{14}C-labeled formate demonstrated the close metabolic interrelationship between various potential donors and acceptors of single C units (Fig. 10). Thus the labeled carbon appears as the β-carbon of serine, as carbons 2 and 8 of the purine ring, and as carbon 2 of the imidazole ring of histidine. The labeled carbon in these positions were not

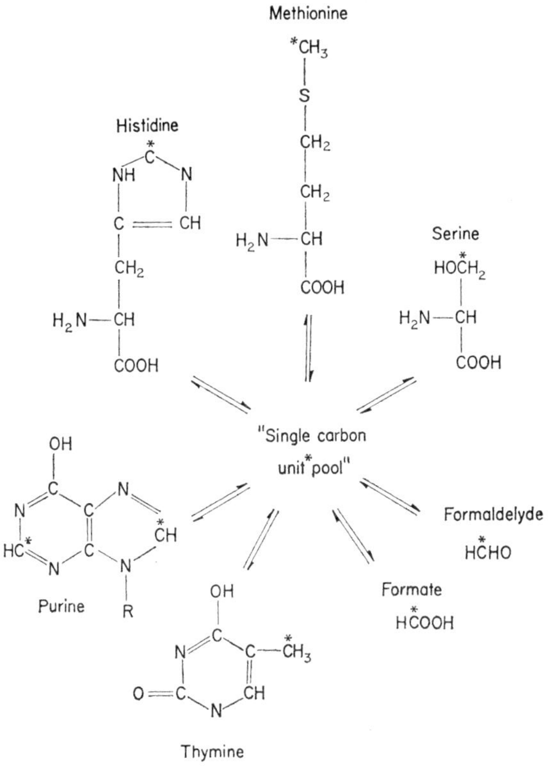

FIG. 10. Carbon units transferred by the folate coenzymes.

only readily interconvertable, but were also in equilibrium with the methyl group of thymine and methionine. All these reactions and interconversions were severely depressed in folate-deficient animals, in bacterial systems lacking folic acid, and under the influence of folic acid antagonists. This aspect has been reviewed by Huennekens and Osborn (1959).

In mammals the primary source or donor of "one-carbon" units is serine, which in turn arises from glucose from which serine is derived.

The major pathways which use these carbon units are concerned with the synthesis of purines, pyrimidines and methionine. The major storage-form of folate is 5-methylH$_4$folate (Donaldson and Keresztesy, 1959). Different reactions involving the folate coenzymes require the transfer of a carbon unit at different states of reduction. The different folate coenzymes are concerned with alteration in the state of reduction of the transferable carbon atom and these compounds, all derivatives of H$_4$folate, are shown in Fig. 11.

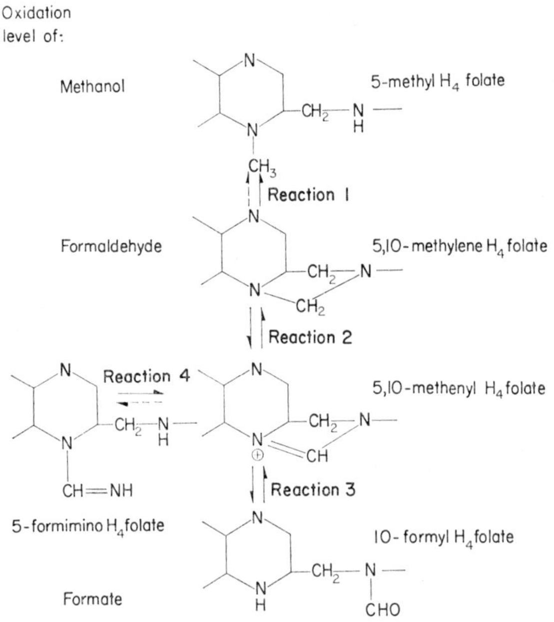

FIG. 11.   Interconversion of the folate coenzymes.

Interconversion of folate coenzymes. The folate-activated conversion of serine to glycine results in the formation of 5,10-methyleneH$_4$folate. This compound is also produced by simple mixing of formaldehyde and H$_4$folate (Kisliuk, 1957). This bridge compound is relatively stable at pH 9.5, but undergoes rapid dissociation at a pH of less than 7.0 (Osborn *et al.*, 1960).

Further reduction of this carbon unit to give 5-methylH$_4$folate (Reaction 1) is catalyzed by the enzyme 5,10-methyleneH$_4$folate reductase. This enzyme has been isolated from both *E. coli* (Cathou and Buchanan,

1963) and from pig liver (Donaldson and Keresztesy, 1962). The hydrogen for the reduction comes from reduced flavin-adenine dinucleotide (FAD), and this in turn is derived from water of the solvent. This flavin-containing enzyme requires reduced nicotinamide-adenine dinucleotide (NADH) as a co-factor. In mammalian systems it has been suggested that this reaction leads to the accumulation of 5-methyltetrahydrofolate; and the release of tetrahydrofolate, on this hypothesis, is achieved only by the transfer of the 5-methyl group to form methionine (Buchanan, 1964).

Oxidation of 5,10-methyleneH$_4$folate to 5,10-methenylH$_4$folate (Reaction 2) is brought about by the enzyme 5,10-methyleneH$_4$folate dehydrogenase. This has nicotinamide-adenine dinucleotide phosphate (NADP) as a co-factor. The enzyme has been purified from yeast (Ramasatri and Blakley, 1962), as well as from beef liver, and chick liver (Osborn and Huennekens, 1957). It has been demonstrated in human red cells by Bertino *et al.* (1962).

Further conversion of 5,10-methenylH$_4$folate to 10-formylH$_4$folate (Reaction 3) occurs via the enzyme 5,10-methenylH$_4$folate cyclohydrolase, and this change can be observed when the reaction is carried out in maleate buffer at pH 7. Once the pH is raised above 8, there is a rapid non-enzymic conversion of 5,10-methenylH$_4$folate to 10-formylH$_4$folate. The enzyme has been extracted from rabbit liver, hog kidney, and other animal tissues (Tabor and Rabinowitz, 1956). Reactions 2 and 3 are reversible.

10-FormylH$_4$folate can also arise directly by condensation of formate (HCOOH) with H$_4$folate. The enzyme formylH$_4$folate synthetase, requires adenosine triphosphate (ATP) as a co-factor, and has been purified 110-fold from human erythrocytes by Bertino *et al.* (1962). The initial product of the reaction of this enzyme from erythrocytes is 10-formyl-H$_4$folate. The activity of the enzyme was greater in reticulocytes than in mature red cells.

The reverse reaction with the release of formate from 10-formylH$_4$folate has been described by Osborn *et al.* (1957), using an enzyme from beef liver, 10-formylH$_4$folate deacylase.

A further source of 5,10-methenylH$_4$folate is from 5-formiminoH$_4$folate which appears as a result of the degradation of *l*-histidine. The conversion 5-formiminoH$_4$folate to 5,10-methenylH$_4$folate (Reaction 4) is catalyzed by formiminoH$_4$folate cyclodeaminase, an enzyme that has been purified from both *Cl. cylindrosporum* (Rabinowitz and Pricer, 1956) and rabbit liver (Tabor and Rabinowitz, 1956). The same reaction can be brought about nonenzymatically in the presence of acid. The changes in absorbancy accompanying these reactions are shown in Fig. 12.

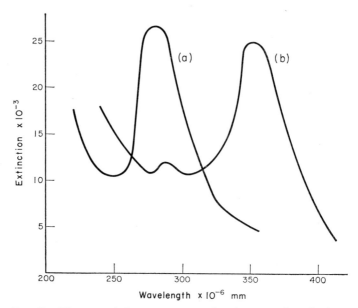

FIG. 12.   The spectral changes accompanying the conversion of 5-formiminoH$_4$folate (a) to 5,10-methenylH$_4$folate (b).

A full account of the interconversion of the folate compounds is contained in the admirable reviews of Rabinowitz (1960) and Friedkin (1963).

Reactions involving the folate coenzymes

Serine-glycine interconversion. The conversion of *l*-serine to glycine (Fig. 13), with release of the β-carbon as a single carbon unit, was suggested by Roepke *et al.*, (1944), and the role of folate in this reaction was demonstrated by Kisliuk and Sakami (1954). The enzyme catalysing the over-all reaction is serine hydroxymethyltransferase, also termed serine hydroxymethylase and serine aldolase, and it results in the formation of 5,10-methyleneH$_4$folate (Blakley, 1954). Serine hydroxymethyltransferase has

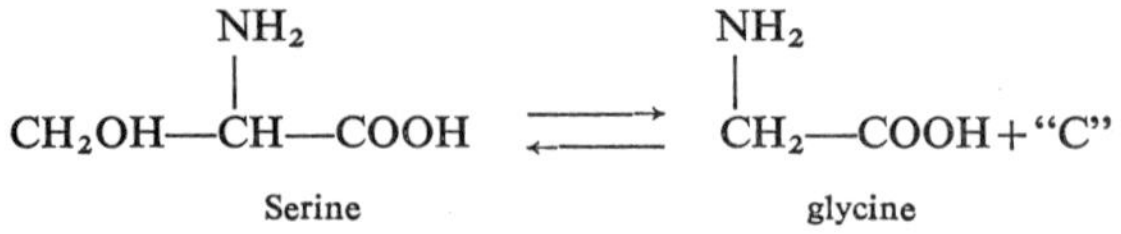

$$\underset{\text{Serine}}{\text{CH}_2\text{OH}-\overset{\overset{\displaystyle\text{NH}_2}{|}}{\text{CH}}-\text{COOH}} \;\rightleftarrows\; \underset{\text{glycine}}{\overset{\overset{\displaystyle\text{NH}_2}{|}}{\text{CH}_2}-\text{COOH} + \text{``C''}}$$

FIG. 13.   Serine–glycine interconversion.

been isolated from the liver of the rabbit, pigeon, guinea pig, sheep, rat, and cow as well as from microorganisms (Rabinowitz, 1960). It has been demonstrated in human red cells by Bertino *et al.* (1962). Not only is there a requirement for H_4folate, NAD, ATP, and also for divalent ions such as Mn^{++} in bacterial systems, but pyridoxal phosphate participates in the reaction (Deodhar and Sakami, 1953; Alexander and Greenberg, 1955; Blakley, 1955). Pyridoxal phosphate is bound to serine hydroxymethyltransferase, and in fact is not separated readily from the enzyme. It is assumed that the reaction proceeds via the attachment of pyridoxal phosphate to serine, and this results in a freeing of the bond between the α and β atoms of serine. The β carbon then links to H_4folate, and glycine is released.

Serine hydroxymethyltransferase has been obtained in a state of relative purity (Schirch and Mason, 1962), its MW has been determined as

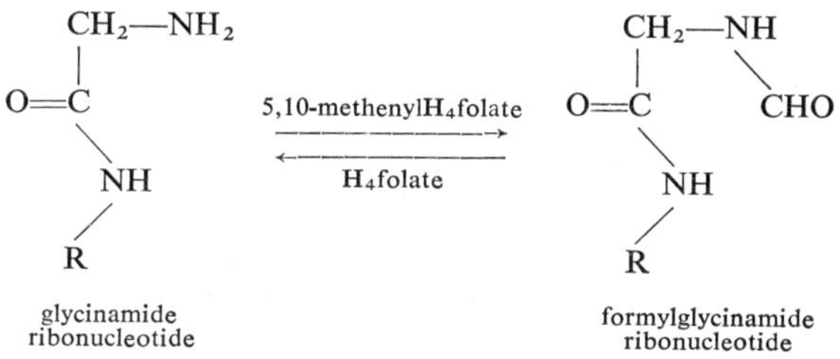

FIG. 14. Action of glycinamide ribonucleotide transformylase (GAR transformylase).

$331,000 \pm 8000$ (Schirch and Mason, 1963), and its absorption spectrum showing a maximum at 430×10^{-6} mm implies that pyridoxal phosphate is bound as a Schiff base.

Purine biosynthesis. Two enzyme preparations which catalyse the incorporation of "activated formate" into purine have been isolated (Goldthwait and Greenberg, 1955). The first of these is glycinamide ribonucleotide transformylase (GAR transformylase). Hartman and Buchanan (1959) demonstrated that the specific formyl donor linking formate to glycine (Fig. 14) in the formation of formylglycinamide ribonucleotide was 5,10-methenylH_4folate. This provides carbon 8 of the purine nucleus.

The second enzyme is 5-amino-4-imidazolecarboxamide ribonucleotide transformylase (AICAR transformylase). This enzyme completes the

D

closure of the purine ring, and the direct formyl donor is specifically
10-formylH$_4$folate, and not 5,10-methenylH$_4$-folate, which is required for
GAR transformylase (Hartman and Buchanan, 1959).

Pyrimidine biosynthesis. The conversion of uracil to thymine involves
the net addition of a methyl group to carbon 5 of the pyrimidine ring
(Fig. 15). This step is mediated by the folate coenzymes, and numerous
studies have shown that formate, formaldehyde, and the β carbon of serine
are better sources of this methyl group than a methyl donor such as
methionine (Huennekens and Osborn, 1959). Further 5-methylH$_4$folate,
the methyl donor in methionine synthesis is ineffective in the methylation
of thymine (Blakley and McDougall, 1962; Pastore and Friedkin, 1962).
The form of pyrimidine taking part in the reaction is deoxyuridine monophosphate (dUMP) and the folate coenzyme is 5,10-methyleneH$_4$folate.

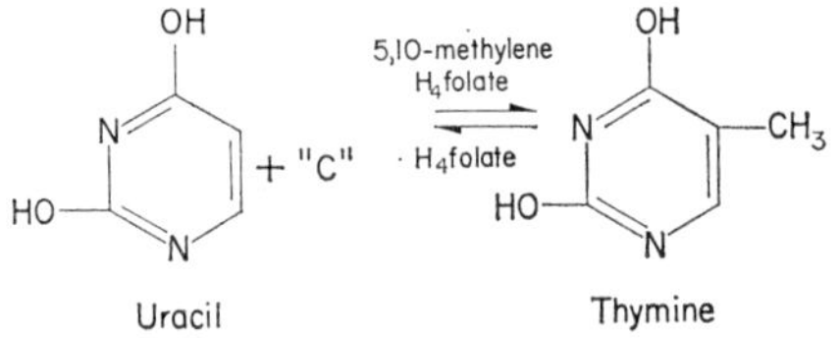

Fig. 15. Methylation of uracil.

The enzyme catalysing the overall reaction to produce thymidine monophosphate has been termed thymidylate synthetase and has been purified
200-fold from calf thymus by Greenberg *et al.* (1961). Hydrogen for the
reduction of the carbon fragment to the methyl form is derived from the
reduced pyrazine ring of H$_4$folate which in the course of the reaction
becomes oxidized to the H$_2$-form. The latter is regenerated via folic acid
reductase.

Methionine biosynthesis. Nutritional studies showed that homocysteine
could replace methionine in rats given a methyl free diet provided that
vitamin B$_{12}$ and folic acid were present (Bennett, 1949). Subsequently
Helleiner and Woods (1956) showed that cell free extracts of *E. coli* were
able to synthesize methionine from serine and homocysteine provided that
pyridoxal phosphate, H$_4$folate and vitamin B$_{12}$ were present (Fig. 16).

```
SH                                    S—CH₃
|                                     |
CH₂                                   CH₂
|          5-methylH₄folate           |
CH₂       ──────────────→             CH₂
|                                     |
CH—NH₂                                CH—NH₂
|                                     |
COOH                                  COOH
```

Homocysteine   Methionine

Fig. 16. Methylation of homocysteine.

The folate coenzyme concerned in the methylation of homocysteine is 5-methylH$_4$folate and the enzyme catalysing the overall reaction has been termed 5-methylH$_4$folate methyl transferase. This enzyme contains a derivative of vitamin B$_{12}$ as a prosthetic group (Foster *et al.*, 1961; Hatch *et al.*, 1961; Kisliuk, 1961). Guest *et al.* (1962) were able to show that the form of vitamin B$_{12}$ concerned was methylcobalamin. Thus the pathway may be visualised as follows (Fig. 17).

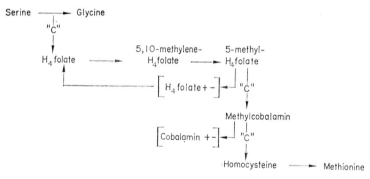

Fig. 17. Possible interrelationship between folate and vitamin B$_{12}$ in methionine synthesis.

In vitamin B$_{12}$ deficiency, as in patients with untreated Addisonian pernicious anemia, elevated serum folate levels were reported by Waters and Mollin (1963). On this hypothesis, this is attributed to failure to form methylcobalamin with consequent accumulation of 5-methylH$_4$folate, and a general trapping of H$_4$folate is the methyl form (Herbert and Zalusky, 1962).

Histidine metabolism. The degradation of histidine in mammalian tissue follows the pathway indicated in Fig. 18, and the role of the folate coenzymes was suggested by the increased urinary excretion of formiminoglutamic acid by folate-deficient rats (Bakerman *et al.*, 1951; Tabor *et al.*, 1953). The carbon in the formimino-(CH NH—) group is derived from

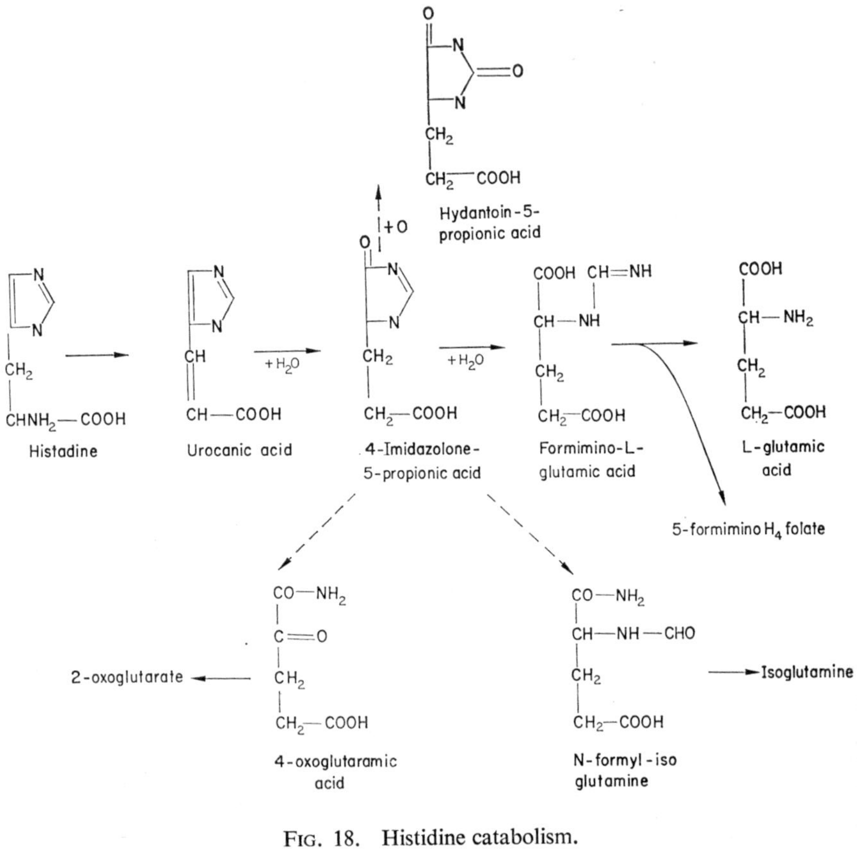

Fig. 18.   Histidine catabolism.

carbon 2 of the imidazole ring of histidine. The enzyme formiminoglutamate formimino transferase catalyses the transfer of the formimino group to H_4folate to give 5-formiminoH_4folate. This enzyme has been detected in a variety of mammalian tissues (Tabor and Wyngarden, 1959).

5-FormiminoH$_4$folate is in turn converted into 5,10-methenylH$_4$folate by the enzyme formiminoH$_4$folate cyclodeaminase.

Other folate-dependent pathways. Many compounds may serve as a source of single carbon units in a less direct way. One of these is the α-carbon of glycine. Studies with ^{14}C-labeled glycine have shown that the α-carbon may supply a carbon unit for the synthesis of purines, thymidine and methionine (Huennekens and Osborn, 1959). A pathway whereby this may take place is as follows. Glycine may condense with succinate to form δ-aminolevulinic acid. The δ-carbon (from glycine) has been shown by Shemin *et al.* (1954) to be a source of single carbon units. The suggestion is that δ-aminolevulinic acid is first deaminated, and then split to yield succinate and formate which via formylH$_4$folate synthetase condenses with H$_4$folate.

Other reactions that have not been adequately studied involve the synthesis of choline and the release of active formaldehyde from sarcosine and dimethyl-glycine (Huenneken and Osborn, 1959).

Degradation of folate coenzymes

When folic acid is incubated with liver slices, there is a decline in the amount of folic acid accompanied by the appearance of an aromatic amine. The reaction is blocked by folic acid antagonists (Futterman and Silverman, 1957; Dinning *et al.*, 1957). The mechanism appears to be enzymatic with reduction of folic acid to H$_4$folate, this step being blocked by aminopterin, followed by cleavage of H$_4$folate in the presence of oxygen to a pteridine and *p*-aminobenzoylglutamate. The administration of tritium labelled folate to man results in the appearance in the urine of a tritium labelled aromatic amine (McLean and Chanarin, 1966).

Estimation of folate compounds

Pteroylglutamic acid in solution may be estimated by its absorbency at 365×10^{-6} mm using the E(1%) 1 cm value of 199 in 0.1 N NaOH (Angier *et al.*, 1946). A subsequent report gave a higher value of 206 at this wavelength (Jukes and Stokstad, 1948).

More often the problem is the estimation of folates in natural materials, and this involves the use of either microbiological assay techniques or growth responses in animals. The preparation of material for assay may require steps to preserve unstable folate compounds. This requires the use of fresh materials, the addition of ascorbic acid, maintenance of a relatively neutral pH and protection from light and from heat.

Organisms used for microbiological assay such as *Streptococcus faecalis* may grow in the presence of non-folate compounds, such as thymine, hypoxanthine, theobromine, guanidine, uric acid, and other compounds (Mitchell and Williams, 1944). Similarly it has been claimed that with *Lactobacillus casei* half the material in food stuffs supporting the growth of this organism are non-folates (Butterworth *et al.*, 1963). Some purification of folates may be achieved by adsorption on to activated charcoal, and subsequent elution. In order to permit complete recovery of folates from the charcoal, it is necessary to pretreat the charcoal with stearic acid to block some of the absorbing sites (Asatoor and Dalgliesh, 1956).

Where it is suspected that folates are present as polyglutamates unavailable to the microbiological assay organisms (and this is the case in assaying food stuff) it is necessary to treat the food extract with enzymes that convert the polyglutamates to monoglutamates (Mims and Laskowski, 1945). Such enzymes are derived from either chicken pancreas or hog kidney. The enzyme preparations may contain substantial amounts of folate, and due allowance must be made for this in the assay procedure. Many of these problems are discussed by Toepfer *et al.* (1951).

Separation of different folate compounds before assay may be achieved by column chromatography on diethylaminoethyl (DEAE)-cellulose (Usdin and Porath, 1957; Toennies and Phillips, 1959; Oliverio, 1961). Folates are eluted with ascorbate phosphate buffer and the eluate fractions assayed microbiologically. Separation of folates may also be achieved by paper chromatography and this procedure can be combined with a bioautographic technique.

Bioautographic technique. Paper chromatograms of the sample under study are prepared. A solid folate-free agar medium is seeded with a folate dependent organism used in folate assay, and the chromatogram strips are placed directly on the agar. This is incubated at 37°, and zones of growth will indicate the site of the folate compounds (Winsten and Eigen, 1950; Clement *et al.*, 1961).

The use of filter paper discs, to which either folic acid or an extract of material being assayed is added, has been developed into a quantitative assay method. The diameter of the zone of growth on a seeded agar plate is proportional to the amount of folate available (Stiffey and Williams, 1954).

The growth response of chicks. Although microbiological assay procedures have largely superseded animal growth techniques, these still have an important function in the assay of the folate content of natural materials since they provide a measure of the availability of the naturally occurring forms of folate compounds. Day-old chicks, divided into groups of 10, are placed on a folate-free basal diet. The chicks are weighed at weekly intervals. A "standard curve" is constructed by noting the growth response of different groups given 0, 0.1, 0.2, 0.4, 1.0, and 2.0 mg of folic acid in solution added to each kilogram of diet. Preferably 2 groups of chicks are each given a supplement of the material under test, which is also mixed with the basal diet. The results can be assessed at the end of a 4-week period (Broquist *et al.*, 1952; Jukes, 1955) by comparing the weight increment of the chicks on the test diet with the weight increment of chicks given standard amounts of folic acid.

Microbiological assay. The choice of microbiological assay organisms will depend on the nature of folate compounds being assayed. Where it is desired to measure pteroylglutamic acid only *Streptococcus faecalis* should be used. This is particularly the case in studies involving the absorption, urinary excretion, and rate of plasma clearance, of either oral or parenteral doses of folic acid in man or experimental animals. *Lactobacillus casei* has the important advantage of utilizing 5-methylH_4folate, as well as tri-glutamates, and is therefore the organism to be used in the assay of folates in animal tissues and food stuffs. *Pediococcus cerevisiae* responds only to reduced forms of folate other than 5-methylH_4folate. The response of the more commonly used assay organisms to various folate analogues is shown in Table 1.

The method of assay used is that described by the Association of Official Agricultural Chemists, United States of America and set out by Toepfer *et al.* (1951), and quoted by Jukes (1955). The same procedure is used in the assay of serum and red cell folate (Baker *et al.*, 1959; Herbert, 1961; Waters and Mollin, 1961). Reduced forms of folate other than 5-methyl-H_4folate are assayed as described by Sauberlich and Baumann (1948).

In the assay of serum folate, it is important to ensure that ascorbic acid in adequate concentration is present in all the tubes in the assay including the aqueous folate standards. A simple way of ensuring this is to add ascorbate to the assay medium in a concentration of 1.0 g per 500 ml medium. Samples of serum for the assay should have dry ascorbate added (5 mg per ml) before storing the sample in the cold, and preferably in the frozen state (Waters and Mollin, 1961).

TABLE 1. THE GROWTH OF THE COMMONLY USED FOLATE-DEPENDENT MICROBIOLOGICAL ASSAY ORGANISMS WITH VARIOUS FOLATE ANALOGS[a]

	P. cerevisiae	S. faecalis	L. casei
pteroic acid (Pte)	−	+	−
10-HCOPte	−	+	−
5-HCOH$_4$Pte	−	+	−
pteroylglutamic acid (PteGlu)	−	+	+
10-HCOPteGlu	−	+	+
H$_2$PteGlu	−	+	+
10-HCOH$_2$PteGlu	−	+	+
H$_4$PteGlu	+	+	+
5-HCOH$_4$PteGlu	+	+	+
10-HCOH$_4$PteGlu	+	+	+
5-HCNHH$_4$PteGlu	+	+	+
5,10-CH$_2$H$_4$PteGlu	+	+	+
5-CH$_3$H$_4$PteGlu	−	−	+
PteGlu$_2$	−	+	+
5-HCOH$_4$PteGlu$_2$	+	+	+
PteGlu$_3$	−	−	+
10-HCOPteGlu$_3$	−	−	+
5-HCOH$_4$PteGlu$_3$	+	−	+
PteGlu$_7$	−	−	−

[a] Johns and Bertino, 1965.

PHYSIOLOGICAL CONSIDERATIONS IN MAN

The folic acid content of food

There are two distinct aspects. The first is how much folate is there in food; the second, how much of this folate is available to man. To neither question do we have a satisfactory answer.

Detailed folate food values have been compiled by Toepfer *et al.* (1951) and Hardinge and Crooks, (1961). The values reported by Santini *et al.* (1962) are generally higher than those obtained by other workers, and they attribute this to the removal, in the preparations of the food extract, of a conjugase inhibitor which interfered with the release of monoglutamates. These workers also suggested that some of the problems in assay of food folate were due to adsorption of free folate onto insoluble celluloses in some types of diet (Luther *et al.*, 1965). Further values for folate content of prepared foods are given by Herbert (1963) and Hurdle (1967). Table 2 lists values for the commoner foodstuffs.

The effect on folate content of preparation of food. Preparation of food, whether in cooking or canning, results in a significant loss of folate activity. Thus the canning of apricots, peaches, and pineapple results in the loss of about 85% of their folate content. On the other hand dried fruits, such as apricots, prunes, and raisins appear to retain their folate content (Hardinge and Crooks, 1961). Cooking of food also results in a significant loss. Thus Cheldelin *et al.* (1943) showed that steaming vegetables such as beet, cabbage, carrots, and potatoes for 20–60 min resulted in a loss of 92–97% of the folate. Similarly meat (beef, pork, bacon) fried in an open pan for 10–15 min showed a decline of 67–95% of their folate content. Fish and chicken lost 62–74% of folate activity in frying. These observations were confirmed by Schweigert *et al.* (1946). Herbert (1963) devised an almost folate-free diet by boiling all ingredients in large quantities of water. On the other hand Hurdle (1967) found that frying eggs, lamb, or chicken did not affect the folate content (assay without conjugase treatment), whereas about 90% of the folate activity of vegetables and cereals (potatoes, cabbage and broccoli) was lost.

Folate intake in man. The folate content of a diet cannot be devised from tables listing the folate content of fresh food, since the bulk of this activity is lost in the preparation of the meal. Denko *et al.* (1946), using a *Str. faecalis* assay, found that folate intake ranged from 43 to 86 mcg per day and Jandl and Lear (1956) reported a value of 1000 to 1500 mcg. Chung *et al.* (1961) found that the daily folate content of a high cost diet was 193 mcg, that of a low cost diet 157 mcg, and that of a poor diet 47 mcg. Jukes (1961) suggested a value of 400 mcg. Santini *et al.* (1962) found that a rural Puerto Rican diet contained about 380 mcg of total folate, and an urban diet about 650 mcg of folate per day. Butterworth *et al.* (1963) found the daily folate value to be 688 mcg, of which 531 mcg were polyglutamate forms. Pace *et al.* (1960) estimated the daily folate intake of American schoolgirls to be 52–97 mcg. Hurdle (1967) found that healthy young controls took 161–297 mcg folate per day, with a mean of 223 mcg. By contrast, elderly people at home took 95–251 mcg (mean 146), and the elderly in hospital 41–190 mcg per day (mean 101). These values were obtained without conjugase treatment. Chanarin *et al.* (1968) assaying 111 diets found a mean total daily folate content of 676 mcg, 160 mcg being "free" folate and 516 mcg polyglutamate.

D*

TABLE 2. FOLATE CONTENT OF FOOD[a] mcg/100 g

	A	B	C	D
Beef	6.0	69.0	—	3.0
Lamb	3.3	—	—	6.0
Chicken breast	3.1	240.0	—	7.0
Chicken leg	2.8	170.0	—	—
Pork	3.2	400.0	—	4.0
Liver – beef	294.0	—	294.0	—
– lamb	276.0	—	—	637.0
– chicken	377.0	360.0	—	—
– pork	221.0	—	—	—
Chicken egg – whole	2–6	—	5.1	30.0
Cow's milk	0.1–0.6	15.0	4–10	8.5
Rice	11–29	210.0	13.7	5.0
Rye	10–45	—	14.6	—
Wheat	6–90	—	195.0	—
Oats	6–29	100.0	22.4	2.0
Corn	1–7	118.0	9.0	—
Flour (wheat)	33.0	29.0	8.0	—
Bread – white	13.8	14.0	15.0	17.0
– whole wheat	27.0	—	30.0	38.0
Yeast (dried)	800–1300	—	3000	—
Honey	3.0	—	—	—
Margarine	—	—	6.8	—
Olive oil	—	—	$\begin{cases} 4.3 \\ 0.39 \end{cases}$	—
Cheese	10–26	—	11–31	6.0
Chocolate	—	—	99.0	12.0
Asparagus	89.0	—	109.0	—
Beans (green)	13–40	38.0	27.5	—
Broccoli	35.0	—	3.5	—
Brussel sprouts	13–33	—	49.0	—
Carrots	5–15	29.0	8.0	3.0
Lettuce	3–58	165.0	21.0	200.0
Onion	6–15	91.0	10.0	15.0
Peas (green)	11–35	—	25.0	—
Potatoes	3–20	75.0	6.8	12.0
Tomatoes	1–15	50.0	8.0	18.0
Mushroom	14–27	—	24.0	17.0
Spinach	58–114	—	75.0	29.0
Fresh apples	0.5	—	2.0	2.0
„ apricot	2.5	—	3.3	—
„ avocado	56.0	46.0	30.0	—
„ banana	10.9	69.0	9.7	27.0
„ grapefruit	2.2	31.0	2.8	11.0
„ grapes	5.0	—	5.2	—
„ melon	5.0	—	6.8	—
„ orange	5.0	38.0	5.1	45.0
„ peach	1–2	—	4.0	—
„ plums	2.9	—	1.0	—

TABLE 2—*continued*

	A	B	C	D
Coffee powder	—	—	0.0	—
Coca cola[b]	—	—	1.0	—
Ginger ale[b]	—	—	1.0	—
Whisky[b]	—	—	1.0	—
Wine[b]	—	—	0.3–1.3	—
Beer (Guinness stout)[b]	—	—	—	75.0

[a] In almost all foodstuffs the values with *L. casei* after digestion with "conjugates" have been given. The quantities (100 g) refer to moist weight.
A. Toepfer *et al.* (1951).
B. Santini *et al.* (1962).
C. Hardinge and Crooks (1961), Herbert (1963), and others.
D. Hurdle (1967). Cooked hospital diet assayed without conjugase treatment.
[b] Values per liter.

Thus, these values show a wide variation. These are probably due to as yet unresolved technological problems in the preparation and assay of the food samples.

The availability of food folate. Assay of the folate content of foodstuffs by microbiological procedures, and by the growth response of animals, appears to give similar results (Jukes, 1961). Nevertheless, more information is required on this point in man. Early observations on the response of pernicious anemia patients to treatment with polyglutamates suggested that only relatively large doses gave an adequate response. Jandl and Lear (1956) claimed that only about 25% of the folate in yeast was absorbed, whereas, after treatment of yeast with a conjugase, the amount absorbed rose to 60%. This was still less than the proportion of folate absorbed when synthetic pteroylglutamic acid was given, when they considered that 95% of the dose was taken up. The apparent discrepancy between the amount of folate in the diet and the small additional amount of pteroylglutamic acid needed to produce a hematological response in tropical sprue (Crosby, 1960) has cast further doubt on the availability to man of much of the material in food measured by microbiological assay techniques. The author has failed to obtain a hematological response in a folate-deficient megaloblastic anemia with the folate equivalent of

100 mcg polyglutamate daily in the form of yeast. The patient then responded to 100 mcg of pteroylglutamic acid daily, by mouth. Thus the availability to man of polyglutamate form of folate is uncertain.

Folate excretion in man. Denko *et al.* (1946) found that the average folate excretion in 7 healthy males was 310 mcg daily (range 226 to 397). The bulk of this was in the feces and only 3 to 5 mcg in the urine. Thus they estimated that the fecal excretion exceeded the dietary intake 5-fold presumably the result of synthesis of folates by bacteria in the large gut. Jandl and Lear (1956) found an average fecal folate content of 219 mcg daily in one subject.

Folate requirement in man. Herbert (1962a) described an experimental study in a male volunteer who subsisted on a relatively folate-free diet until the appearance of early megaloblastic changes in the blood and marrow 19 weeks after the start of the study. On the basis of the folate content of liver in folate-replete subjects (6.9 mcg per g) and that in patients with megaloblastic anemia (1.0 mcg per g) (Chanarin *et al.*, 1966), the liver folate should have declined from about 10 to 1.5 mg during this period. This is approximately a fall of 65 mcg a day. Nevertheless in the absence of direct measurement of hepatic folate in such a patient this value is only a wide approximation of requirement. An initial hepatic folate value of 12 mcg per g would approximate to a fall of 140 mcg per day.

Attempts have been made to determine the amount of folate required to restore to normal a function dependent on the folate coenzymes or to maintain serum folate levels.

Thus Herbert (1962b) suggested that a supplement of 50 mcg a day was adequate in preventing a fall in the serum folate level in volunteers taking a relatively folate-free diet. However, all 3 volunteers had lower serum folate values towards the end of the study than at the beginning, and this was least marked in the volunteer given a supplement of 100 mcg each day. Thus, this limited but valuable study suggests that 50 mcg daily was too small, and that the correct amount needed to maintain serum folate levels was in excess of 100 mcg daily.

A few observations have also been made on the amount of folate required to restore normal formiminoglutamic acid excretion. Chanarin (unpublished observations) found that a normal formiminoglutamic acid excretion was restored in two patients with gluten-sensitive enteropathies and megaloblastic anemia due to folic acid deficiency given 10 mcg pteroylglutamic acid daily by injection. Similar results were obtained in two patients given 20 mcg folate each day, one with megaloblastic anemia due to folic acid deficiency after partial gastrectomy, and the second with untreated Addisonian pernicious anemia. Hansen and Weinfeld (1962) found that the urinary formiminoglutamic acid excretion was restored to normal in 3 out of 7 patients with folic acid deficiency given 200 mcg daily, and that 3 others showed a considerable decline of formiminoglutamic acid excretion in the period of study (6–9 days), on the same dose of folic acid. On the other hand some patients have a persistently elevated urocanic acid and formiminoglutamic acid excretion, despite relatively large amounts of oral and parenteral folic acid (Chanarin, 1963).

The amount of folic acid required to produce a hematological response in patients with megaloblastic anemia due to folic acid deficiency has attracted much interest. Jandl and Lear (1961) initially suggested that 200–300 mcg daily "constituted adequate daily therapy for an adult." Subsequently Marshall and Jandl (1956) found that a daily parenteral dose of 400 mcg of folic acid induced an adequate reticulocyte response in 3 patients with folic-acid deficiency, but failed to do so in 3 patients with Addisonian pernicious anemia in relapse. Thus they suggested that 400 mcg daily was "physiologic". Hansen and Weinfeld (1962) obtained satisfactory responses with parenteral doses of 100–200 mcg folic acid. Thirkettle *et al.* (1964) obtained suboptimal responses (reticulocyte peak on day 12 in 3 out of 4 cases) with 200 mcg folic acid daily. Izak *et al.* (1963) found that 10 mcg folic acid daily was inadequate in producing a response in megaloblastic anemia due to folate deficiency, but 100 mcg daily by injection produced as good a response as did a dose of 500 mcg. However, in some patients smaller doses of folic acid have proved effective; 50 mcg (Zalusky and Herbert, 1961); 25 mcg (Sheehy *et al.*, 1961; Druskin *et al.*, 1962); 5 mcg (Velez *et al.*, 1963). On the other hand, where there is evidence of an increased requirement for folic acid, much larger doses may be required to restore normoblastic hematopoiesis (Lindenbaum and Klipstein, 1963).

Considerably more information is required on mans' requirement for folic acid. Nevertheless it is likely that this quantity is of the order of 100–200 mcg per day. The amount of folic acid that restores to normal a particular folate-dependent pathway, or induces a hematological response, may not necessarily be the same as that required under normal physiological circumstances, and we need to know the daily amount that will maintain normal folate status, including normal hepatic stores. This type of information is better obtained by nutritional studies on human volunteers than in observing hematological responses in patients with megaloblastic anemia.

In normal pregnancy, an oral supplement of 100 mcg folate each day will maintain the red cell and serum folate throughout pregnancy (Chanarin, Rothman and Ward, unpublished observations).

The absorption of folic acid

Polyglutamate folate analogues are probably cleaved to monoglutamate forms in the intestinal cells in man by the folic acid conjugase enzymes which are optimally active at pH 4.5 (Perry and Chanarin, 1968; Hoffbrand and Peters, 1969; Butterworth *et al.*, 1969). Monoglutamate forms of folate are reduced to the tetrahydro-form, methylated and 5 methyltetrahydrofolate passes to the blood (Perry and Chanarin, 1970).

Anderson *et al.* (1960) found that normal control subjects absorbed a mean of 79% of a 200 mcg dose of folic acid. A similar percentage of an oral dose of 40 mcg per kg of body weight was taken up. Polyglutamates are not as well absorbed as simpler forms (Jandl and Lear, 1956). Perry and Chanarin (1968) suggested that about one-third of yeast polyglutamate was absorbed by man and Butterworth *et al.* (1969) found that between 37 to 67% of synthetic polyglutamate of varying chain length was absorbed.

Like other water soluble vitamins folates are probably absorbed in the upper gut (Cox *et al.*, 1958) but extensive disease of the ileum may be associated with impaired folate absorption (Chanarin, 1960; Chanarin and Bennett, 1962). Furthermore, patients with resection of the jejunum alone (for diverticulitis) may absorb folate normally.

Biliary excretion of folic acid

Baker *et al.* (1965b) found that the folate content of duodenal juice was 2–13 times as high as that in serum and that this was due to the high folate content of bile. Tritium labeled folic acid given intravenously appeared in high concentration in the bile 30 min after injection. Thus, it appears likely that folic acid undergoes an enterohepatic circulation, and Herbert (1965) has suggested that the quantity of folate involved in this circulation is about 0.1 mg each day. The folate content of bile exceeds that of serum both in patients with folate deficiency and in vitamin B_{12} deficiency.

Folate content of body fluids and tissues in man

Serum. The level of 5-methylH$_4$folate in serum or plasma may be assayed microbiologically (Baker *et al.*, 1959; Herbert, 1961; Waters and Mollin, 1961). Serum folate is probably loosely bound to plasma proteins (Johns *et al.*, 1961). Considerable variation in the range of serum folate values in healthy subjects have been obtained in different centers. The lower limits of 18 reported series range from 2.5 to 8.0 ng per ml, and the upper limits from 7.4 to 45 ng per ml. Nevertheless, the mean is 4.8 ng per ml for the lower limit, and 16.0 for the upper limit (Mollin and Hoffbrand, 1965). Differences of technique undoubtedly play a major part in this variability. It is desirable to add ascorbate to sera prior to storage in the cold to prevent oxidation of the unstable 5-methylfolate. Food has only a minor effect on serum folate levels (Cooper and Lowenstein, 1964), although an exceptionally large meal of liver may produce an elevated serum folate level (Herbert, 1964; Cooper and Lowenstein, 1964). Mollin and Hoffbrand (1965) have reported similar increases after oral yeast.

Red blood cells. The red blood cells contain more than 30 times as much folate as the serum (Toennies *et al.*, 1956), and, as in serum, the form of folate appears to be almost entirely 5-methylfolate. The amount of folate present has been expressed in terms of whole blood, after a correction for variation in the red cell mass has been made, or preferably in terms of the folate content of 1.0 ml of packed red blood cells. For whole blood, Izak *et al.* (1961) reported values in normal subjects of 50–160 ng per ml, Grossowicz *et al.* (1962) reported values of 47–149 ng per ml, and Hansen and Weinfeld (1962) 23–94 ng per ml. When expressed in terms of the folate content of red cells, reported values are 180–880 ng per ml of packed cells (Cooper and Lowenstein, 1964), and 184–655 ng per ml (Mollin and Hoffbrand, 1965). The rise in red cell folate associated with a reticulocyte response (Cooper and Lowenstein, 1964) suggests that the reticulocytes may have a higher folate content than mature erythrocytes.

Whole blood folate in infants has been found to be half that present in adults, viz. a mean of 39 ng per ml, as compared to a mean of 89 ng per ml in adults (Matoth *et al.*, 1964). Strelling *et al* (1966) found that whole blood folate in normal infants at birth was about 250 ng per ml, and this fell steadily to reach about 30 ng per ml at 12 weeks of age. The level rose to 50 ng per ml at 36 weeks.

The folate in red cells is unavailable to microbiological assay organisms until the haemolysate has been allowed to react with plasma (Toennies *et al.*, 1956; Usdin *et al.*, 1956). The inference is that red cell folate is present as a polyglutamate, and that plasma contains a "conjugase" that releases forms of folate available for microbiological assay. Chromatography of red cell folate revealed a single peak of folate activity, which was identified as 5-methylH$_4$folate (McLean and Chanarin, unpublished observations). This material is bound to protein (Iwai *et al.*, 1964), and incubation may help to release folate from its protein link. More recently Foster and Harding (personal communication) identified a polyglutamate in human red cells.

Cerebrospinal fluid. The folate concentration in cerebrospinal fluid is approximately 3 times that found in serum, the range being from 17 to 41 ng per ml (Herbert and Zalusky, 1961).

Liver. Romaine (1960) assayed the folate content of liver samples obtained at autopsy, from patients dying of various forms of heart disease. The folate content ranged from 3.6 to 12.1 mcg per g of liver with a mean of 5.8 mcg. Chanarin *et al.* (1966) assayed liver samples obtained at laparotomy. Six patients with normal serum folate levels, and normal urinary excretion of formiminoglutamic acid, had hepatic folate levels between 5.2 to 10.0 mcg per g, with a mean of 6.9. Leevy *et al.* (1965a) obtained a mean value of 7.0 mcg per g in percutaneous biopsy specimens in 5 patients with normal serum folate values.

Hepatic folate in man is almost entirely in the form of 5-methylfolate (McLean and Chanarin, 1966); but, as with red cells, incubation results in a release of forms active for *Str. fecalis* and *P. cerevisiae* (Girdwood, 1952).

Leucocytes. Butterworth *et al.* (1957) measured the folate content of leucocytes after treatment with conjugase, and found folate concentrations of 46–97 mcg per ml of leucocytes.

PHARMACOLOGY

Urinary excretion of folic acid

An oral or parenteral dose of folic acid of the order of 200–300 mcg is rapidly removed from the circulation to the tissues in man with no accumulation in serum or loss in the urine (Chanarin and Bennett, 1962c). Such doses are presumably physiological in amount, in so far as they are within the capacity of the tissues to dispose of them.

Larger doses of folic acid tend to accumulate in the blood, and be excreted into the urine. Thus, with an 0.5 mg oral dose about 12% is recovered from the urine, and this increases to 22%, with a 1.0 mg dose; 43% with a 2.0 mg dose; 49% with a 5 mg dose, and 77% with a 15 mg dose (Jukes *et al.*, 1947). With doses of 5 mg or less, the greater part of the urinary excretion is complete in 6–8 hr, but with larger doses high blood levels and urinary excretion persist for 12–24 hr. In patients with impaired renal function, high blood folate levels may persist for days (Chanarin and Bennett, 1962c). With parenteral doses of folic acid of the order of 15 mcg per kg of body weight, there is a good relationship between the serum folate levels 15 min after the injection and the amount of folate appearing in the urine (Chanarin and Bennett, 1962c).

Pteroylglutamic acid that is filtered through the glomerulus is actively reabsorbed by the renal tubule (Condit and Grob, 1958; Goresky *et al.*, 1963). A significant amount of the folate reabsorbed by the renal tubule is retained within the tubular cell. Tubular reabsorption is complete with small doses of folic acid, but as the dose is increased the proportion reabsorbed diminishes. With larger doses of oral or parenteral folate, not only does pteroylglutamic acid appear in the urine, but 10-formylfolate and 5-methylH$_4$folate as well (McLean and Chanarin, 1966).

Toxic reactions to folic acid in animals

The toxicity of folic acid was investigated by Harned *et al.* (1946). In animals, folic acid did not affect blood pressure, respiration, or blood sugar levels, and had little action on the isolated intestine. Five mg per kg given intraperitoneally each day for 2 months to rats and rabbits produced no unfavourable reactions. At a dose level of 50–75 mg per kg, minor changes were present in the kidney tubules. The LD$_{50}$ for mice was 600 mg per kg, for rats 500 mg per kg, for rabbits 410 mg per kg, and for guinea pigs 120 mg per kg. Death was due to precipitation of folate crystals in the renal tubules.

Toxic reactions to folic acid in man

Sensitivity. A few examples of sensitivity to folic acid have been reported (Mitchell *et al.*, 1949; Chanarin *et al.*, 1957). An oral or parenteral dose of folic acid in these patients was followed by a pruritic erythematous skin reaction most pronounced on the limbs, general malaise, and bronchospasm. Intradermal tests with folic acid and aminopterin gave positive results, but folate analogs having a subsituent in the 5 position (such as folinic acid or methotrexate) were negative.

Syncope. Rarely does an intravenous injection of a solution of folic acid result in vertigo, syncope, and a marked drop of blood pressure. Recovery is complete in a few minutes. Although Heinle *et al.* (1947) suggested that this occurred after the rapid injection of large doses of folic acid of the order of 150 mg, the same reaction may occur with about 1.0 mg of folic acid in a volume of 1.0 ml.

Precipitation of epileptic attacks. Although Hawkins and Meynell (1958) found that epileptic patients with megaloblastic anemia showed considerable improvement, with diminution in the number of seizures after folic acid therapy, this is not always the case. Thirteen out of 26 treated epileptics given folate showed an increase in the frequency of fits. This was accompanied in 22 of these patients by an improvement in their mental state (Reynolds, 1967). Rarely folate may precipitate status epilepticus in such patients (Chanarin *et al.*, 1960).

Aggravation of vitamin B_{12} deficiency. The reports by Vilter *et al.*, (1945), and Moore *et al.* (1945), that hematological and clinical remissions were brought about in patients with Addisonian pernicious anemia treated with folic acid, were followed by the observations that in a high proportion of these patients the remissions were not sustained. This relapse affected the nervous system, the blood as well as the gastrointestinal tract. After 3 years, at least 80% of patients with pernicious anemia given folate showed evidence of relapse (Schwartz *et al.*, 1950). Indeed, it is remarkable that this relapse had not extended to all such patients, and marrow examination in patients in apparent remission would have been of interest. However, even many in this group did not feel as well on folate as they had been while receiving liver injections, and asked to be restored to the injection regime. Only 12 out of 85 patients remained apparently well.

Neurological relapse. (Meyer, 1947; Vilter *et al.*, 1947; Heinle and Welch, 1947; Hall and Watkins, 1947; Heinle *et al.*, 1947; Davidson, 1948; Ross *et al.*, 1948; Bethell and Sturgis, 1948; Israëls and Wilkinson, 1949). An increasingly high incidence of neurological relapse in patients with pernicious anemia given folate occurs with time. The earliest evidence of relapse is found about 3 months after the start of folic acid therapy, and in a group of 20 patients followed up for 3 years by Israëls and Wilkinson (1949) 80% showed abnormalities. This frequency of neurological relapse is higher than that recorded by most observers. In a group of 70 patients followed up for 2 years, the incidence of neurological relapse was 45% (Schwartz *et al.*, 1950). Not surprisingly there is no obvious relation between relapse and the dose of folic acid, since all doses were relatively large. There is only a suggestion that those with evidence of neurological disorder before the commencement of folate therapy showed a higher incidence of relapse than those without preceding nerve involvement. Thus 13 out of 43 patients (30%) with peripheral nerve or cord involvement showed a further deterioration of their neurological status, while on folate therapy as compared to 19 out of 89 patients (21%) who did not have nervous involvement at the start of treatment.

Neurological relapse occurring while on folate therapy usually involves peripheral nerves, frequently the posterior columns, and least of all the lateral columns of the cord. In some, changes were profound, with marked mental disorder, and loss of sphincter control, as in the patient described by Fuld (1950) who was given folate for 15 months. In a few cases the onset has been described as "explosive", coming on about 3 months after the start of folate therapy, and characterized by sudden and rapidly progressive development of paraesthesia, loss of reflexes and of vibration sense (Heinle and Welch, 1947), or by the rapid development of severe spastic paraplegia (Bethell and Sturgis, 1948).

On the other hand, in some patients peripheral neuritis disappeared after folate therapy, and in some there was a return of taste (Meyer, 1947), and an improvement in gait. This (often temporary) improvement was noted in at least 17 out of 121 patients.

Neurological relapse on folate therapy may also occur in patients with post-gastrectomy vitamin B_{12} deficiency (Ross *et al.*, 1948; Beebe and Meneely, 1949), and in patients with intestinal malabsorption, such as idiopathic steatorrhoea, who are unable to absorb vitamin B_{12} and are maintained on oral folate (Chanarin, unpublished observations). Neurological relapse has also been reported in patients with pernicious anemia treated with pteroyltriglutamic acid (Meyer *et al.*, 1951), and in patients receiving folate in polyvitamin preparations (Baldwin and Dalassio, 1961).

Neurological damage induced by folate therapy remits in the usual way to therapy with vitamin B_{12}, i.e. where symptoms and signs are of short duration, response can be anticipated. Where they are of long duration, the prognosis is uncertain. Eight out of 23 cases maintained on folate by Schwartz *et al.* (1950) failed to respond after 6 months of liver therapy.

Hematological relapse. A return of anemia with megaloblastic hemato-poiesis in the marrow may also occur in patients with vitamin B_{12} deficiency maintained on folate therapy. This takes place in about 25% of patients at the end of 12 months, and in about 45% at the end of 2 years of folate therapy (Schwartz *et al.*, 1950).

Other features. Glossitis appears in about 5% of vitamin B_{12} deficient subjects given folate. Other patients lose the sensation of well-being that accompanied an earlier remission induced by liver extracts. Some patients may lose weight (Schwartz *et al.*, 1950).

CLINICAL EFFECT OF FOLATE DEFICIENCY

The effects of folate deprivation may arise from a gross decline of the amount of this vitamin in the body, or more acutely by the administration of folate antagonists, which interfere with the metabolic function of the folate-coenzymes. These effects have been studied in a wide variety of species including rats (Wright and Welch, 1943b), chicks (Hutchings *et al.*, 1941), turkeys (Richardson *et al.*, 1945) ducks (Hegsted and Stare, 1945), mice (Cerecedo and Mirone, 1947), guinea pigs (Wooley and Sprince, 1945), mink (Schaefer *et al.*, 1946), dogs (Krehl *et al.*, 1946), foxes (Schaefer *et al.*, 1947), and insects such as the mosquito, *Aedes aegyptii* (Goldberg *et al.*, 1945).

The most detailed studies have been on the effects of folate deficiency in the monkey (May *et al.*, 1949; May *et al.*, 1952; Sundberg *et al.*, 1952), and in swine (Cartwright *et al.*, 1948: Cartwright *et al.*, 1952; Heinle *et al.*, 1948).

The clinical effects of folate deficiency are due to the inhibition of syn-thesis of nucleic acid in proliferating cells. The rate of cell proliferation is high in hematopoietic tissue, in the mucosal surfaces of the mouth and gastro-intestinal tract, in the skin and the gonads. It is low in hepatic and nerve tissue.

Acute folate "deficiency" in man

Gastro-intestinal tract. Painful lesions on lips, tongue, and buccal mucosa may commence as small, shallow, white or yellow red edged spots, and these may ulcerate. There may be anorexia, nausea accompanied by colic type of abdominal pain, and vomiting. In animals and in man, the small gut may show atrophic degeneration of villi which come to resemble the villus atrophy of gluten sensitive enteropathy. This may be followed by ulceration (Williams, 1961; Trier, 1961).

Skin. Dermatitis, often limited to the hands and feet, may occur, as does loss of hair (Van Scott and Reinertson, 1959).

Reproductive system. Transitory azoospermia and amenorrhoea have been reported (Van Scott and Reinertson, 1959), and in early pregnancy fetal malformation and fetal death may occur (Thiersch, 1952). The response of epithelial tissue to estrogen administration does not take place when folate deficiency is present (Hertz, 1948).

Hematopoiesis. A megaloblastic type of hematopoiesis develops in the marrow, and both macrocytic red cells and neutrophil polymorphs with hypersegmented nuclei appear in the peripheral blood. The changes may progress to pancytopenia with a low platelet count, and to severe marrow hypoplasia.

"Chronic" folate deficiency

Clinical syndromes in which folate deficiency may appear are frequently associated with deficiency of other substances, and the importance of lack of any particular food factor in the pathogenesis of the syndrome may be uncertain. Nevertheless, there are a number of features that can be ascribed to folate deficiency, and which improve when therapy with folate is instituted.

Gastrointestinal tract. A smooth, red, often painful tongue due to atrophy of the lingual papillae (although frequently seen in both vitamin B_{12} and in iron deficiency) is a frequent accompaniment of a megaloblastic anemia responding only to folate therapy. Angular stomatitis is common.

Intestinal malabsorption is an important factor in producing folate deficiency; nevertheless, many of the clinical and laboratory features of disorders such as tropical sprue are considerably ameliorated by folate therapy (Darby, 1947). Thus, folate deficiency, however initiated, may in turn further interfere with gut function, possibly by inadequate renewal of intestinal epithelium.

Skin. Dry, roughened skin may be found, and may proceed to eczematoid eruption. These changes are due to folate deficiency. However, widespread disorders of the skin *per se* are frequently associated with biochemical evidence of folate deficiency (Knowles *et al.*, 1963a). In such cases, folate deficiency results if the increased requirement for folate consequent on rapid renewal of skin surfaces exceeds the amount of folate available from dietary sources.

Reproductive system. Amenorrhoea and sterility is frequent in women with long-standing folate deficiency, as may occur in intestinal malabsorption.

Nervous system. It is uncertain whether folic acid deficiency *per se* produces neurological changes. Nevertheless, amelioration of neurological signs have been observed after folate therapy. An improvement usually transient may on occasion be found in patients with pernicious anemia given folate. Improvement of peripheral neuritis, and even of cord involvement, has been reported in patients with folate deficiency, often epileptics, given folate (Long *et al.*, 1963; Anand, 1964; Hansen *et al.*, 1964; Grant *et al.*, 1965). Abnormalities of the electroencephalogram are usual in severe megaloblastic anemia due to folate deficiency (Laidlaw, J. personal communication).

Hematopoiesis. The changes are those of a megaloblastic anemia, and a detailed account may be found in any standard text on Hematology (Wintrobe, 1961).

Folate deficiency without megaloblastic hematopoiesis

Biochemical evidence of folate deficiency is frequent among patients admitted to hospital wards, although their blood and marrows appear normal (Chanarin, 1964a; Leevy *et al.*, 1965a). Do such patients suffer any clinical consequences from what are presumably depleted folate stores? Luhby and Cooperman (1962) have reported a decline in transfusion requirements of thallesemic infants given folate. Watson-Williams (1962) found 5 patients with sickle-cell anemia associated with normoblastic hematopoiesis, retardation of growth, and delayed puberty. Oral folate therapy produced a marked spurt of growth, and in all 4 females regular menstruation commenced.

BIOCHEMICAL EFFECTS OF FOLATE DEFICIENCY

Serum folate levels

Healthy subjects have serum folate levels between 5 to 16 ng per ml of serum. The majority (but not all) patients with megaloblastic anemias due to folate deficiency have values of less than 3 ng per ml. However, many patients with megaloblastic anemia have values between 3 and 5, and a few have apparently normal serum folate concentrations (Chanarin, 1964a).

Reduced serum folate values are frequent in patients who are admitted to hospital with a variety of disorders. Low values were found in 18% of such patients by Mollin and Hoffbrand, (1965), in 32% by Chanarin (1964a), and in 45% by Leevy *et al.* (1965a). Such patients frequently have low hepatic folate stores (Leevy *et al.*, 1965a), although in a few patients the low serum folate values were accompanied by normal hepatic folate stores (Chanarin *et al.*, 1966). Mollin and Hoffbrand (1965) found low serum folate values in 68% of patients with Crohn's disease, 65% of patients with rheumatoid arthritis, and 80% of patients with carcinomatosis. The great majority of these patients did not have a megaloblastic anemia.

Elevated serum folate values, i.e. above 16 ng per ml, are seen in about 15% of patients with Addisonian pernicious anemia (Waters and Mollin, 1961). More important, however, is the discrepancy that exists between the serum folate values in untreated pernicious anemia patients, which are usually normal, and the low folate content of the red cells, which thus indicates the presence of folate deficiency. It has been suggested that the highest serum folate values are found in the least anemic pernicious anemia patients, and in particular in those patients with neurological involvement (Waters and Mollin, 1963). Elevated serum folate values have also been found in patients with anatomical abnormalities of the small gut (Hoffbrand *et al.*, 1966).

The serum folate concentration declines at a relatively early stage in the development of folate deficiency, and may decline within 2 weeks of dietary deprivation of folate (Herbert, 1962a). However, at this early stage of dietary deprivation, the serum folate level can hardly reflect tissue stores, since far longer than 2 weeks is required to produce a major fall in hepatic folate.

Red cell folate levels

The red cell folate level is less sensitive to changes of folate status than either the serum folate level or the urinary excretion of formiminoglutamic acid, presumably because of the relatively slow rate of red cell turnover, and because red cell folate is not in equilibrium with folate in other tissues. Nevertheless, the red cell folate is usually reduced in folate deficiency states (Izak *et al.*, 1961; Kende *et al.*, 1963; Lowenstein *et al.*, 1963; Hansen, 1964; Mollin and Hoffbrand, 1965). It is also low in patients with Addisonian pernicious anemia in relapse (Hansen and Weinfeld, 1962; Cooper and Lowenstein, 1964), and indeed there is a correlation between the degree of anemia and the decline of red cell folate (Mollin and Hoffbrand, 1965). A similar relationship between the degree of anemia in vitamin B_{12} deficiency and the folic acid clearance test has been noted (Chanarin *et al.*, 1958a).

Hepatic folate levels

Grossly reduced hepatic folate concentrations are found in patients with megaloblastic anemia due to folate deficiency. Thus 6 patients with liver disease due to alcoholism were found to have hepatic folate values of 1.0 mcg per g, using material obtained by liver biopsy (Leevy *et al.*, 1965a; Chanarin *et al.*, 1966). All these patients had low serum folate levels, and those studied by Chanarin *et al.* (1966) presented with a megaloblastic anemia. There is generally a good correlation between serum folate values and hepatic folate in patients with liver disease and alcoholism. However, Chanarin *et al.* (1966) found that in only half of a group of patients did a low serum folate or indeed an elevated formiminoglutamic acid excretion reflect reduced hepatic folate stores.

Romaine (1960) measured hepatic folate in post-mortem material, and found an average value of 3.5 mcg per g in patients dying of carcinamatosis, and an average of 1.9 mcg per g in patients with leukemia. Patients dying of heart disease had a mean value of 5.8 mcg per g of liver.

Leucocyte folate values

Butterworth *et al.* (1957) found reduced leucocyte folate values in 12 patients with folate deficiency due to tropical sprue. These ranged from 24 to 66 mcg per ml.

Urinary formiminoglutamic acid excretion

Bakerman *et al.* (1951) identified an unstable precursor of glutamic acid in the urine of rats on a folate deficient diet. This compound was identified as formiminoglutamic acid by Seegmiller *et al.* (1954). Broquist (1956) showed that this compound appeared in the urine of leukemic children given folate antagonists, and Luhby (1957) showed that there was also an increased excretion in a patient with megaloblastic anemia in pregnancy. Nevertheless, the failure of many patients with folate deficiency to exhibit an increased output of this compound in the urine led Luhby *et al.* (1959) to put this metabolic pathway under stress by giving large oral doses of histidine from which formiminoglutamic acid is derived. Under these circumstances the majority of nonpregnant subjects with folate deficiency excreted increased amounts of formiminoglutamic acid in the urine.

Formiminoglutamic acid is stable at an acid pH, and undergoes rapid hydrolysis in the presence of alkali, to form glutamic acid, ammonia, and carbon-dioxide. The conversion to glutamic acid also results in the appearance of a free —NH_2 group, so that the compound now stains with ninhydrin. These properties of formiminoglutamic acid have given rise to a host of ingenious methods for its detection, and these have been reviewed by Luhby and Cooperman (1964). All methods that are of value require the collection of a urine sample into some acid for at least 8 hr after an oral dose of histidine. A convenient dose is 15 g of *l*-histidine monohydrochloride given as a single dose. Blood and urinary histidine levels in normal subjects reach their maximum in the first 3 hr after the oral dose (Fig.19), and are followed by a rise in formiminoglutamic acid excretion after the third hour (Chanarin *et al.*, 1963).

The most widely used method to detect formiminoglutamic acid in urine is that of electrophoresis on paper, followed by exposure to ammonia, and thereafter ninhydrin (Knowles *et al.*, 1960; Kohn *et al.*, 1961). This method being qualitative, reflects concentration of the material in urine, and is inadequate for more critical studies. Detectable amounts of formiminoglutamic acid are considered to be abnormal. The most useful methods for the estimation of forminoglutamic acid are enzymatic. The simplest and the method of choice is that described by Chanarin and Bennett (1962a). A more sensitive but more complex method is described by Tabor and Wyngarden (1958). Both methods involve the enzymatic transfer of the formimino-group to H_4folic acid and the conversion of this compound to 5,10-methenylH_4folic acid by acidification. The concentration of the compound is read by its absorbency at 350×10^{-6} mm.

Healthy subjects excrete 1–17 mg (mean 9 mg) of formiminoglutamic acid in the urine, following a single oral dose of 15 g of histidine (Chanarin and Bennett, 1962a). The same result is obtained if the histidine is given as three 5 g doses, and urine collected over 24 hr (Grasbeck *et al.*, 1961).

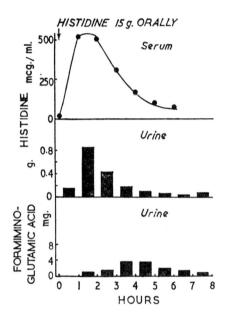

FIG. 19. The serum histidine level and urinary histidine and formimino-glutamic acid excretion after an oral dose of 15 g of histidine in a normal subject.

Patients with folate deficiency with some notable exceptions excrete increased amounts of formiminoglutamic acid in the urine, and this may vary from over 20 mg to 1500 mg in 8 hr. The exceptions are patients with megaloblastic anemia in pregnancy, only half of whom have an elevated urinary formiminoglutamic acid excretion (Chanarin *et al.*, 1963). This is due to changes in the metabolism of aminoacids such as histidine in pregnancy with increased urinary loss, and increased incorporation into protein (Berry *et al.*, 1963; Chanarin *et al.*, 1965a). Normal values may also be found in patients developing megaloblastic anemia while receiving anticonvulsant drugs (Reynolds *et al.*, 1966).

Patients with vitamin B_{12} deficiency such as Addisonian pernicious anemia have an increased excretion of formiminoglutamic acid (Fig. 20),

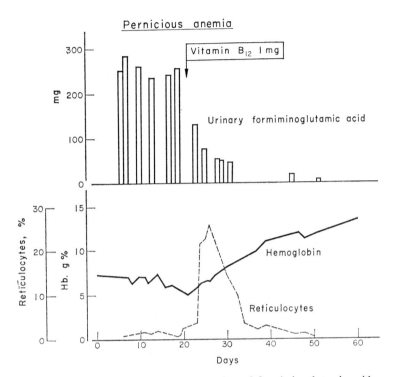

Fig. 20. The change in urinary excretion of formiminoglutamic acid after 15 g of oral histidine in a patient with Addisonian pernicious anemia treated with vitamin B_{12}.

and this returns to within the normal range after therapy with vitamin B_{12} alone (Chanarin, 1963).

A return of normal formiminoglutamic acid excretion takes place within 3 to 5 days of the start of folate therapy, although in some cases an abnormal excretion may persist for a longer period (Chanarin, 1963).

Urinary excretion of imidazole compounds

Not only do increased quantities of formiminoglutamic acid appear in the urine in patients with megaloblastic anemia, but other imidazole compounds that are derived from histidine may be excreted. The most important are urocanic acid and hydantoin-5-propionic acid, the latter being derived from 4-imidazolone-5-propionic acid (Brown and Kies, 1959), which is the immediate precursor substance of formiminoglutamic acid.

Indeed, if the block to histidine breakdown occurs at the stage of conversion of urocanic acid to imidazolone-propionic acid, so that urocanic acid accumulates, then it is impossible for formiminoglutamic acid to be formed. In some cases it seems that high levels of formiminoglutamic acid may depress the levels of enzymes such as urocanase, so that formiminoglutamic acid is no longer formed, and there is a pile-up of the precursor compounds. Thus, patients in whom high levels of urocanate excretion alternated with formiminoglutamic acid excretion have been described (Chanarin, 1963). In others, the excretion of formiminoglutamic acid may disappear, and be replaced by a predominantly urocanate excretion (Chanarin *et al.*, 1963)

It has been suggested that urocanate excretion is particularly common in patients with hepatic impairment (Merrit *et al.*, 1962; Knowles *et al.*, 1963b). However, most patients who excrete significant amounts of formiminoglutamic acid also excrete urocanic acid to a greater or lesser extent (Bennett and Chanarin, 1961, 1962), and may also excrete other imidazoles as well (Middleton, 1965).

Metabolism of ^{14}C-labeled histidine in man

Fish *et al.* (1963) injected 0.5 mg of histidine labeled with ^{14}C in the carbon 2 position of the imidazole ring, and measured the excretion of [14]CO_2 in the breath over the next hour. In normal subjects, and in patients with vitamin B_{12} deficiency, the maximum [14]CO_2 output occurred 20–50 min after the intravenous injection, and total excretion in 1 hr ranged from 0.71 to 1.34 % of the dose. In patients with folate deficiency, the maximum output took place 140–240 min after the dose, and after 1 hr 0.06–0.22 % was excreted in the breath. Patients showing reticulocyte responses following therapy with vitamin B_{12} or folate also showed a maximum excretion in the first hour, but the total amount of [14]CO_2 was 0.06–0.35 %. These results demonstrate a reduction in the amount of the labeled carbon entering the single carbon unit pool, and hence a reduction in the amount of that carbon ultimately disposed of as CO_2. It is not known whether differences between vitamin B_{12} deficient subjects and control subjects could be brought out by increasing the amount of the histidine load.

Serine-glycine metabolism

Butterworth *et al.* (1958) studied the absorption of glycine in patients with tropical sprue, and its conversion to serine. Measuring both serum glycine and serum serine levels after an oral dose of 25 g of glycine, they found some impairment of glycine absorption, but no impairment of conversion to serine. Probably this approach was not sufficiently sensitive to demonstrate any failure in serine-glycine interconversion in these folate-deficient patients.

Urinary excretion of aminoimidazolecarboxamide ribonucleotide (AICAR)

This compound is formylated to yield a purine structure. Luhby and Cooperman (1962) reported an increased excretion in the urine of this compound in patients with pernicious anemia in relapse. Herbert *et al.* (1964) found an increased output in folate deficiency and in hepatic cirrhosis.

Urinary excretion of formic acid

This compound, which may contribute carbon units to the single carbon unit pool, appears in the urine of folate-deficient rats (Rabinowitz and Tabor, 1958). Hiatt *et al.* (1958) demonstrated an increased output of formic acid in the urine of leukemic children receiving therapy with folate antatonists.

Urinary excretion of hydroxyphenol derivatives

Swendseid *et al.* (1943) showed that there was an elevated urinary excretion of hydroxyphenol compounds in untreated pernicious anemia, which declined after therapy. This was confirmed by Abbott and James (1950). This also applies to patients with folate deficiency, to folate deficient rats, and to patients receiving folate antagonists (Goodfriend and Kaufman, 1961).

Although folic acid is active in the conversion of phenylalanine to tyrosine (Fig. 21) in liver extracts, pteridine compounds lacking the *p*-amino-benzoyl-glutamate portion were considerably more active

(Kaufman, 1958). Pteridines with methyl substituents in the 6 and 7 positions showed greatest activity (Ellenbogen *et al.*, 1965). The abnormal phenylalanine-tyrosine metabolism in folate deficiency suggests that these pteridine cofactors may arise from dietary folates, or that conditions leading to folate deficiency also lead to deficiency of those pteridines.

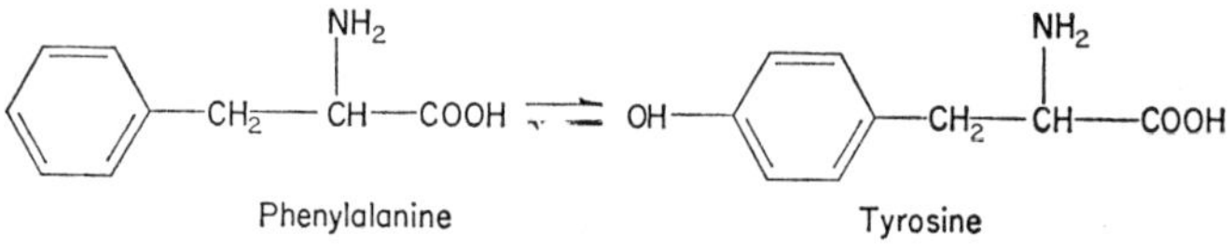

Phenylalanine   Tyrosine

FIG. 21.   Phenylalanine-tyrosine interconversion.

Serum levels of lactic acid dehydrogenase

Hess and Gehm (1955) found an increased serum lactic acid dehydrogenase activity in Addisonian pernicious anemia. The levels found in patients with frank megaloblastic hematopoiesis are considerably higher than that found in any other disorder. Thus whereas controls have less than 500 units of activity per liter of serum the values in megaloblastic anemia ranged from 1500 to 11,000 units (Anderssen, 1964).

Fleming and Elliott (1964) also noted markedly elevated lactic acid dehydrogenase activity as well as serum α-hydroxybutyrate dehydrogenase activity in patients with severe megaloblastic anemia in pregnancy. The values were normal in pregnant women with early megaloblastic changes, and normal values were also noted in epileptic patients showing evidence of early megaloblastic changes in the marrow (Reynolds *et al.*, 1966). Treatment produced a rapid fall of lactic acid dehydrogenase activity within 3 days, although strictly normal values were not attained for more than 2 weeks (Anderssen, 1964). The origin of the serum enzyme is uncertain, but it is likely that it is derived directly from effete marrow cells (Libnoch *et al.*, 1966).

Urinary excretion of parenteral folic acid

Patients with folic acid deficiency retain a larger proportion of a parenteral dose of folic acid than do control subjects, and less is excreted into the urine (Spray *et al.*, 1951; Swendseid *et al.*, 1952; Girdwood, 1953).

With a daily parenteral dose of 15 mcg of folic acid per kg body weight, more folate is retained in the first 2 days in normal subjects than on subsequent days, when the urinary excretion reaches a plateau (Chanarin and Bennett, 1962b). In folate deficiency a greater proportion of folate is retained for about 4–5 days. A further phase of increased folate retention was noted after 6–8 days of daily injections (Fig. 22). The explanation for this is uncertain.

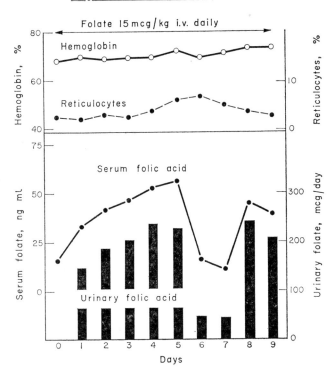

FIG. 22. The serum folate levels and urinary excretion of folate following a daily injection of 15 mcg of folate per kg body weight, in a patient with megaloblastic anemia in pregnancy.

Plasma clearance of parenteral folic acid

When small doses of parenteral folic acid are given intravenously to patients with folate deficiency, the folate is cleared from the plasma to the tissues more rapidly in these patients than in healthy subjects (Spray and Witts, 1953ab; Chanarin *et al.*, 1958a). Thus using an intravenous dose of 15 mcg per kg of body weight Chanarin *et al.* (1958a) found that the serum folate level with *Str. fecalis* as the test organisms 15 min after the injection ranged from 21 to 80 ng per ml (mean 40 ng). The 15-min serum folate level was almost invariably lower than this in folate deficiency (Fig. 23), and was frequently zero at this time. A relatively slow folate clearance was observed only in patients with paroxymal nocturnal hemoglobinuria (Chanarin *et al.*, 1959a). Herbert and Zalusky (1962) have

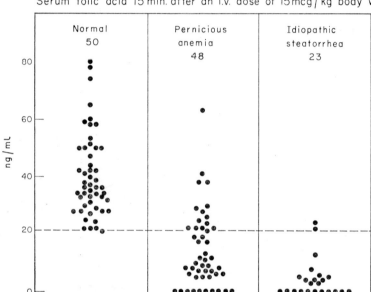

FIG. 23. The serum folate level 15 min after an i.v. dose of 15 mcg folate per kg in normal subjects, in 48 patients with untreated Addisonian pernicious anemia and 23 patients with megaloblastic anemia and idiopathic steatorrhoea. The megaloblastic anemia in the last group was due to folate deficiency.

suggested that in untreated Addisonian pernicious anemia, there is a reaccumulation in the plasma of the injected folate in the 5-methyl form. This has not been confirmed (Chanarin and McLean, 1967).

Effect of folate deficiency on the serum vitamin B_{12} concentration

Wilson and Pitney (1955) noted a decline in the serum vitamin B_{12} level of monkeys on folate deficient diets. Similarly, the development of megaloblastic anemia due to the action of the folic acid antagonist, pyrimethamine, was accompanied by a marked decline in the serum vitamin B_{12} concentration (Chanarin, 1964b). A relatively low serum vitamin B_{12} concentration is not infrequently encountered in patients with folate deficiency, although these patients are able to absorb vitamin B_{12} in a normal manner. Treatment with folic acid (Fig. 24) produces a rapid rise in the serum vitamin B_{12} level (Mollin and Ross, 1956; Mollin *et al.*, 1961; Johnson *et al.*, 1962). This effect is due to redistribution of vitamin B_{12} throughout different body compartments, and not to any effect on vitamin B_{12} absorption.

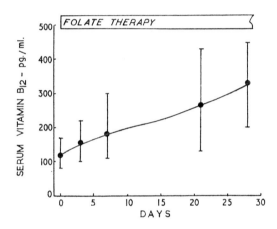

Fig. 24. The mean and range of the serum vitamin B_{12} level in 20 patients with megaloblastic anemia due to folate deficiency following therapy (after Mollin *et al.*, 1961).

Effect of folate deficiency on intestinal absorption

A transient malabsorption of vitamin B_{12} has been found in patients with megaloblastic anemia due to anticonvulsant drugs. In these cases the absorption of vitamin B_{12} was found to be normal when the test was repeated after folate therapy (Lees, 1961; Reynolds *et al.*, 1965). In some of these patients, xylose absorption was impaired before folate therapy, and was found to be normal after therapy. A general improvement of intestinal absorption occurs in patients with tropical sprue given folate therapy (Darby, 1947).

E

IRON AND FOLATE METABOLISM

Iron deficiency and folate deficiency frequently coexist in pregnancy, in those taking poor diets, associated with hookworm infestation, and not uncommonly after partial gastrectomy. In these conditions the peripheral blood and marrow may show evidence of iron deficiency only. Following adequate iron therapy, macrocytes may appear in the peripheral blood, and megaloblasts may become evident in the marrow (Pedersen *et al.*, 1957; Tasker, 1959). Thus, when both iron and folic acid are lacking, the morphological picture is dominated by iron deficiency.

There is some evidence that iron deficiency may also be a factor in producing the folate deficiency state. Thus Chanarin *et al.* (1965) found that pregnant women not receiving iron supplements ultimately showed not only the highest incidence of iron deficiency anemia, but also the highest incidence of megaloblastic anemia at the end of pregnancy, and the lowest serum folate values as compared to control groups receiving iron. Velez *et al.* (1965), studying patients with iron deficiency and megaloblastic marrow changes, found that normoblastic hematopoiesis was restored by iron therapy alone. These patients were maintained on low dietary folate intakes throughout the study. Increased urinary formiminoglutamic acid excretion has been reported in simple iron deficiency in man (Chanarin *et al.*, 1962e), and in the rat (Vitale *et al.*, 1965). Finally Vitale *et al.* (1965) have produced some evidence that the enzyme, formimino-transferase was low in the liver of folate-deficient rats, and they suggested that the production of this enzyme was impaired in iron deficiency.

Detailed observations on iron metabolism in untreated patients with pernicious anemia were made by Finch *et al.* (1956), and it is probable that these observations are equally applicable to megaloblastic anemia due to folate deficiency. The serum iron level was usually elevated (Rath and Finch, 1949), and the elevated serum iron levels fall precipitously to subnormal levels 24–48 hr after the start of folate therapy (Hawkins, 1955).

Tracer iron was cleared rapidly from the plasma, and accumulated rapidly in the marrow in untreated megaloblastic anemia. There was impaired utilization of ^{59}Fe, as judged by the depressed incorporation of iron into red cells (Finch *et al.*, 1949), and an accumulation of iron in the liver 7–10 days following the tracer dose. However, the rate of delivery of labeled cells to the blood was approximately normal i.e. at about 4 days (Finch *et al.*, 1956).

VITAMIN B_{12} AND FOLATE METABOLISM

The precise biochemical pathways in mammals in which the vitamin B_{12} coenzymes participate remain uncertain, and hence any discussion on the relation between folate and vitamin B_{12} remains speculative.

Much of the evidence indicating the intimate biochemical link between vitamin B_{12} and folate has been discussed. Deficiency of either vitamin may lead to identical changes in blood and marrow, i.e. those of a megaloblastic anemia. Patients with vitamin B_{12} deficiency respond hematologically to treatment with folic acid. Furthermore, patients with folate deficiency may on occasion respond to treatment with vitamin B_{12} (Zalusky *et al.*, 1962; Alperin, 1964). Patients with vitamin B_{12} deficiency, such as untreated Addisonian pernicious anemia, show profound abnormalities of folate metabolism, suggesting the presence of true folate deficiency. They may retain increased amounts of parenteral folic acid (Spray *et al.*, 1951), and clear parenteral folate very rapidly from blood

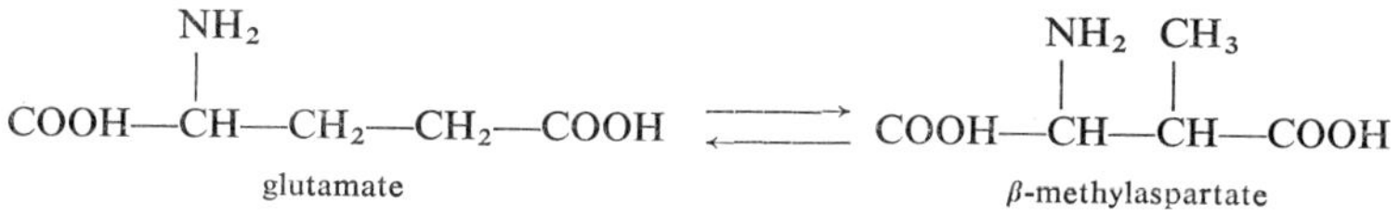

$$\underset{\text{glutamate}}{\text{COOH}-\underset{\underset{\text{NH}_2}{|}}{\text{CH}}-\text{CH}_2-\text{CH}_2-\text{COOH}} \rightleftharpoons \underset{\beta\text{-methylaspartate}}{\text{COOH}-\underset{\underset{\text{NH}_2}{|}}{\text{CH}}-\underset{\underset{\text{CH}_3}{|}}{\text{CH}}-\text{COOH}}$$

Fig. 25. Action of glutamate isomerase.

to the tissues (Chanarin *et al.*, 1958a). The urinary formiminoglutamic acid excretion is usually increased, the red cell folate is abnormally low and at least in vitamin B_{12} deficient sheep the hepatic folate is low (Dawbarn *et al.*, 1958). Folate deficiency may depress the serum vitamin B_{12} level, and, conversely, vitamin B_{12} deficiency may elevate the serum folate level.

Vitamin B_{12} coenzyme has been shown to participate in reactions involving the following enzymes (Weissbach and Dickerman, 1965).

(1) Glutamate isomerase which converts glutamate to β-methylaspartate (Fig. 25).

(2) Glycol dehydrase converting, e.g. 1,2-propandiol to propionaldehyde (Fig. 26).

$$\underset{\text{propanediol}}{\text{CH}_2\text{OH}-\text{CHOH}-\text{CH}_3} \xrightarrow{-\text{H}_2\text{O}} \underset{\text{propionaldehyde}}{\text{CHO}-\text{CH}_2-\text{CH}_3}$$

Fig. 26. Action of glycol dehydrase.

(3) Methylmalonyl isomerase converting succinyl coenzyme A to methylmalonyl coenzyme A (Fig. 27).

None of these three reactions appear to involve the folate coenzymes, and only the third has been identified in mammals. Methylmalonic acid

$$CO-SCoA-CH_2-CH_2-COOH \; \rightleftharpoons \; CO-SCoA-\overset{\overset{\displaystyle CH_3}{\displaystyle |}}{CH}-COOH$$

Succinyl coenzyme A   Methylmalonylcoenzyme A

FIG. 27.   Action of methylmalonyl isomerase.

is excreted in the urine in increased amounts in untreated Addisonian pernicious anemia (Cox and White, 1962).

(4) More recently it has been suggested that cobamide coenzymes are implicated in the reduction of ribotides to deoxyribotides in *Lactobacillus leichmannii* (Blakley and Barker, 1964), although there is no evidence for such a reaction in mammalian tissue.

The demonstration that both vitamin B_{12} and folate participate in methionine synthesis has focused attention on this series of reactions. The methyl donor in methionine synthesis is methylfolate, but final transfer of the methyl group is via methylcobalamin. In untreated Addisonian pernicious anemia, the serum level of methylfolate may be maintained despite reduced tissue folate stores such as that in the red cell. Herbert and Zalusky (1962) have claimed that, following parenteral folate given to pernicious anemia patients in relapse, there is an initial disappearance of the parenteral dose from the serum followed by its reappearance as *L. casei* active material, presumably methylfolate. Further it has been suggested that folate in the form of 5-methylfolate can be mobilized only by donating the methyl group to cobalamin, and thereafter to homocysteine to form methionine. In vitamin B_{12} deficiency there is thus a trapping of available folate in the 5-methyl form (Buchanan, 1964). This hypothesis would account for some of the known facts, but is dependent on the assumption that folate from 5-methylfolate can only be regenerated via vitamin B_{12} in man.

DIAGNOSIS OF FOLATE DEFICIENCY

In patients with megaloblastic hematopoiesis

Exclusion of vitamin B_{12} deficiency. A normal serum vitamin B_{12} level in a patient with megaloblastic anemia indicates that the megaloblastic hematopoiesis, with rare exceptions such as orotic aciduria (Huguley *et al.*,

1959), is due to folate deficiency. Even when the serum vitamin B_{12} level is low, normal vitamin B_{12} absorption should also be interpreted as excluding vitamin B_{12} deficiency as the cause of the megaloblastic process, except in the case of very strict vegetarians taking no form of animal protein at all in their diet. It is all the more important to adopt this approach in the diagnosis of problems in megaloblastic anemias, because of the unfortunate consequences that can follow folate therapy in patients with primary vitamin B_{12} deficiency.

Tests which assess folate function directly. These tests are of less value, because not only can they be abnormal in Addisonian pernicious anemia, but may be abnormal in patients who do not have any hematological abnormality. Thus, the results of tests such as serum and red cell folate assays, and the urinary excretion of formiminoglutamic acid, should be looked upon as confirmatory, and on occasion they may even be normal in a patient still responding hematologically to therapy with folic acid. Because these tests can be abnormal in Addisonian pernicious anemia, considerable caution is required before interpreting such results as indicating a double deficiency of both vitamin B_{12} and folate. Although this may often prove true in a biochemical sense, it is rare, for example, for pernicious anemia patients showing abnormal folate tests to require therapeutic folic acid in addition to vitamin B_{12} in order to achieve a full remission.

Diagnosis by the hematological response. An optimal response to folate therapy at a dose level of less than 200 mcg daily is evidence of folate deficiency and similarly an optimal response to a dose of 2–3 mcg of vitamin B_{12} daily is evidence of vitamin B_{12} deficiency. The only certain evidence of clinically significant deficiency of both folate and vitamin B_{12} is the production of a reticulocyte response with each of these substances, the second substance being given when the reticulocytes have returned to base line levels while continuing the first hematinic.

Suboptimal reticulocyte responses have little diagnostic significance, and may occur following oral histidine (Rundles and Brewer, 1958; Chanarin, 1963; MacGibbon and Mollin, 1965), oral serine (Butterworth *et al.*, 1960); oral choline (Davis and Brown, 1947), as well as to uracil, thymine and methionine (Vilter *et al.*, 1950).

In a patient with normoblastic hemopoiesis. Here the diagnosis of folate deficiency depends on the results of tests such as the assay of the serum and red cell folate, and the urinary excretion of formiminoglutamic acid after an oral histidine load. Abnormal results may not always parallel the state of the tissue stores, but it is likely that red cell folate assay may prove of greater value than either serum folate estimation or urinary formiminoglutamic acid excretion.

CLINICAL DISORDERS ASSOCIATED WITH MEGALOBLASTIC ANEMIA AND FOLATE DEFICIENCY

Megaloblastic anemia requiring folate therapy arises:

(1) When the folate intake is deficient, either because of an inadequate diet, or because of intestinal malabsorption.

(2) When the requirement for folate is increased beyond that taken in from dietary sources. This increased folate requirement is usually due to an increased cell turn over.

(3) When there is interference with the folate coenzymes, e.g. by drugs such as methotrexate, pyrimethamine, drugs used in the treatment of epilepsy, and by alcohol.

Nutritional megaloblastic anemia

An inadequate dietary intake of folate remains a major etiological factor in folate deficiency in many parts of the world. Even in the more affluent parts of the world this state of affairs is not uncommon among elderly people with inadequate means (Gough *et al.*, 1963; Forshaw *et al.*, 1964; Read *et al.*, 1965). The diagnosis should be entertained only after careful exclusion of other causes of folate deficiency.

Intestinal malabsorption

Impaired intestinal absorption of dietary folate is common to a number of disorders the most important of which are coeliac disease of childhood, adult coeliac disease, or idiopathic steatorrhoea or non-tropical sprue, and tropical sprue. The impairment of folate absorption is only part of a general intestinal malabsorption, wherein abnormal absorption of fat, glucose, xylose, iron, calcium, fat-soluble vitamins such as A, D, and K, and water-soluble vitamins such as cobalamin and ascorbic acid, may be demonstrated. A megaloblastic process is almost the rule in patients presenting with tropical sprue (Carmichael-Low, 1928; Mansen-Bahr and Willoughby, 1930); it is present at some time in more than half the patients with non-tropical sprue (Innes, 1948; Cooke *et al.*, 1948; Estren, 1957); and was found in 8 out of 19 children with coeliac disease by Dormandy *et al.* (1963). Folate malabsorption can be demonstrated in almost all these patients (Doig and Girdwood, 1960; Chanarin and Bennett, 1962), and about from half to two-thirds also have impaired absorption of vitamin B_{12} (Mollin *et al.*, 1957).

Although impaired folate absorption can be demonstrated in more than half the patients with Crohn's disease (Chanarin and Bennett, 1962), megaloblastic anemia is usually due to vitamin B_{12} deficiency, because the ileum is so frequently diseased, resected, or bypassed in this order. Similarly in the disorders that have been grouped under the heading of anatomical abnormalities of the small gut (small intestinal diverticulosis, strictures, resections, fistulae, etc.), megaloblastic anemia is almost invariably due to vitamin B_{12} deficiency, and not to folate deficiency.

Impaired absorption has been described in patients with reticuloses (Pitney *et al.*, 1960), and is certainly altered in normal pregnancy, the serum folate levels after an oral dose of folate reaching only half that found in controls (Chanarin *et al.*, 1959b).

A number of methods are available for the assessment of folate absorption.

(1) The urinary excretion of folate following a 5 mg parenteral dose and a 5 mg oral dose is measured microbiologically, and the result expressed as follows

$$\frac{\text{folate output after 5 mg orally}}{\text{folate output after 5 mg parenterally}} \times 100$$

The ratio is normally greater than 75%, and less in malabsorption states (Girdwood, 1956).

(2) The serum folate level is measured microbiologically with *Str. faecalis* after an oral dose of 40 mcg of folate per kg of body weight. The test is preceded by a parenteral dose of 15 mg of folate given 36 hr before the oral dose, in order to overcome temporarily any tissue depletion of folate, and thus to provide a fairly standard rate of clearance from the plasma of absorbed folate. Normal subjects have a peak serum folate value of greater than 50 ng per ml in the first or second hour after the dose (Chanarin *et al.*, 1958b; Chanarin and Bennett, 1962d), and this is almost

invariably reduced in idiopathic steatorrhoea (Fig. 28), and frequently reduced in other malabsorption syndromes.

(3) The radioactivity appearing in the urine after an oral dose of 40 mcg of tritium-labeled folic acid per kg of body weight is measured. The oral

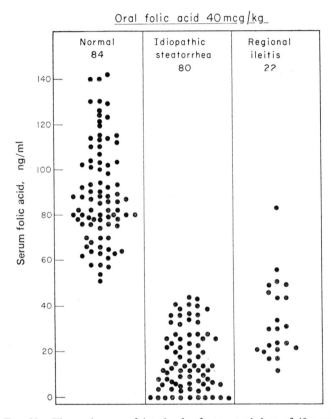

FIG. 28.   The peak serum folate levels after an oral dose of 40 mcg of folate per kg of body weight.

dose is accompanied by an injection of 15 mg of non-radioactive folic acid. In this way more than 25% of the radioactivity is excreted in the urine in controls, and usually less than this in patients with intestinal malabsorption (Anderson *et al.*, 1960; Belcher *et al.*, 1960).

Megaloblastic anemia in pregnancy

In Great Britain, megaloblastic hematopoiesis has been found in more than 2% of all pregnant women (Giles and Shuttleworth, 1958). The frequency is far greater in countries with poor nutritional standards, and the paucity of reports concerning this disorder from countries like the United States of America and Australia suggest a relatively low incidence in those parts. The diagnosis should be suspected when anemia persists

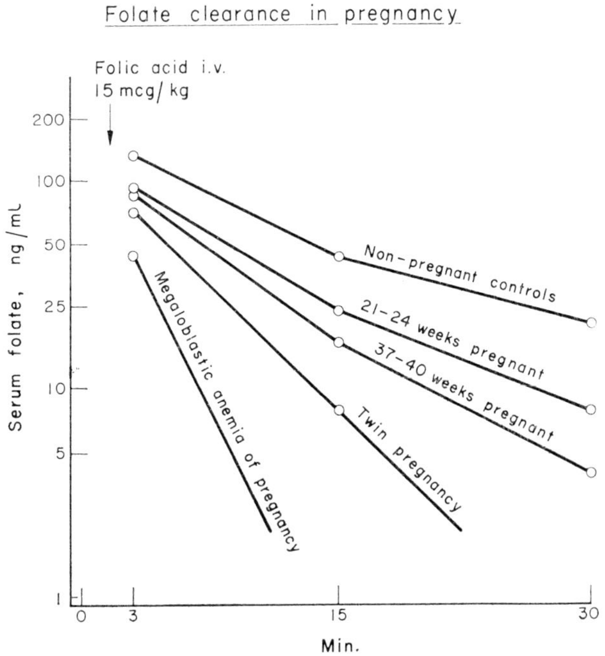

Folate clearance in pregnancy

FIG. 29. The "mean" folate clearance in various groups of pregnant women given 15 mcg of folate per kg intravenously (Chanarin *et al.*, 1959b).

in spite of adequate iron therapy, or when the stained peripheral blood film shows more than 3% of 5-lobed neutrophils, accompanied by occasionally large red cells. The diagnosis should be confirmed by examination of the marrow.

Normal pregnancy is accompanied by a progressive fall in the serum concentration of both vitamin B_{12} and folate, and in the last few weeks

E*

about 5% of women in pregnancy have abnormally low serum vitamin B_{12} levels, and about 50% low serum folate levels (Heinrich, 1954; Boger *et al.*, 1956; Solomons *et al.*, 1962; Chanarin *et al.*, 1965b). Similarly, whole blood folate declines in pregnancy (Izak *et al.*, 1961; Hansen, 1964), and the rate of clearance of intravenous folate becomes progressively more rapid as pregnancy approaches term (Fig. 29). In the last 4 weeks of pregnancy about 60% of normal pregnant women have a rapid folate clearance (Chanarin *et al.*, 1959b). These observations suggest a high incidence of subclinical folate deficiency in pregnancy.

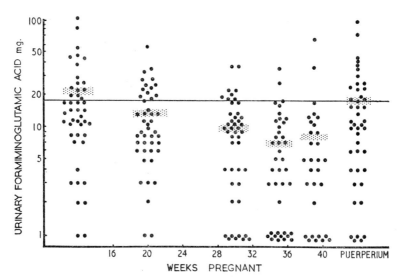

FIG. 30.   Urinary formiminoglutamic acid excretion after 15 g histidine
in normal pregnancy.

The urinary excretion of formiminoglutamic acid is an unsatisfactory index of folate deficiency in pregnancy because of altered metabolism of histidine throughout pregnancy (Berry *et al.*, 1963). Thus the formiminoglutamic acid excretion declines from a mean of 21 mg before the 16th week to 7 mg at 35 weeks (Fig. 30), and may be normal in about half the patients with megaloblastic anemia in pregnancy. This has been attributed to: (1) slow intestinal absorption of histidine during pregnancy; (2) loss of histidine in the urine, owing to a lowered renal threshold; (3) transfer of histidine to the fetus; and (4) probably increased utilization for protein synthesis (Page *et al.*, 1954; Chanarin *et al.*, 1963; Chanarin *et al.*, 1965a).

Megaloblastic anemia in pregnancy is almost invariably due to folate deficiency. The exception to this rule occurs in pregnancy in patients who also have tropical sprue with malabsorption of vitamin B_{12} (Baker *et al.*, 1962). In the absence of a specific gastric or intestinal cause for vitamin B_{12} malabsorption, the absorption of this vitamin is normal in pregnancy (Badenoch *et al.*, 1955). The declining vitamin B_{12} level in pregnancy should not be regarded as denoting any tendency to vitamin B_{12} deficiency, and vitamin B_{12} malabsorption must continue for at least 3 years before significant tissue depletion of vitamin B_{12} appears. Rather the low serum concentrations of vitamin B_{12} in pregnancy reflect active transfer of vitamin B_{12} to the fetus accompanied by some hemodilution. Because folate deficiency *per se* causes a fall in serum vitamin B_{12} levels, low serum vitamin B_{12} levels are particularly frequent in megaloblastic anemia in pregnancy (Mollin and Ross, 1954; Ball and Giles, 1964). Furthermore, because of the high frequency of abnormal results of tests that assess folate function in pregnancy, such tests are of little aid in the diagnosis of megaloblastic anemia in pregnancy.

The cause of the folate deficiency in pregnancy is probably the increased requirement for this vitamin, owing to the rapid growth of the fetus. The incidence of megaloblastic anemia is considerably greater in twin pregnancy, where, if untreated, at least 1 in 10 women may show evidence of a megaloblastic process.

Megaloblastic anemia during lactation

In women taking a relatively poor diet, prolonged lactation imposes additional burdens on their folate stores, and megaloblastic anemia appearing many months after the end of the pregnancy is common (Metz, 1958). Shapiro *et al.* (1965) compared two groups of Bantu women after delivery, one group receiving only iron supplements, and the other iron with additional folic acid. The mean folate clearance (15 min serum level) remained 22–24 ng per ml in the group not given folate, but rose steadily in the folate-supplemented group. The serum folate level showed the same behaviour. The urinary formiminoglutamic acid excretion rose in the group not given folate, but fell in the supplemented group. Thus lactation for a period of 1 year resulted in the development of folate deficiency which was prevented by folate supplements.

Megaloblastic changes in neoplastic disease and leukemia

Megaloblastic anemia associated with carcinoma was recorded by Erlich and Lazarus (1898). A megaloblastic form of hematopoiesis is frequent in patients with neoplastic disorders, such as reticulosarcomas, myeloma, as well as the acute leukemias. This is probably due to an increased requirement for folate by the tumour, and possibly also to diminished dietary intake. However, it is rare for a well-marked anemia to result only from folate deficiency in such patients. Treatment with folate will restore normoblastic hematopoiesis, but will seldom improve the hemoglobin level, and on occasion, as in acute leukemia, may produce a deterioration in the patients general condition. Presumably this is because folate deficiency acts as a limiting factor in the growth of the neoplasm as well as a limiting factor for the growth of normal marrow. Serum folate levels are usually low in patients with neoplastic disorders, whether they are megaloblastic or not (Bertino et al., 1963; Magnus, 1963; Rama-Rao et al., 1963), the urinary formiminoglutamic acid excretion is elevated (Chanarin, 1963; Dymock, 1964), and the folate clearance is abnormally rapid (Chanarin et al., 1958b).

Drugs used in treatment of these disorders, such as folate and purine antagonists, themselves produce a megaloblastic form of hematopoiesis. Finally, Addisonian pernicious anemia may be present in patients who also have a neoplastic process.

Megaloblastic hematopoiesis complicating a hemolytic anemia

Chronic hemolysis, as in patients with hemoglobinopathies or hereditary spherocytosis, leads to an increased folate requirement, and frequently biochemical evidence of folate deficiency. These patients clear parenteral folate rapidly from the plasma (Chanarin et al., 1959a), the serum folate level may be low (Lindenbaum and Klipstein, 1963), and urinary formiminoglutamic acid may be elevated (Chanarin, 1963). Thus, it is not surprising that megaloblastic anemia is a frequent complication, and this should be suspected when there is an unexpected decline in hemoglobin concentration, with a fall in the reticulocyte count. Published case reports have been listed by Lindenbaum and Klipstein (1963), and these indicate the frequency with which either an intercurrent infection or pregnancy, by imposing an additional burden on folate metabolism, triggers off the onset of a megaloblastic anemia in these patients. Megaloblastic arrest is particularly common in association with sickle cell anemia (Jonsson et al., 1959; MacIver and Went, 1960; Pierce and Rath, 1962; Watson-Williams,

1962). The diagnosis is confirmed by demonstrating megaloblasts in the marrow, and the *status quo* is restored by oral folate therapy.

Megaloblastic anemia due to anticonvulsant drugs

The association of megaloblastic anemia and drugs used in the treatment of epilepsy was noted by Mannheimer *et al.* (1952), and Badenoch (1954). It is presumed that these drugs in some way interfere with folate metabolism, but biochemical data in support is lacking (Hamfelt and Wilmanns, 1965). The drugs involved are principally diphenylhydantoin (Dilantin, Phenytoin, Epanutin) and primidone (Mysoline), and these are given usually in combination with other drugs such as phenobarbitone and other barbiturates. Published case reports have been listed by Klipstein (1963). The studies of Hawkins and Meynell (1958), Klipstein (1963), and Reynolds *et al.* (1966) indicate that early megaloblastic changes are present in the blood and marrow of up to 40% of epileptic subjects receiving anticonvulsant drugs. In a small number of cases the megaloblastic anemia becomes severe, and it has been suggested that this is due to additional dietary folate deficiency. The serum folate level is usually (but not always) low; the urinary formiminoglutamic acid excretion may be normal. Occasionally there may be a marked reduction of the serum vitamin B_{12} level (Kidd and Mollin, 1957), despite usually normal vitamin B_{12} absorption. In these cases folate therapy produces a rapid rise in the serum vitamin B_{12} level to normal within 1–2 weeks.

Studies in a patient with erythroid aplasia due to Dilantin administration suggested that there was an inhibition of deoxyribose nucleic acid synthesis, possibly due to interference of formation of deoxyribotides (Yunis *et al.*, 1965).

Cirrhosis, alcohol and megaloblastic anemia

Leevy *et al.* (1965b) found reduced serum folate values in 47% of alcoholics with cirrhosis, in 40% of alcoholics with fatty livers, and in 30% of alcoholics with histologically normal livers. Assay of the folate content of liver biopsy samples gave values of 0–3.5 mcg per g of liver (mean 1.6) in cirrhosis, and values of 0–8.1 (mean 4.6) in those with histologically normal livers. A major factor in producing folate deficiency in those patients is a grossly deficient diet consisting largely of carbohydrate. However, the study by Sullivan and Herbert (1964) showed that alcohol acts as a direct toxin in inducing a megaloblastic form of hematopoiesis.

Bertino *et al.* (1965) suggested that the effect of alcohol is directly on tetrahydrofolate formylase. The relationship between cirrhosis and folate deficiency has been studied by Herbert *et al.* (1963), and by Klipstein and Lindenbaum (1965).

It is unusual to find megaloblastic anemia in non-alcoholic patients with liver disease, and there is little evidence that megaloblastic anemia is more frequent in such patients than in the general population. Similarly megaloblastic anemia in patients with hemochromatosis (Koszewski, 1952) is usually associated with excessive alcohol consumption.

Chronic myelofibrosis and megaloblastic anemia

Chronic myelofibrosis is characterized by a leuco-erythroblastic blood picture, usually massive sphenomegaly, and failure to aspirate marrow for study. Eventually marrow failure and pancytopenia supervenes in the majority of cases. It is not widely recognized that an important cause of marrow failure in these patients is megaloblastic hematopoiesis due to folate deficiency. The difficulty in establishing the diagnosis is partly due to inability to obtain marrow for examination. Nevertheless, it is often possible to express a drop of fluid from the marrow needle, which should be spread, and this may show the usual features of megaloblastic hematopoiesis. Alternately, both megaloblasts and giant metamyelocytes may be recognized in buffy coat preparations. In particular the onset of thrombocytopenia should lead to search for a megaloblastic process.

Chanarin *et al.* (1958b) described an example of megaloblastic anemia in myelofibrosis, and noted that four other patients with chronic myelofibrosis who were normoblastic also had an abnormally rapid folate clearance. Thus, it seems likely that folate deficiency is usual in this group of patients. Further cases were described by Forshaw *et al.* (1964), Chanarin (1964a), and Mollin and Hoffbrand (1965). Chanarin, Mollin, and Szur (unpublished observations) studied 15 patients with chronic myelofibrosis, and found evidence of megaloblastic hematopoiesis in 8 of them. The explanation for the presumably increased folate requirement in these patients is uncertain.

Megaloblastic hematopoiesis in sideroblastic anemia

This form of anemia is characterized by the simultaneous occurrence of normochromic and hypochromic cells in the peripheral blood, and by the presence of many iron granules often arranged as a ring about the nucleus of the erythroblasts (Rundles and Falls, 1946; Dacie *et al.*, 1959). The descriptive term "refractory normoblastic anemia" is unfortunate, since more than half the cases show morphological evidence of megaloblastic hematopoiesis(MacGibbon and Mollin, 1965), and 80% show biochemical evidence of folate deficiency. More than one third show a hematological response to therapy with folic acid. Others fail to respond to folate, but may respond to pyridoxine.

Megaloblastic features are also prominent in patients with sideroblastic anemia due to the administration of antituberculous drugs, such as isoniazid, cycloserine, and pyrizinamide (Verwilghen *et al.*, 1965). Normoblastic hematopoiesis in these patients is restored by withdrawal of the drug.

Rarely a patient who presents primarily with a megaloblastic anemia, e.g. due to alcoholism, may in addition have a dimorphic blood picture and prominent sideroblasts in the marrow. Such cases respond completely to therapy with folic acid, with the disappearance of ringed sideroblasts from the marrow.

Megaloblastic anemia of childhood

Megaloblastic anemia in young children may be due to failure to absorb vitamin B_{12}, either because of congenital failure to elaborate intrinsic factor, or to gastric atrophy in older children (Juvenile autoimmune pernicious anemia), or because of an intestinal lesion (Spurling *et al.*, 1964). Further megaloblastic anemia may be due to some of the disorders discussed such as the hemoglobinopathies and coeliac disease.

Megaloblastic anemia in infants being reared on goat's milk was recognised by Parsons (1933). Goat's milk has an extremely low folate content. Megaloblastic anemia was noted in infants fed on dried milk that had a very low ascorbate content (Aldrich and Nelson, 1947), and this anemia disappeared when ascorbate was added to the dried milk preparations (Zuelzer and Rutzky, 1953). The most important group of megaloblastic anemias in infants arise in association with Kwashiorkor, in association with malnutrition and with infection. Walt *et al.* (1956) found that megaloblastic anemia was present in 5.4% of all pediatric admission to a hospital for Bantu children in South Africa. MacIver and Back (1960) found that megaloblastic anemia constituted 6.3% of all pediatric admissions in Jamaica. The megaloblastic anemia was due to folate deficiency, and good responses were obtained with folate therapy.

The cause of the folate deficiency was uncertain, but malnutrition was considered to be important. The role of infection was difficult to evaluate, but was a frequent accompaniment in most of the children.

Strelling *et al.* (1966) have reported a high incidence of megaloblastic hematopoiesis in premature infants.

Other disorders associated with megaloblastic anemia due to folate deficiency

Scurvy is frequently associated with a megaloblastic anemia which may respond to ascorbate therapy alone (Brown, 1955). Other cases may respond to small doses of folate (Zalusky and Herbert, 1961).

Megaloblastic anemia following partial gastrectomy is due to vitamin B_{12} deficiency in 80% of cases, but in the remaining 20% it is due to folate deficiency. The diagnosis of folate deficiency is probable when (1) the serum vitamin B_{12} concentration is normal (Mollin and Hines, 1964), (2) the absorption of vitamin B_{12} is normal irrespective of the serum vitamin B_{12} level, (3) the gastric juice contains either hydrochloric acid or when its intrinsic factor concentration exceeds 10 units per ml of gastric juice (Ardeman and Chanarin, 1966), and (4) the patient is receiving vitamin B_{12} therapy.

Malaria prophylaxis with pyrimethamine (Daraprim) may give rise to a megaloblastic anemia (Laing, 1957). The effect of this drug on folate metabolism in man has been studied (Chanarin, 1964b).

There is possibly an increased incidence of megaloblastic anemia due to folate deficiency in patients with rheumatoid arthritis, although the majority of such patients with megaloblastic anemia prove to have Addisonian pernicious anemia (Mollin *et al.*, 1963; Partridge and Duthie, 1963; Gough *et al.*, 1964).

FOLATE THERAPY

Folate compounds for clinical use are available as follows:

(1) Tablets containing 5 mg of pteroylglutamic acid.

(2) Solution containing 15 mg in 1.0 ml volume of pteroylglutamic acid as the sodium salt for parenteral injection.

(3) Solution of folinic acid (5-formyltetrahydropteroylglutamic acid) as a mixture of 1.5 mg of the active *l*-isomer and 1.5 mg of the inactive *d*-isomer as the calcium salts in 1.0 ml volume for parenteral injection.

(4) Tablets containing both iron salts and pteroylglutamic acid and intended for administration during pregnancy. These may contain the following:

Ferrous gluconate	300 mg;	folic acid	5 mg.
Ferrous gluconate	300 mg;	folic acid	3 mg.
Ferrous gluconate	250 mg;	folic acid	5 mg.
Ferrous gluconate	30 mg;	folic acid	50 mcg.
Iron aminoates	350 mg;	folic acid	50 mcg.
Ferrous sulphate	194 mg;	folic acid	1.7 mg.
Ferrous fumarate	200 mg;	folic acid	100 mcg.

Oral administration of 5 mg of folic acid once or twice a day is more than adequate, and even patients with severe intestinal malabsorption appear to take up sufficient folic acid with this dose. Failure to respond hematologically is rarely, if ever, due to failure of adequate absorption, but rather to incorrect diagnosis, or to complicating factors preventing a normal hematological response. Thus, the indication for parenteral folate as a therapeutic agent is rare in a patient who is able to swallow tablets. Folinic acid must be given by injection, since it is unstable at an acid pH such as may be encountered in normal gastric juice. It should be used specifically to overcome the toxic effects of folic acid antagonists such as methotrexate which inactivate the enzyme, folate reductase. Injections containing 1.5 mg of the active form should be given 2 or 3 times daily until there is clinical improvement.

THE RESPONSE OF A PATIENT WITH MEGALOBLASTIC ANEMIA TO FOLATE THERAPY

The hematological response of a patient with megaloblastic anemia to specific therapy has been evaluated in great detail in relation to the therapy of pernicious anemia with liver extracts. The specific response to folate therapy is identical.

In an optimal response there is a restoration of normoblastic hemopoiesis, with a virtual disappearance of megaloblasts from the marrow after 48 hr. However, giant metamyelocytes persist up to 12 days. The character of the response is assessed by the number of reticulocytes

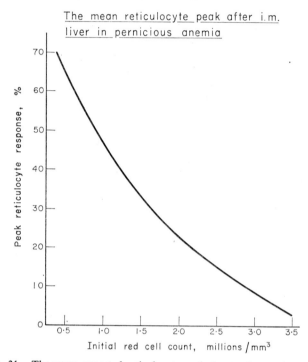

FIG. 31. The mean expected reticulocyte peak due to therapy in megalo-blastic anemia.

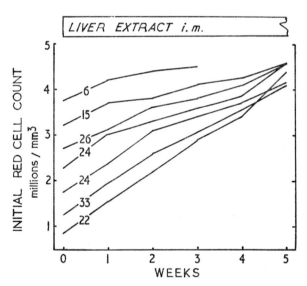

FIG. 32. The expected rise in the red cell count following therapy in megaloblastic anemia. The numbers refer to the number of patients with pernicious anemia treated in each group.

produced, which should reach their expected peak (Fig. 31) on either day 5, 6, or 7, day 0 being the day folate therapy was commenced. The height of the reticulocyte peak depends on the initial severity of the anemia (Sturgis and Isaacs, 1938). This should be followed by a rise in the red cell count, and an increase in the hemoglobin concentration. The red cell count should reach, and probably exceed 3.0 million per mm^3 three weeks after the start of therapy (Bethell, 1935) (Fig. 32). The platelet count rises with the rise in the reticulocyte count, and reaches a plateau after 10 days.

Failure to achieve an optimal response must be investigated. It may be that either the diagnosis of folate deficiency is incorrect, or that there is a further complicating disorder such as renal failure, an infection such as pyelonephritis or respiratory tract infection, an associated neoplasm or leukemic process. It is rare for associated iron deficiency to prevent an adequate reticulocyte response, although iron deficiency may be a limiting factor in the subsequent increase of the red cell mass.

REFERENCES

(a) BOOKS, REVIEWS, AND MONOGRAPHS

BELCHER, E. H., ANDERSON, B., CHANARIN, I. and MOLLIN, D. L. (1960). Clinical and experimental studies with H^3 folic acid in megaloblastic anaemias. In: *Radioaktive Isotope in Klinik und Forschung*, pp. 184–192. FELLINGER, K. and HÖFER, R. (Ed.). Bad Gastein. Urban and Schwartzenberg, München.

BETHELL, F. H. (1935). Quoted by STURGIS, C. C. and ISAACS, R. (1938). Pernicious anaemia. In: *Handbook of Hematology*, vol. III, p. 2267. DOWNEY, H. (Ed.). Hamish Hamilton, London.

CHANARIN, I. (1959). Diagnosis of folic acid deficiency. In: *Proc. 7th Congr. Europ. Soc. Haemat.*, London, Karger, Basel.

DARBY, W. J. (1947). The physiological effects of pteroylglutamates in man with particular reference to pteroylglutamic acid (PGA). *Vitam. and Horm.* vol. 5, 119–161. HARRISS, R. S. and THIMANN, K. V. (Ed.). Acad. Press, New York.

DELMONTE, L. and JUKES, T. H. (1962). Folic acid antagonists in cancer chemotherapy. *Pharmacol. Rev.*, **14**: 91–135.

ERLICH, P. and LAZARUS, A. (1898). *Die Anamie* Vienna. Translated by W. MYERS as *Histology of the blood, normal and pathological.* Cambridge, 1900.

ESTREN, S. (1957). The blood and bone marrow in idiopathic sprue. In: *The malabsorption syndrome*, pp. 130–142. ALDERSBERG, D. (Ed.). Grune and Stratton, N.Y.

FRIEDKIN, M. (1963). Enzymatic aspects of folic acid. In: *Ann. Rev. Biochem.* vol. 32, pp. 185–214. SNELL, E. E., LUCK, J. M. (Ed.). Annual Reviews Inc., Palo Alto, California.

GOLDTHWAIT, D. A. and GREENBERG, G. R. (1955). Some methods for the study of *de novo* synthesis of purine nucleotides. In: *Methods in Enzymology*, vol. 2, pp. 504–519. COLEWICK, S. P. and KAPLAN. N. O. (Ed.). Academic Press, New York.

HANSEN, H. A. (1964). *On the diagnosis of folic acid deficiency.* Almquist and Wiksell, Stockholm.

HUENNEKENS, F. M. and OSBORN, M. J. (1959). Folic acid coenzymes and one-carbon metabolism. In: *Advances in Enzymology*, vol. 21, pp. 396–397. NORD, F. F. (Ed.) pp. 396–397. Interscience Publishers Inc., New York.

JOHNS, D. G. and BERTINO, J. R. (1965). Folates and megaloblastic anaemia: A review. *Clin. pharm. Therap.* 6: 372–392.

JUKES, T. H. (1955). Assay of compounds with folic acid activity. In: *Methods of Biochemical analysis*, vol. 2, GLICK, D. (Ed.) pp. 121–151. Interscience Publ., New York.

JUKES, T. H. and STOKSTAD, E. L. R. (1948). Pteroylglutamic acid and related compounds. *Physiol. Rev.*, 28: 51–106.

LOWENSTEIN, L., BRUNTON, L., COOPER, B. A., MILAD, A. A. and HSIEH, Y. (1963). The relation of erythrocyte and serum *L. casei* folate activity to folate deficiency in certain megaloblastic anaemias. In: *Proc. 9th Cong. Europ. Soc. Haemat.*, pp. 364–375. Lisbon, S. Karger, Basel.

LUHBY, A. L. and COOPERMAN, J. M. (1964). Folic acid deficiency in man and its interrelationship with vitamin B_{12} metabolism. In: *Advances in Metabolic disorders.* LEVINE, R. and LUFT, R. (Ed.) pp. 236–334. Academic Press, New York.

METZ, J. (1958). Megaloblastic anaemia in a malnourished population. In: *Proc. 7th Internat. Congr. Int. Soc. Haemat. Rome*, 1958, pp. 339.

MOLLIN, D. L. and HOFFBRAND, A. V. (1965). The diagnosis of folate deficiency. In: *Vitamin B_{12} and folic acid*, pp. 1–18. BJORKMAN, S. E. (Ed.). Munksgaard, Copenhagen.

MOLLIN, D. L. and ROSS, G. I. M. (1956). The pathophysiology of vitamin B_{12} deficiency in the megaloblastic anaemias. In: *Vitamin B_{12} und Intrinsic Factor. First European Symposium Hamburg* pp. 413–430. HEINRICH, H. C. (Ed.). F. Enke,Stuttgart.

MOLLIN, D. L., WATERS, A. H. and HARRISS, E. (1961). Clinical aspects of the metabolic interrelationships between folic acid and vitamin B_{12}. In: *Vitamin B_{12} und Intrinsic Factor. Second European Symposium, Hamburg*, pp. 737–755. HEINRICH, H. C. (Ed.). F. Enke, Stuttgart.

RABINOWITZ, J. C. (1960). Folic acid. In: *The Enzymes*, vol. 2, pp. 185–251. BOYER, P.D., LARDY, H. and MYRBACK, K. (Ed.). Academic Press, New York.

STIFFEY, A. V. and WILLIAMS, W. L. Quoted by JUKES, T. H. (1955). Assay of compounds with folic acid activity. In: *Methods of Biochemical Analysis*, vol. 2, pp. 141–146. GLICK, D. (Ed.). Interscience Publ., New York.

STOKSTAD, E. L. R. (1954). Pteroylglutamic acid. In: *The Vitamins*, vol. III, pp. 163–166. SEBRELL, W. H., JR. and HARRISS, R. S. (Ed.). Academic Press, New York.

STURGIS, C. C. and ISAACS, R. (1938). Pernicious anemia. In: *Handbook of Hematology.* Vol. III, p. 2261. DOWNEY, H. (Ed.). Hamish Hamilton, London.

TOEPFER, E. W., ZOOK, E. G., ORR, M. L. and RICHARDSON, L. R. (1951). *Folic acid content of foods. Microbiological assay by standardized methods and compilation of data from the literature.* Agriculture Handbook No. 29, U.S. Dept. of Agriculture, Washington, 25.

WEISSBACH, H. and DICKERMAN, H. (1965). Biochemical role of vitamin B_{12}. *Physiol. Rev.*, **45**: 80–97.

WINTROBE, M. M. (1961). *Clinical Hematology.* Henry Kimpton, London.

ZUELZER, W. W. and RUTZKY, J. (1953). Megaloblastic anaemia of infancy. In: *Advances in Pediatrics*, vol. VI, pp. 243–306. LEVINE, S. Z. (Ed.). The Year Book Publ., Chicago.

Folic Acid and Derivatives 137

(b) ORIGINAL PAPERS

ABBOTT, L. D. and JAMES, W. G. (1950). Effect of vitamin B_{12} on the urinary phenol fractions in pernicious anaemia. *J. lab. clin. Med.*, **35**: 35–42.
ALDRICH, R. A. and NELSON, E. N. (1947). Megaloblastic anaemia in infants. *Lancet*, **67**: 399–402.
ALEXANDER, N. and GREENBERG, D. M. (1955). Studies on the biosynthesis of serine. *J. biol. Chem.*, **214**: 821–837.
ALPERIN, J. B. (1964). Effect of vitamin B_{12} therapy in a patient with folic acid deficiency. *Amer. J. clin. Nutr.*, **15**: 117–23.
ANAND, M. P. (1964). Iatrogenic megaloblastic anaemia with neurological complications. *Scot. med. J.*, **9**: 388–90.
ANDERSON, D., BELCHER, E. H., CHANARIN, I. and MOLLIN, D. C. (1960). The urinary and faecal excretion of radioactivity after oral doses of 3H-folic acid. *Brit. J. Haemat.*, **6**: 439–55.
ANDERSSEN, N. (1964). The activity of lactic dehydrogenase in megaloblastic anaemia. *Scand. J. Haemat.*, **1**: 212–9.
ANGIER, R. B., BOOTHE, J. H., HUTCHINGS, B. L., MOWAT, J. H., SEMB, J., STOKSTAD, E. L. R., SUBBA ROW, Y., WALLER, C. W., COSULICH, D. B., FAHRENBACH, M. J., HUTQUIST, M. E., KUH, E., NORTHEY, E. H., SEEGER, D. R., SICKELS, J. P. and SMITH, J. H., JR. (1946). Synthesis of a compound identical with the *L. casei* factor isolated from liver. *Science*, **102**: 227–8.
ARDEMAN, S. and CHANARIN, I. (1966). Intrinsic factor concentration after partial gastrectomy. *Gut*, in press.
ASATOOR, A. and DALGLIESH, C. E. (1956). The use of deactivated charcoals for the isolation of aromatic substances. *J. chem. Soc.*, 2291–9.
BADENOCH, J. (1954). The use of labelled vitamin B_{12} and gastric biopsy in the investigation of anaemia. *Proc. R. Soc. Med.*, **47**: 426–31.
BADENOCH, J., CALLENDER, S. T., EVANS, J. R., TURNBULL, A. L. and WITTS, L. J. (1955) Megaloblastic anaemia of pregnancy and the puerperium. *Brit. med. J.*, **i**: 1245–7.
BAKER, H., FRANK, O., FEINGOLD, S., ZIFFER, H., GELLENE, R. A., LEEVY, C. M. and SOBOTKA, H. (1965a). The fate of orally and parenterally administered folates. *Amer. J. clin. Nutrit.*, **17**: 88–95.
BAKER, H., HERBERT, V., FRANK, O., PASHER, I., HUTNER, S. H., WASSERMAN, L. R. and SOBOTKA, H. (1959). A microbiologic method for detecting folic acid deficiency in man. *Clin. Chem.*, **5**: 275–80.
BAKER, S. J., JACOB, E., RAJAN, K. T. and SWAMINATHAN, S. P. (1962). Vitamin B_{12} deficiency in pregnancy and puerperium. *Brit. med. J.*, **i**: 1658–61.
BAKER, S. J., KUMAR, S. and SWAMINATHAN, S. P. (1965b). Excretion of folic acid in bile. *Lancet*, **i**: 685.
BAKERMAN, H. A., SILVERMAN, M. and DAFT, F. S. (1951). Influence of succinylsulfathiazole and folic acid on glutamic acid excretion. *J. biol. Chem.*, **188**: 117–23.
BALDWIN, J. N. and DALASSIO, D. J. (1961). Folic acid therapy and spinal-cord degeneration in pernicious anaemia. *New Eng. J. Med.*, **264**: 1339–42.
BALL, E. W. and GILES, C. (1964). Folic acid and vitamin B_{12} levels in pregnancy and their relation to megaloblastic anaemia. *J. clin. Path.*, **17**: 165–4.
BÁNHIDI, Z. G. and ERICSON, L.-E. (1953). Bioautographic separation of vitamin B_{12} and various forms of folinic acid occurring in some brown and red seaweeds. *Acta Chem. Scand.*, **7**: 713–20.
BEEBE, R. T. and MENEELY, J. K. (1949). Pernicious anaemia following gastrectomy. *New York State of J. Med.*, **49**: 2437–38.
BENNETT, M. C. (1949). Some observations on the role of folic acid in utilization of homocystine by the rat. *Science*, **110**: 589–90.

138 *Hematopoietic Agents*

BENNETT, M. C. and CHANARIN, I. (1961). Urinary excretion of urocanic acid in megaloblastic anaemia. *Lancet*, ii: 1095.

BENNETT, M. C. and CHANARIN, I. (1962). Urinary excretion of urocanic acid and formiminoglutamic acid. *Nature, Lond.*, **196**: 271–2.

BERRY, V., BOOTH, M. A., CHANARIN, I. and ROTHMAN, D. (1963). Urinary formiminoglutamic acid excretion in pregnancy. *Brit. med. J.*, ii: 1103–04.

BERTINO, J. R., SIMMONS, B. and DONOHUE, D. M. (1962). Purification and properties of the formate-activating enzyme from erythrocytes. *J. biol. Chem.*, **237**: 1314–18.

BERTINO, J. R., GABRIO, B. W. and HUENNEKENS, F. M. (1961). Increased activity of leucocyte dihydrofolic reductase in amethopterin-treated patients. *Clin. Res.*, **9**: 103.

BERTINO, J. R., HELLMAN, S. and IANNOTT, A. T. (1963). Low levels of serum folate in patients with carcinoma of the head and neck. *Cancer Chemotherapy Reps.*, **28**: 21–3.

BERTINO, J. R., WARD, J., SARTORELLI, A. C. and SIBER, R. (1965). An effect of ethanal on folate metabolism. *J. clin. Invest.*, **44**: 1028.

BETHELL, F. H. and STURGIS, C. C. (1948). The relation of therapy in pernicious anaemia to changes in the nervous system. Early and late results in a series of cases observed for periods of not less than ten years, and early results of treatment with folic acid. *Blood*, **3**: 57–67.

BETHELL, F. H., MEYERS, M. C., ANDREWS, G. A., SWENDSEID, M. E., BIRD, O. D. and BROWN, R. A. (1947). Metabolic function of pteroylglutamic acid and its hexaglutamyl conjugate. I. Hematologic and urinary excretion studies on patients with macrocytic anemia. *J. lab. clin. Med.*, **32**: 3–22.

BIRD, O. D., ROBBINS, M., VANDERBELT, J. M. and PFIFFNER, J. J. (1946). Observations on vitamin Bc conjugase from hog kidney. *J. biol. Chem.*, **163**: 649–59.

BLAKLEY, R. L. and BARKER, H. A. (1964). Cobamide stimulation of the reduction of ribotides to deoxyribotides in Lactobacillus leichmannii. *Biochem. biophys. Res. Commun.*, **16**: 391–7.

BLAKLEY, R. L. (1954). The interconversion of serine and glycine: role of pteroylglutamic acid and other cofactors. *Biochem. J.*, **58**: 448–52.

BLAKLEY, R. L. (1955). The interconversion of serine and glycine: participation of pyridoxal phosphate. *Biochem. J.*, **61**: 315–23.

BLAKLEY, R. L. and McDOUGALL, B. M. (1962). The biosynthesis of thymidylic acid. III. Purification of thymidylate synthetase and its spectrophotometric assay. *J. biol. Chem.*, **237**: 812–18.

BOGER, W. P., WRIGHT, L. D., BECK, G. D. and BAYNE, G. M. (1956). Vitamin B_{12}: correlation of serum concentrations and pregnancy. *Proc. Soc. exp. biol. Med.*, **92**: 140–3.

BROQUIST, H. P., BROCKMAN, J. A., JR., FAHRENBACH, M. J., STOKSTAD, E. L. R. and JUKES, T. H. (1952). Comparative biological activity of Leucovorin and pteroylglutamic acid. *J. Nutr.*, **47**: 93–103.

BROQUIST, H. P., KOHLER, A. R., HUTCHISON, D. J. and BURCHENAL, J. H. (1953). Studies on the enzymatic formation of citrovorum factor by *steptococcus faecalis*. *J. biol. Chem.*, **202**: 59–66.

BROQUIST, H. P. (1956). Evidence for the excretion of formiminoglutamic acid following folic acid antagonist therapy in acute leukaemia. *J. Amer. chem. Soc.*, **78**: 6205–6.

BROWN, A. (1955). Megaloblastic anaemia associated with adult scurvy: Report of a case which responded to synthetic ascorbic acid alone. *Brit. J. Haemat.*, **1**: 345–51.

BROWN, D. D. and KIES, M. W. (1959). The mammalian metabolism of L-histidine. I. The enzymatic formation of L-hydantoin-5-propionic acid. *J. biol. Chem.*, **234**: 3182–7.

BROWN, G. M., WEISMAN, R. A. and MOLNAR, D. A. (1961). The biosynthesis of folic acid. I. Substrate and cofactor requirements for enzymatic synthesis by cell-free extracts of escherichia coli. *J. biol. Chem.*, **236**: 2534–43.

BUCHANAN, J. M. (1964). The function of vitamin B_{12} and folic acid. *Medicine*, **43**: 697–709.

BUTTERWORTH, C. E., Jr., BAUGH, C. M. and KRUMDIECK, C. (1969). A study of folate absorption and metabolism in man utilizing carbon-14-labeled polyglutamates synthesized by the solid phase method. *J. clin. Invest.*, **48**: 1131–1142.

BUTTERWORTH, C. E., NADEL, H., PEREZ-SANTIAGO, E., SANTINI, R. and GARDNER, F. H. (1957). Folic acid absorption, excretion and leukocyte concentration in tropical sprue. *J. lab. clin. Med.*, **50**: 673–81.

BUTTERWORTH, C. E., SANTINI, R. and PEREZ-SANTIAGO, E. (1958). The absorption of glycine and its conversion to serine in patients with sprue. *J. clin. Invest.*, **37**: 20–27.

BUTTERWORTH, C. E., SOLER, J. SANTINI, R. and PEREZ-SANTIAGO, E. (1960). Certain aspects of glycine and histidine metabolism in patients with sprue. *Blood*, **15**: 60–70.

BUTTERWORTH, C. E., SANTINI, R. and FROMMEYOR, W. B. (1963). The pteroylglutamate components of American diets as determined by chromatographic fractionation. *J. clin. Invest.*, **42**: 1929–39.

CARMICHAEL-LOW, G. (1928). Sprue. An analytical study of 150 cases. *Quart. J. Med.*, **21**: 523–34.

CARTWRIGHT, G. E., TATTING, B., KURTH, D. and WINTROBE, M. M. (1952). Experimental production of nutritional macrocytic anemia in swine. V. Hematologic manifestations of a combined deficiency of vitamin B_{12} and pteroylglutamic acid. *Blood*, **7**: 992–1004.

CARTWRIGHT, G. E., FAY, J., TATTING, B. and WINTROBE, M. M. (1948). Pteroylglutamic acid deficiency in swine; effects of treatment with pteroylglutamic acid, liver extract and protein. *J. lab. clin. Med.*, **33**: 397–416.

CATHOU, R. E. and BUCHANAN, J. M. (1963). Enzymatic synthesis of the methyl group of methionine. V. Studies with 5,10-methylenetetrahydrofolate reductase from *Escherichia coli. J. biol. Chem.*, **238**: 1746–51.

CERECEDO, L. R. and MIRONE, L. (1947). The beneficial effect of folic acid (*Lactobacillus casei* factor) on lactation in mice maintained on highly purified diets. *Arch. Biochem.*, **12**: 154–5.

CHANARIN, I. (1964a). Studies on urinary formiminoglutamic acid excretion. *Proc. R. Soc. Med.*, **57**: 384–8.

CHANARIN, I. (1964b). Studies in drug-induced megaloblastic anaemia. *Scand. J. Haemat*; **1**: 280–8.

CHANARIN, I. (1963). Urocanic acid and formiminoglutamic acid excretion in megaloblastic anaemia and other conditions: the effect of specific therapy. *Brit. J. Haemat.*, **9**: 141–57.

CHANARIN, I. (1960). Folic-acid absorption tests. *Brit. med. J.*, **ii**: 1160.

CHANARIN, I., ANDERSON, B. B. and MOLLIN, D. L. (1958b). The absorption of folic acid. *Brit. J. Haemat.*, **4**: 156–66.

CHANARIN, I. and BENNETT, M. C. (1962a). A spectrophotometric method for estimating formimino-glutamic acid and urocanic acid. *Brit. med. J.*, **i**: 27–29.

CHANARIN, I. and BENNETT, M. C. (1962b). The plasma clearance of daily doses of folic acid in megaloblastic anaemia. *Brit. J. Haemat.*, **8**: 95–109.

CHANARIN I. and BENNETT, M. C. (1962c). The disposal of small doses of intravenously injected folic acid. *Brit. J. Haemat.*, **8**: 28–35.

CHANARIN, I. and BENNETT, M. C. (1962d). Absorption of folic acid and d-xylose as tests of small intestinal function. *Brit. med. J.*, **i**: 985–9.

CHANARIN, I., BENNETT, M. C. and BERRY, V. (1962e). Urinary excretion of histidine derivatives in megaloblastic anaemia and other conditions and a comparison with the folic acid clearance test. *J. clin. Path.*, **15**: 269–73.

CHANARIN, I., DACIE, J. V. and MOLLIN, D. L. (1959a). Folic-acid deficiency in haemolytic anaemia. *Brit. J. Haemat.*, **5**: 245–56.

CHANARIN, I., FENTON, J. C. B. and MOLLIN, D. L. (1957). Sensitivity to folic acid. *Brit. med. J.*, **i**: 1162–3.

CHANARIN, I., HUTCHINSON, M., McLEAN, A. and MOULE, M. (1966). Hepatic folate in man. *Brit. med. J.*, **i**: 396–9.

CHANARIN, I., LAIDLAW, J., LOUGHRIDGE, L. W. and MOLLIN, D. L. (1960). Megaloblastic anaemia due to phenobarbitone. The convulsant action of therapeutic doses of folic acid. *Brit. med. J.*, **i**: 1099–102.

CHANARIN, I., MACGIBBON, B. M., O'SULLIVAN, W. J. and MOLLIN, D. L. (1959b). Folic acid deficiency in pregnancy. The pathogenesis of megaloblastic anaemia of pregnancy. *Lancet*, **ii**: 634–9.

CHANARIN, I. and McLEAN, A. (1967). Origin of serum and urinary methyltetrahydrofolate in man. Some observations on the methylfolate blood hypothesis in Addisonian pernicious anaemia. *Clin. Sci.*, **32**: 57–66.

CHANARIN, I., MOLLIN, D. L. and ANDERSON, B. B. (1958a). The clearance from the plasma of folic acid injected intravenously in normal subjects and patients with megaloblastic anaemia. *Brit. J. Haemat.*, **4**: 435–46.

CHANARIN, I., MOLLIN, D. L. and ANDERSON, B. B. (1958b). Folic deficiency and the megaloblastic anaemias. *Proc. R. Soc. Med.*, **51**: 31–37.

CHANARIN, I., ROTHMAN, D. and BERRY, V. (1965b). Iron deficiency and its relation to folic-acid status in pregnancy: Results of a clinical trial. *Brit. med. J.*, **i**: 480–5.

CHANARIN, I., ROTHMAN, D., ARDEMAN, S. and McLEAN, A. (1965a). Studies on histidine and urocanate metabolism in pregnancy. *Clin. Sci.*, **28**: 377–84.

CHANARIN, I., ROTHMAN, D., PERRY, J. and STRATFULL, D. (1968). Normal dietary folate, iron, and protein intake, with particular reference to pregnancy. *Brit. med. J.*, **2**: 394–397.

CHANARIN, I., ROTHMAN, D. and WATSON-WILLIAMS, E. J. (1963). Normal formiminoglutamic acid excretion in megaloblastic anaemia in pregnancy. Studies in histidine metabolism in pregnancy. *Lancet*, **i**: 1068–72.

CHELDELINE, V. H., WOODS, A. M., and WILLIAMS, R. J. (1943). Loss of B vitamins due to cooking of foods. *J. Nutr.*, **26**: 477–85.

CHUNG, A. S. M., PEARSON, W. N., DARBY, W. J., MILLER, O. N. and GOLDSMITH, G. A. (1961). Folic acid, vitamin B_6, pantothenic acid, and vitamin B_{12} in human dietaries. *Amer. J. clin. Nutr.*, **9**: 573–82.

CLEMENT, D. H., NICHOL, C. A. and WELCH, A. D. (1961). A case of juvenile pernicious anemia: Study of the effects of folic acid and vitamin B_{12}. *Blood*, **17**: 618–31.

CONDIT, P. T. and GROB, D. (1958). Studies on the folic acid vitamins. I. Observations on the metabolism of folic acid in man and on the effect of aminopterin. *Cancer*, **11**: 525–36.

COOKE, W. T., FRAZER, A. C., PEENEY, A. L. P., SAMMONS, H. G. and THOMPSON, M. D. (1948). Anomalies of intestinal absorption of fat. II. The haematology of idiopathic steatorrhoea. *Quart. J. Med.*, **17**: 19–24.

COOPER, B. A. and LOWENSTEIN, L. (1964). Relative folate deficiency of erythrocytes in pernicious anemia and its correction with cyanocobalamin. *Blood*, **24**: 502–21.

COSULICH, D. B., SMITH, J. M., JR. and BROQUIST, H. P. (1952a). Diastereoisomers of leucovorin. *J. Amer. chem. Soc.*, **74**: 4215–16.

COSULICH, D. B., ROTH, B., SMITH, J. M., HULTQUIST, M. E. and PARKER, R. P. (1952b). Chemistry of leucovorin. *J. Amer. chem. Soc.*, **74**: 3252–63.

COX, E. V., MEYNELL, M. J., COOKE, W. T. and GADDIE, R. (1958). The folic acid excretion test in the steatorrhoea syndrome. *Gastroenterology*, **35**: 390–7.

COX, E. V. and WHITE, A. M. (1962). Methylmalonic acid excretion: An Index of vitamin B_{12} deficiency. *Lancet*, **2**: 853–7.

CROSBY, W. H. (1960). The daily dose of folic acid. *J. chron. Dis.*, **12**: 583–5.

DACIE, J. V., SMITH, M. D., WHITE, J. C. and MOLLIN, D. L. (1959). Refractory normo-blastic anaemia: A clinical and haematological study of seven cases. *Brit. J. Haemat.*, **5**: 56–82.

DAVIDSON, L. S. P. (1948). Pteroylglutamic acid (folic acid). Therapeutic indications and limitations. *Edinburgh med. J.*, **55**: 400–11.

DAVIS, L. J. and BROWN, A. (1947). The erythropoietic activity of choline chloride in megaloblastic anaemias. *Blood*, **2**: 407–25.

DAWBARN, M. C., HINE, D. C. and SMITH, J. (1958). Effect of vitamin B_{12} deficiency and citrovorum factor. *Aust. J. exp. biol.*, **36**: 541–6.

DAY, D. L., LANGSTON, W. C. and SHUKERS, C. F. (1936). Leucopenia and anemia in the monkey resulting from dietary deficiency. *J. biol. Chem.*, **114**: XXV.

DENKO, C. W., GRUNDY, W. E., PORTER, J. W., BERRYMAN, G. H., FRIEDEMANN T. D. and YOUMAN J. B. (1946). The excretion of B-complex vitamins in the urine and faeces of seven normal adults. *Arch. Biochem.*, **10**: 33–40.

DEODHAR, S. and SAKAMI, W. (1953). Biosynthesis of serine. *Fed. Proc.*, **12**: 195–6.

DINNING, J. S., SIME, J. T., WORK, P. S., ALLEN, B. and DAY, P. L. (1957). The metabolic conversion of folic acid and citrovorum factor to a Diazotizable amine. *Arch. Biochem. Biophys.*, **66**: 114–9.

DOCTOR, V. M. and COUCH, J. R. (1953). Occurrence and properties of a conjugated form of Leucoustoc citrovorum factor. *J. biol. Chem.*, **200**: 223–31.

DOIG, A. and GIRDWOOD, R. H. (1960). The absorption of folic acid and labelled cyano-cobalamin in intestinal malabsorption. *Quart. J. med.*, **29**: 333–74.

DONALDSON, K. O. and KERESZTESY, J. C. (1959). Naturally occurring forms of folic acid. I. "Prefolic A". *J. biol. Chem.*, **234**: 3235–40.

DONALDSON, K. O. and KERESZTESY, J. C. (1962). Naturally occurring forms of folic acid. II. Enzymatic conversion of methylenetetrahydrofolic acid to prefolic A-methyl-tetrahydrofolate. *J. biol. Chem.*, **237**: 1298–304.

DORMANDY, K. M., WATERS, A. H. and MOLLIN, D. L. (1963). Folic acid deficiency in coeliac disease. *Lancet*, i: 632–5.

DRUSKIN, M. S., WALLEN, M. H. and BONAGURA, L. (1962). Anticonvulsant-associated megaloblastic anaemia. Response to 25 micrograms of folic acid administered by mouth daily. *New Eng. J. Med.*, **267**: 483–5.

DYMOCK, J. W. (1964). Urinary excretion of urocanic acid and formiminoglutamic acid in neoplastic disease. *Lancet*, ii: 475.

ELLENBOGEN, L., TAYLOR, R. J. and BRUNDAGE, C. B. (1965). On the role of pteridines as cofactors for tyrosine hydroxylase. *Biochem. biophys. Res. Comm.*, **19**: 708–15.

FINCH, C. A., COLEMAN, D. H., MOTULSKY, A. G., DONOHUE, D. M. and REIFF, R. H. (1956). Erythrokinetics in pernicious anemia. *Blood*, **11**: 807–20.

FINCH, C. A., GIBSON, J. G., PEACOCK, W. C. and FLUHARTY, R. G. (1949). Iron meta-bolism. Utilization of intravenous radioactive iron. *Blood*, **4**: 905–27.

FISH, M. B., POLLYCOVE, M. and FLEICHTMEIR, T. V. (1963). Differentiation between vitamin B_{12}-deficient and folic acid-deficient megaloblastic anaemia with C^{14}-histidine. *Blood*, **21**: 447–61.

FLEMING, A. F. and ELLIOTT, B. A. (1964). Serum enzyme tests for megaloblastic erythropoiesis in anaemia in pregnancy. *Brit. med. J.*, ii: 1108–11.

FLYNN, E. H., BOND, T. J., BARDOS, T. J. and SHIVE, W. J. (1951). A synthetic compound with folinic acid activity. *J. Amer. chem. Soc.*, **73**: 1979–82.

FORSHAW, J., HARWOOD, L. and WEATHERALL, D. J. (1964). Folic acid deficiency and megaloblastic erythropoises in myelofibrosis. *Brit. med. J.*, i: 671–2.

FORSHAW, J., MOORHOUSE, E. H. and HARWOOD, L. (1964). Megaloblastic anaemia due to dietary deficiency. *Lancet*, i: 1004–8.

FOSTER, M. A., JONES, K. M. and WOODS, D. D. (1961). The purification and properties of a factor containing vitamin B_{12} concerned in the synthesis of methionine by Escherichia coli. *Biochem. J.*, **80**: 519–31.

FRIEDKIN, M., CRAWFORD, E. J., HUMPHREYS, S. R. and GOLDIN, A. (1962). The association of increased dihydrofolate reductase with amethopterin resistance in mouse leukemia. *Cancer Res.*, **22**: 600–6.

FULD, H. (1950). Effect of vitamin B_{12} on neuropathy in pernicious anaemia treated with folic acid. *Brit. med. J.*, **ii**: 147–8.

FUTTERMAN, S. and SILVERMAN, M. (1957). The "inactivation" of folic acid by liver. *J. biol. chem.*, **224**: 31–40.

GILES, C. and SHUTTLEWORTH, E. M. (1958). Megaloblastic anaemia of pregnancy and the purperium. *Lancet*, **ii**: 1341–7.

GIRDWOOD, R. H. (1952). The occurrence of growth factors for Lactobacillus leichmannii, streptococcus faecalis and leuconostoc citrovorum in the tissues of pernicious anaemia patients and controls. *Biochem. J.*, **52**: 58–63.

GIRDWOOD, R. H. (1953). Folic-acid excretion studies in the investigation of malignant disease. *Brit. med. J.*, **ii**: 741–5.

GIRDWOOD, R. H. (1956). The megaloblastic anaemias, their investigation and classification. *Quart. J. Med.*, **25**: 87–119.

GOLDBERG, L., DE MEILLON, B. and LAVOIPIERRE, M. (1945). The nutrition of the larva of *Aedes aegypti L.* II. Essential water-soluble factors from yeast. *J. exp. biol.*, **21**: 90–6.

GOODFRIEND, T. L. and KAUFMAN, S. (1961). Phenylalanine metabolism and folic acid antagonists. *J. clin. Invest.*, **40**: 1743–50.

GORDON, M., RAVEL, J. M., EAKIN, R. E. and SHIVE, W. (1948). Formylfolic acid a functional derivative of folic acid. *J. Amer. chem. Soc.*, **70**: 878–9.

GORESKY, C. A., WATANABE, H. and JOHNS, D. G. (1963). The renal excretion of folic acid. *J. clin. Invest.*, **42**: 1841–9.

GOUGH, K. R., McCARTHY, C. F., READ, A. E., MOLLIN, D. L. and WATERS, A. H. (1964). Folic acid deficiency in rheumatoid arthritis. *Brit. med. J.*, **i**: 212–7.

GOUGH, K. R., READ, A. E., McCARTHY, C. F. and WATERS, A. H. (1963). Megaloblastic anaemia due to nutritional deficiency. *Quart. J. Med.*, **32**: 243–56.

GRANT, H. C., HOFFBRAND, A. V. and WELLS, D. G. (1965). Folate deficiency and neurological disease. *Lancet*, **ii**: 763–7.

GRÄSBECK, R., BJÖRKSTEN, F. and NYBERG, W. (1961). Formiminoglutaminsyra i urin vid folsyrabrist. *Nord. Med.*, **66**: 1343–8.

GREENBERG, D. M., NATH, R. and HUMPHREYS, G. K. (1961). Purification and properties of thymidylate synthetase from calf thymus. *J. biol. Chem.*, **236**: 2271–6.

GROSSOWICZ, N., MANDELBAUM-SHAVIT, F., DAVIDOFF, R. and ARONOVITCH, J. (1962). Microbiologic determination of folic acid derivatives in blood. *Blood*, **20**: 609–16.

GUEST, J. R., FRIEDMAN, S., WOODS, D. D. and SMITH, E. L. (1962). A methyl analogue of cobamide coenzyme in relation to methionine synthesis by bacteria. *Nature, Lond.*, **195**: 340–2.

HAKALA, M. T., ZAKREWSKI, S. F. and NICHOL, C. A. (1960). Mechanism of resistance of amethopterin in sarcoma 180 (S-180) cells in culture. *Proc. Amer. Ass. Cancer Res.*, **3**: 115.

HALL, B. E. and WATKINS, C. H. (1947). Experience with pteroylglutamic acid (synthetic folic) acid in the treatment of pernicious anaemia. *J. lab. clin. Med.*, **32**: 622–34.

HAMFELT, A. and WILMANNS, W. (1965). Inhibition studies on folic acid metabolism with drugs suspected to act on the myeloproliferative system. *Clin. chim. Acta*, **12**: 144–52.

HANSEN, H. A., NORDVIST, P. and SOURANDER, P. (1964). Megaloblastic anemia and neurologic disturbances combined with folic acid deficiency. Observations on an epileptic patient treated with anticonvulsants. *Acta. med. Scand.*, **176**: 243–51.

HANSEN, H. A. and WEINFELD. A. (1962). Metabolic effects and diagnostic value of small doses of folic acid and B_{12} in megaloblastic anaemias. *Acta. med. Scand.*, **172**: 427–43.

HARDINGE, M. G. and CROOKS, H. (1961). Lesser known vitamins in foods. *J. Amer. dietet. Ass.*, **38**: 240–5.

HARNED, B. K., CUNNINGHAM, R. W., SMITH, H. D. and CLARK, M. C. (1946). Pharmacological studies of pteroylglutamic acid. *Ann. N. Y. Acad. Sci.*, **48**: 289–98.

HARTMAN, S. C. and BUCHANAN, J. M. (1959). Biosynthesis of the purines XXVI. The identification of the formyl donors of the transformylation reaction. *J. biol. Chem.*, **234**: 1812–16.

HATCH, F. T., LARRABEE, A. R., CATHOU, R. E. and BUCHANAN, J. M. (1961). Enzymatic synthesis of the methyl group of methionine. I. Identification of the enzymes and cofactors involved in the system isolated from *Escherichia coli*. *J. biol. Chem.*, **236**: 1095–104.

HAWKINS, C. F. (1955). Value of serum iron levels in assessing effects of haematinics in the macrocytic anaemias. *Brit. med. J.*, **i**: 383–5.

HAWKINS, C. F. and MEYNELL, M. J. (1958). Macrocytosis and macrocytic anaemia caused by anticonvulsant drugs. *Quart. J. Med.*, **27**: 45–63.

HEGSTED, D. M. and STARE, F. J. (1945). Nutritional studies with the duck. I. Purified rations for the duck. *J. Nutr.*, **30**: 37–44.

HEINLE, R. W., DINGLE, J. T. and WEISBERGER, A. S. (1947). Folic acid in the maintenance of pernicious anaemia. *J. lab. clin. Med.*, **32**: 970–81.

HEINLE, R. W. and WELCH, A. D. (1947). Folic acid in pernicious anaemia. Failure to prevent neurologic relapse. *J. Amer. Med. Ass.*, **133**: 739–41.

HEINLE, R. W., WELCH, A. D. and PRITCHARD, J. A. (1948). Essentially of both the antipernicious anaemia factor of liver and pteroylglutamic acid for hematopoiesis in swine. *J. lab. clin. Med.*, **33**: 1647.

HEINRICH, H. C. (1954). Die biochemischen Grundlagen der Diagnostik und Therupie der vitamin B_{12}-Mangelzustände (B_{12}-Hypo-und Avitaminosen) des Menschen und der Haustiere. II. Untersuchungen zum vitamin B_{12}-Stoffwechsel des Menshchen Während der Gravidität und Lactation. *Klin. Wschr.*, **32**: 205–9.

HEISLER, C. R. and SCHWEIGERT, B. S. (1955). Conversion of pteroylglutamic acid to citrovorum factor by cell-free extracts of *Lactobacillus casei*. *Fed. Proc.*, **14**: 436–7.

HELLEINER, C. W. and WOODS, D. D. (1956). Cobalamin and the synthesis of methionine by cell-free extracts of *Escherichia coli*. *Biochem. J.*, **63**: 26P.

HERBERT, V. (1961). The assay and nature of folic acid activity in human serum. *J. clin. Invest.*, **40**: 81–91.

HERBERT, V. (1962a). Experimental nutritional folate deficiency in man. *Trans. Ass. Amer. Phys.*, **65**: 307–20.

HERBERT, V. (1962b). Minimal daily adult folate requirement. *Arch. int. Med.*, **110**: 649–52.

HERBERT, V. (1963). A palatable diet for producing experimental folate deficiency in man. *Amer. J. clin. Nutr.*, **12**: 17–20.

HERBERT, V. (1964). Studies of folate deficiency in man. *Proc. R. Soc. Med.*, **57**: 377–84.

HERBERT, V. (1965). Excretion of folic acid in bile. *Lancet*, **i**: 913.

HERBERT, V., LARRABEE, A. R. and BUCHANAN, J. M. (1962). Studies on the identification of a folate compound of human serum. *J. clin. Invest.*, **41**: 1134–8.

HERBERT, V., STREIFF, R., SULLIVAN, L. and MCGEER, P. (1964). Accumulation of a purine intermediate (amino-imidazolecarboxamide) (AIC) in megaloblastic anaemias associated with vitamin B_{12} deficiency, folate deficiency with alcoholism and liver disease. *Fed. Proc.*, **23**: 188.

HERBERT, V. and ZALUSKY, R. (1961). Selective concentration of folic acid activity in cerebrospinal fluid. *Fed. Proc.*, **20**: 453.

HERBERT, V. and ZALUSKY, R. (1962). Interrelations of vitamin B_{12} and folic acid metabolism; folic acid clearance studies. *J. clin. Invest.*, **41**: 1263–76.

HERBERT, V., ZALUSKY, R. and DAVIDSON, C. S. (1963). Correlation of folate deficiency with alcoholism and associated macrocytosis, anaemia and liver disease. *Ann. intern. Med.*, **58**: 977–88.

HERTZ, R. (1948). Interference with oestrogen induced tissue growth in the chick genital tract by a folic acid antagonist. *Science*, **107**: 300.

HESS, B. and GEHM, B. (1955). Uber die Milchsäuredehydrogenase im menschlichen Serum. *Klin. Wschr.*, **33**: 91–3.

HIATT, H. H., RABINOWITZ, J. C., TOCH, R. and GOLDSTEIN, M. (1958). Effects of folic acid antagonist therapy on urinary excretion of formic acid by humans. *Proc. Soc. exp. biol. Med.*, **92**: 144–7.

HOFFBRAND, A. V. and PETERS, T. J. (1969). The subcellular localization of pteroyl polyglutamate hydrolase and folate in guinea pig intestinal mucosa. *Biochim. Biophys. Acta*, **192**: 479–485.

HOFFBRAND, A. V., TABAQCHALI, S. and MOLLIN, D. L. (1966). High serum-folate levels in intestinal blind-loop syndrome. *Lancet*, i: 1339–42.

HOGAN, A. G. and PARROT, E. M. (1939). Anemia in chicks due to vitamin deficiency. *J. biol. Chem.*, **128**: xlvi–xlvii.

HOLLAND, B. R. and MEINKE, W. W. (1949). The serine requirement of Streptococcus faecalis R as a function of the basal medium. *J. biol. Chem.*, **178**: 7–15.

HUGULEY, C. M. J., BAIN, J. A., RIVERS, S. L. and SCOGGINS, R. (1959). Refractory megaloblastic anemia associated with excretion of orotic acid. *Blood*, **14**: 615–34.

HURDLE, A. D. F. (1967). The folate content of a hospital diet. Ph.D. Thesis, University of London.

HUTCHINGS, B. L., BOHONOS, N., HEGSTED, D. M., ELVEHJEM, V. A. and PETERSON, W. H. (1914b). Relation of a growth factor required by Lactobacillus casei to the nutrition of the chick. *J. biol. Chem.*, **140**: 681–82.

HUTCHINGS, B. L., BOHONOS, N. and PETERSON, W. H. (1941a). Growth factors for bacteria. XIII. Purification and properties of an eluate factor required by certain lactic acid bacteria. *J. biol. Chem.*, **141**: 521–28.

HUTCHINGS, B. L., STOKSTAD, E. L. R., BOHONOS, N., SLOANE, N. H. and SUBBA ROW, Y. (1948a). The isolation of the fermentation Lactobacillus casei factor. *J. Amer. chem. Soc.*, **70**: 1–3.

HUTCHINGS, B. L., STOKSTAD, E. L. R., MOWAT, J. H., BOOTHE, J. H., WALLER, C. W., ANGIER, R. B., SEMB, J. and SUBBA ROW, Y. (1948b). Degradation of the fermentation L. casei factor. *J. Amer. chem. Soc.*, **70**: 10–13.

INNES, E. M. (1948). The blood and bone marrow in the sprue syndrome. A study of 63 cases. *Edinburgh Med. J.*, **55**: 282–92.

ISRAËLS, M. C. G. and WILKINSON, J. F. (1949). Risk of neurological complications in pernicious anaemia treated with folic acid. *Brit. med. J.*, ii: 1072–5.

IWAI, K., LUTTNER, P. M. and TOENNIES, G. (1964). Blood folic acid studies. VII. Purification and properties of the folic acid precursors of human erythrocytes. *J. biol. Chem.*, **239**: 2365.

IZAK, G., RACHMILEWITZ, M., SADOVSKY, A., BERCOVICI, B., ARONOVITCH, J. and GROSSOWICZ, N. (1961). Folic acid metabolities in whole blood and serum in anemia of pregnancy. *Amer. J. clin. Nutr.*, **9**: 473–7.

IZAK, G., RACHMILEWITZ, M., ZAN, S. and GROSSOWICZ, N. (1963). The effect of small doses of folic acid in nutritional megaloblastic anemia. *Amer. J. clin. Nutr.*, **13**: 369–77.

JAENICKE, L., ENGLISH, J. P., GUEST, J. and HUENNEKENS, F. M. (1965). Nomenclature and symbols for folic acid and related compounds. *Biochim. biophys. Acta*, **107**: 11–13.

JANDL, J. H. and LEAR, A. A. (1956). The metabolism of folic acid in cirrhosis. *Ann. intern. Med.*, 45: 1027–44.

JOHNS, D. G., SPERTI, S. and BURGEN, A. S. V. (1961). The metabolism of tritiated folic acid in man. *J. clin. Invest.*, 40: 1684–95.

JOHNSON, S., SWAMINATHAN, S. P. and BAKER, S. J. (1962). Changes in serum vitamin B_{12} levels in patients with megaloblastic anaemia treated with folic acid. *J. clin. Path.*, 15: 274–7.

JONSSON, U., ROATH, O. S. and KIRKPATRICK, C. I. F. (1959). Nutritional megaloblastic anemia associated with sickle cell states. *Blood*, 14: 535–47.

JUKES, T. H. (1961). Concerning the daily dose of folic acid. *J. chron. Dis.*, 14: 283.

JUKES, T. H., FRANKLIN, A. L., STOKSTAD, E. L. R. and BOEHNE, J. W. (1947). The urinary excretion of pteroylglutamic acid and certain related compounds. *J. lab. clin. Med.*, 32: 1350–5.

KAUFMAN, S. (1958). A new cofactor required for the enzymatic conversion of phenylalanine to tyrosine. *J. biol. Chem.*, 230: 931–9.

KAZENKO, A. and LASKOWSKI, M. (1948). On the specificity of chicken pancreas conjugase (γ-glutamic acid carboxypeptidase). *J. biol. Chem.*, 173: 217–21.

KENDE, G., RAMOT, B. and GROSSOWICZ, N. (1963). Blood folic acid and vitamin B_{12} activities in healthy infants and in infants with nutritional anaemias. *Brit. J. Haemat.*, 9: 328–35.

KERESZTESY, J. C., RICKES, E. L. and STOKES, J. L. (1943). A new growth factor for *Streptococcus lactis*. *Science*, 97: 465.

KERESZTESY, J. C. and SILVERMAN, M. (1951). Crystalline citrovorum factor from liver. *J. Amer. chem. Soc.*, 73: 5510.

KIDD, P. and MOLLIN, D. L. (1957). Megaloblastic anaemia and vitamin B_{12} deficiency after anticonvulsant therapy. *Brit. med. J.*, ii: 974–6.

KISLIUK, R. L. (1957). Studies on the mechanism of formaldehyde incorporation into serine. *J. biol. Chem.*, 227: 805–14.

KISLIUK, R. L. (1961). Further studies on the relationship of vitamin B_{12} to methionine synthesis in extracts of Escherichia coli. *J. biol. Chem.*, 236: 817–22.

KISLIUK, R. L. and SAKAMI, W. (1954). The stimulation of serine biosynthesis in pigeon liver extracts by tetrahydrofolic acid. *J. Amer. chem. Soc.*, 76: 1456–7.

KLIPSTEIN, F. A. (1963). Subnormal serum folate and macrocytosis associated with anticonvulsant drug therapy. *Blood*, 23: 68–86.

KLIPSTEIN, F. A. and LINDENBAUM, J. (1965). Folate deficiency in chronic liver disease. *Blood*, 25: 443–56.

KNOWLES, J. P., SHUSTER, S. and WELLS, G. C. (1963a). Folic acid deficiency in patients with skin disease. *Lancet*, i: 1138–9.

KNOWLES, J. P., SHALDON, S. and FLEMING, A. (1963b). Folic acid metabolism in liver disease. *Clin. Sci.*, 24: 39–45.

KNOWLES, J. P., PRANKARD, T. A. J. and WESTALL, R. G. (1960). Simplified method for detecting formiminoglutamic acid in urine as a test of folic-acid deficiency. *Lancet*, ii: 347–8.

KOHN, J., MOLLIN, D. L. and ROSENBACH, L. M. (1961). Conventional voltage electrophoresis for formiminoglutamic acid determination in folic acid deficiency. *J. clin. Path.*, 14: 345–50.

KOSZEWSKI, B. J. (1952). The occurrence of megaloblastic erythropoiesis in patients with haemochromatosis. *Blood*, 7: 1182–95.

KREHL, W. A., TORBET, N., DE LA HUERGA, J. and ELVEHJEM, C. A. (1946). Relation of synthetic folic acid to Niacin deficiency in dogs. *Arch. Biochem.*, 11: 363–369.

KYEDA, K. and RABINOWITZ, J. C. (1963). Fluorescence properties of tetrahydrofolate and related compounds. *Anal. Biochem.*, 6: 100–8.

LAING, S. R. S. (1957). Refractory anaemia, a problem in diagnosis and epidemiology in a tea garden in Assam. *J. trop. Med. Hyg.*, **60**: 131–6.

LAMPEN, J. O. and JONES, M. J. (1947). The growth-promoting and antisulfonamide activity of a p-aminobenzoic acid, pteroylglutamic acid and related compounds for *Lactobacillus arabinosus* and *Streptobacterium plantarum*. *J. biol. Chem.*, **170**: 133–46.

LARRABEE, A. R., ROSENTHAL, S., CATHOU, R. E. and BUCHANAN, J. M. (1961). A methylated derivative of tetrahydrofolate as an intermediate of methionine biosynthesis. *J. Amer. chem. Soc.*, **83**: 4094–5.

LEES, F. (1961). Radioactive vitamin B_{12} absorption in the megaloblastic anaemia caused by anticonvulsant drugs. *Quart. J. Med.*, **30**: 231–48.

LEEVY, C. M., CARDI, L., FRANK, O., GELLENE, R. and BAKER, H. (1965a). Incidence and significance of hypovitaminemia in a randomly selected municipal hospital population. *Amer. J. clin. Nutrit.*, **17**: 259–71.

LEEVY, C. M., BAKER, H., TENHOVE, W., FRANK, O. and CHERRICK, G. R. (1965b). B-complex vitamins in liver disease of the alcoholic. *Amer. J. clin. Nutr.*, **16**: 339–46.

LIBNOCH, J. A., YAKULIS, V. J., and HELLER, P. (1966). Lactate dehydrogenase in megaloblastic bone marrow. *Amer. J. clin. Path.*, **45**: 302–5.

LINDENBAUM, J. and KLIPSTEIN, F. A. (1963). Folic acid deficiency in sickle-cell anaemia. *New Eng. J. Med.*, **269**: 875–82.

LONG, M. T., CHILDRESS, R. H., BOND, W. H. (1963). Megaloblastic anemia associated with the use of anticonvulsant drugs. *Neurology, Minniap.*, **13**: 697–702.

LUHBY, A. L. (1957). Observations on the excretion of formiminoglutamic acid in folic acid deficiency in man. *Clin. Res. Proc.*, **5**: 8–9.

LUHBY, A. L., COOPERMAN, J. M. and TELLER, D. N. (1959). Histidine metabolic loading test to distinguish folic acid deficiency from vitamin B_{12} in megaloblastic anaemias. *Proc. Soc. exp. Biol. Med.*, **101**: 350–2.

LUHBY, A. L. and COOPERMAN, J. M. (1962). Aminoimidazole carboxamide excretion in vitamin B_{12} and folic acid deficiencies. *Lancet*, **2**: 1381–2.

LUHBY, A. L. and COOPERMAN, J. M. (1962). Am noimidazole carboxamide excretion in vitamin B_{12} and folic acid deficiencies. *Lancet*, **2**: 1381–2.

LUTHER, L., SANTINI, R., BREWSTER, C., PEREZ-SANTIAGO, E. and BUTTERworth, C. E. (1965). Folate binding by insoluble components of American and Puerto Rican diets. *Alabama J. Med. Sci.*, **2**: 389–93.

McDOUGALL, B. M. and BLAKLEY, R. L. (1960). Mechanism of the action of thymidylate synthetase. *Nature, Lond.*, **188**: 944.

MACGIBBON, B. H. and MOLLIN, D. L. (1965). Sideroblastic anaemia: Observations on seventy cases. *Brit. J. Haemat.*, **11**: 59–69.

MACIVER, J. E. and BACK, E. H. (1960). Megaloblastic anaemia of infancy in Jamaica. *Arch. Dis. Childh.*, **35**: 134–45.

MACIVER, J. E. and WENT, L. N. (1960). Sickle-cell anaemia complicated by megaloblastic anaemia of infancy. *Brit. med. J.*, **i**: 775–9.

McLEAN, A. and CHANARIN, I. (1966). Urinary excretion of 5-methyltetrahydrofolate in man. *Blood* (In press).

McLEAN, A. and CHANARIN, I. (1966). In preparation.

MAGNUS, E. M. (1963). Low serum folic-acid in malignancy. *Lancet*, **ii**: 302.

MANNHEIMER, E., PAKESCH, F., REIMER, E. E. and VETTER, H. (1952). Die hämatologischen Komplikationen der Epilepsiebehandlung mit Hydantoinkörpern. *Med. Klin.*, **47**: 1397–401.

MANSON-BAHR, P. and WILLOUGHBY, H. (1930). Studies on sprue with special reference to treatment. Based upon an analysis of 200 cases. *Quart. J. Med.*, **23**: 411–42.

MARSHALL, R. A. and JANDL, J. H. (1960). Responses to "physologic" doses of folic acid in the megaloblastic anemias. *Arch. int. Med.*, **105**: 352–60.

MATOTH, Y., PINKAS, A., ZAMIR, R., MOOALLEM, F. and GROSSOWICZ, N. (1964). 1. Blood levels of folic and folinic acid in healthy infants. *Pediatrics*, **33**: 507–11.

MAY, M., BARDOS, T. J., BARGER, F. L., LANSFORD, M. RAVEL, J. M., SUTHERLAND, G. L. and SHIVE, W. (1951). Synthetic and degradative investigations of the structure of folinic acid-SF. *J. Amer. chem. Soc.*, **73**: 3067–75.

MAY, C. D., HAMILTON, A. and STEWART, C. T. (1952). Experimental megaloblastic anaemia and scurvy in the monkey. IV. Vitamin B_{12} and folic acid compounds in the diet, liver, urine and feces and effects of therapy. *Blood*, **7**: 978–91.

MAY, C. D., NELSON, E. N. and SALMON, R. J. (1949). Experimental production of megaloblastic anaemia: an interrelationship between ascorbic acid and pteroylglutamic acid. *J. lab. clin. Med.*, **34**: 1724–5.

MERRIT, A. D., RUCKNAGEL, D. L., SILVERMAN, M. and GARDINER, R. C. (1962). Urinary urocanic acid in man: the identification of urocanic acid and N-formiminoglutamic acid after oral histidine in patients with liver disease. *J. clin. Invest.*, **41**: 1472–83.

MEYER, L. M. (1947). Folic acid in the treatment of pernicious anaemia. *Blood*, **2**: 50–61.

MEYER, L. M., RITZ, N. D., FINK, H. and MILBERG, M. S. (1951). Treatment of pernicious anaemia with pteroyltriglutamic acid (Teropterin). *Acta med. Scand.*, **140**: 307–16.

MIDDLETON, J. E. (1965). Detection by paper chromatography of imidazoles, including hydantein-5-propionic acid, in urine after histidine dosage. *J. clin. Path.*, **18**: 605–10.

MIMS, V. and LASKOWSKI, M. (1945). Studies on vitamin Bc conjugase from chicken pancreas. *J. biol. Chem.*, **160**: 493–503.

MIMS, V. TOTTER, J. R. and DAY, P. L. (1944). A method for the determination of substances enzymatically convertible to the factor stimulating *Streptococcus lactis R. J. biol. Chem.*, **155**: 401–5.

MITCHELL, D. C., VILTER, R. W. and VILTER, C. F. (1949). Hypersensitivity to folic acid. *Ann. intern. Med.*, **31**: 1102–05.

MITCHELL, H. K., SNELL, E. E. and WILLIAMS, R. J. (1941). The concentration of "folic acid". *J. Amer. chem. Soc.*, **63**: 2284.

MITCHELL, H. K. and WILLIAMS, R. J. (1944). Folic acid. III. Chemical and physiological properties. *J. Amer. chem. Soc.*, **66**: 271–4.

MOLLIN, D. L., BOOTH, C. C. and BAKER, S. J. (1957). The absorption of vitamin B_{12} in control subjects, in Addisonian pernicious anaemia and in the malabsorption syndrome. *Brit. J. Haemat.*, **3**: 412–28.

MOLLIN. D. L. and HINES, J. D. (1964). Observations on the nature and pathogenesis of anaemia following partial gastrectomy. *Proc. R. Soc. Med.*, **57**: 575–80.

MOLLIN, D. L., WATERS, A. H., GOUGH, K. R. and READ, A. E. (1963). Macrocytic anaemia in rheumatoid arthritis. *Brit. med. J.*, **i**: 609.

MOORE, C. V., BIERBAUM, O. S., WELCH, A. D. and WRIGHT, L. D. (1945). The activity of synthetic Lactobacillus casei factor ("folic acid") as an antipernicious anemia substance. *J. lab. clin. Med.*, **30**: 1056–69.

NICHOL, C. A. and WELCH, A. D. (1950). Synthesis of citrovorum factor from folic acid by liver slices: augmentation by ascorbic acid. *Proc. Soc. exp. biol. Med.*, **74**: 52–5.

NIMMO-SMITH, R. H., LASCALLES, J. and WOODS, D. D. (1948). The synthesis of "folic acid" by *Streptobacterium plantarum* and its inhibition by sulphonamides. *Brit. J. exp. Path.*, **29**: 264–81.

O'DELL, B. L., VANDENBELT, J. M., BLOOM, E. S. and PFIFFNER, J. J. (1947). Hydrogenation of vitamin Bc (pteroylglutamic acid) and related pterines. *J. Amer. chem. Soc.*, **69**: 250–3.

OLIVERIO, V. T. (1961). Chromatographic separation and purification of folic acid analogs. *Analyt. chem.*, **33**: 263–5.

OSBORN, M. J. and HUENNEKENS, F. M. (1957). Participation of anhydroleucovorin in the hydroxymethyltetrahydrofolic dehydrogenase system. *Biochim. biophys. Acta*, **26**: 646–7.

OSBORN, M. J. and HUENNEKENS, F. M. (1958). Enzymatic reduction of dihydrofolic acid. *J. biol. Chem.*, **233**: 969–74.

OSBORN, M. J., HATEFI, Y., KAY, L. D. and HUENNEKENS, F. M. (1957). Evidence for the enzymic deacylation of N^{10}-formyltetrahydrofolic acid. *Biochim. biophys. Acta*, **26**: 208–10.

OSBORN, M. J., TALBERT, P. T. and HUENNEKENS, F. M. (1960). The structure of "active" formaldahyde (N^5,N^{10}-methylenetetrahydrofolic acid). *J. Amer. chem. Soc.*, **82**: 4921–7.

PACE, J. K., STIER, L. B., TAYLOR, D. D. and GOODMAN, P. A. (1960). Intake and urinary excretion of folic acid by 36 preadolescent girls. *Fed. Proc.*, **19**: 415.

PAGE, E. W., GLENDENNING, M. B., DIGNAM, W. and HARPER, H. A. (1954). The causes of histidinuria in normal pregnancy. *Amer. J. Obstet. Gynec.*, **68**: 110–8.

PARSONS, L. G. (1933). Studies in the anaemias of infancy and early childhood. *Arch. Dis. Childh.*, **8**: 85–94.

PARTRIDGE, R. E. H. and DUTHIE, J. J. R. (1963). Incidence of macrocytic anaemia in rheumatoid arthritis. *Brit. med. J.*, **i**: 89–91.

PASTORE, E. J. and FRIEDKIN, M. (1962). The enzymatic synthesis of thymidylate. II. Transfer of tritium from tetrahydrofolate to the methyl group of thymidylate. *J. biol. Chem.*, **23**: 3802–10.

PEDERSEN, J., LUND, J., OHLSEN, A. and KRISTENSEN, H. P. O. (1957). Partial megaloblastic erythropoiesis in elderly patients, achlorhydric patients with mild anaemia. *Lancet*, **i**: 448–53.

PERRY, J. and CHANARIN, I. (1968). Absorption and utilization of polyglutamyl forms of folate in man. *Brit. med. J.*, **4**: 546–549.

PERRY, J. and CHANARIN, I. (1970). Intestinal absorption of reduced folate compounds in man. *Brit. J. Haemat.*, **18**: 329–339.

PFIFFNER, J. J., BINKLEY, S. B., BLOOM, E. S., BROWN, R. A., BIRD, O. D., EMMETT, A. D., HOGAN, A. G. and O'DELL, B. L. (1943). Isolation of the antianemia factor (vitamin Bc) in crystalline form from liver. *Science*, **97**: 404–5.

PFIFFNER, J. J., CALKINS, D. G., BLOOM, E. S. and O'DELL, B. L. (1946). On the peptide nature of vitamin Bc conjugate from yeast. *J. Amer. chem. Soc.*, **68**: 1392.

PIERCE, L. E. and RATH, C. E. (1962). Evidence for folic acid deficiency in genesis of anemic sickle cell crisis. *Blood*, **20**: 19–32.

PITNEY, W. R., JOSKE, R. A. and MACKINNON, N. L. (1960). Folic acid and other absorption tests in lymphosarcoma, chronic lymphocytic leukaemia, and some related conditions. *J. clin. Path.*, **13**: 440–7.

RABINOWITZ, J. C. and PRICER, W. E. (1956). Formimino-tetrahydrofolic acid and methenyltetrahydrofolic acid as intermediates in the formation of N^{10}-formyltetrahydrofolic acid. *J. Amer. chem. Soc.*, **78**: 5702–4.

RABINOWITZ, J. C. and TABOR, H. (1958). The urinary excretion of formic acid and formiminoglutamic acid in folic acid deficiency. *J. biol. Chem.*, **233**: 252–5.

RAMA-RAO, P. B., LAGERTOF, B., EINHORN, J. and REIZENSTEIN, P. (1963). Low serum folic-acid in malignancy. *Lancet*, **ii**: 1192–3.

RAMASASTRI, B. V. and BLAKLEY, R. L. (1962). 5,10-methylenetetrahydrofolic dehydrogenase from Bakers' yeast. *J. biol. Chem.*, **237**: 1982–8.

RATH, C. E. and FINCH, C. A. (1949). Serum iron transport measurements of iron binding capacity of serum in man. *J. clin. Invest.*, **28**: 79–85.

RAUEN, H. M., STAMM, W. and KIMBEL, K. H. (1952). N(12)-formyl-Folsäure als fermentatives Umwandlungsprodukt der Folsäure. *Z. physiol. Chem.*, **289**: 80–4.

READ, A. E., GOUGH, K. R., PARDOE, J. L. and NICHOLAS, A. (1965). Nutritional studies on the entrants to an old people's home, with particular reference to folic-acid deficiency. *Brit. med. J.*, **ii**: 843–8.

REYNOLDS, E. H. (1967). Effects of folic acid on the mental state and fit frequency of drug-treated epileptic patients. *Lancet*, **i**: 1086–8.

REYNOLDS, E. H., HALLPIKE, J. F., PHILLIPS, B. M. and MATTHEWS, D. M. (1965). Reversible absorptive defects in anticonvulsant megaloblastic anaemia. *J. clin. Path.*, **18**: 593–8.

REYNOLDS, E. H., SUTTON, J., MATTHEWS, D. M. and CHANARIN, I. (1966). The effects of anticonvulsant therapy on haemopoiesis and folic acid metabolism. *Quart. J. med.*, (in press).

RICHARDSON, L. R., HOGAN, A. G. and KEMPSTER, H. L. (1945). The requirement of the turkey poult for vitamin Bc. *J. Nutr.*, **30**: 151–7.

ROEPKE, R. R., LIBBY, R. L. and SMALL, M. H. (1944). Mutation or variation of *Escherichia coli* with respect to growth requirements. *J. Bact.*, **48**: 401–12.

ROMAINE, M. K. (1960). The folic acid activity of human livers as measured with *Lactobacillus casei*. *J. Vitaminl.*, **6**: 196–201.

ROSS, J. F., BELDING, H. and PAEGEL, B. L. (1948). The development and progression of subacute combined degeneration of the spinal cord in patients with pernicious anaemia treated with synthetic pteroylglutamic (folic) acid. *Blood*, **3**: 68–90.

ROTH, B., HULTQUIST, M. E., FAHRENBACH, M. J., COSULICH, D. B., BROQUIST, D. B., BROCKMAN, H. P., SMITH, J. M., PARKER, R. P., STOKSTAD, E. L. R. and JUKES, T.H. (1952). Synthesis of leucovorin. *J. Amer. chem. Soc.*, **74**: 3247–52.

RUNDLES, R. W. and BREWER, S. S. (1958). Hematologic responses in pernicious anaemia to orotic acid. *Blood*, **13**: 99–115.

RUNDLES, R. W. and FALLS, H. F. (1946). Hereditary (? sex-link) anemia. *Amer. J Med. Soc.*, **211**: 641–58.

SANTINI, R., BERGER, F. M., SHEEHY, T. W., AVILES, J. and DAVILA, I. (1962). Folic acid activity in Puerto Rican Foods. *J. Amer. Diet Ass.*, **14**: 562–7.

SANTINI, R., PEREZ-SANTIAGO, E., WALKER, L. and BUTTERWORTH, C. E. (1966). Folic acid conjugase in normal human plasma and in the plasma of patients with tropical sprue. *Amer. J. clin. Nutr.*, **19**: 342–4.

SAUBERLICH, H. E. (1949). The effect of folic acid upon the urinary excretion of the growth factor required by leuconstoc citrovorum. *J. biol. Chem.*, **181**: 467–73.

SAUBERLICH, H. E. (1952). Comparative studies with the natural and synthetic citrovorum factor. *J. biol. Chem.*, **195**: 337–49.

SAUBERLICH, H. E. and BAUMANN, C. A. (1948). A factor required for the growth of lenconstoc citrovorum. *J. biol. Chem.*, **176**: 165–73.

SCHAEFER, A. E., WHITEHAIR, C. K. and ELVEHJEM, C. A. (1946). Purified rations and the importance of folic acid in mink nutrition. *Proc. soc. exp. biol. Med.*, **62**: 169–74.

SCHAEFER, A. E. and WHITEHAIR, C. K. and EVEHJHEM, C. A. (1947). Purified rations and the requirement of folic acid for foxes. *Arch. Biochem.*, **12**: 349–57.

SCHIRCH, L. and MASON, M. (1962). Serine transhydroxymethylase: spectral properties of the enzyme-bound pyridoxal-5-phosphate. *J. biol. Chem.*, **237**: 2578–81.

SCHIRCH, L. G. and MASON, M. (1963). Serine transhydroxymethylase. *J. biol. Chem.*, **238**: 1032–7.

SCHWARTZ, S. O., KAPLAN, S. R. and ARMSTRONG, B. E. (1950). The long-term evaluation of folic acid in the treatment of pernicious anaemia. *J. lab. clin. Med.*, **35**: 894–8.

SCHWEIGERT, B. S., POLLARD, A. E. and ELVEHJEM, C. A. (1946). The folic acid content of meats and the retention of this vitamin during cooking. *Arch. Biochem.*, **10**: 107–111.

F

SEEGMILLER, J. E., SILVERMAN, M., TABOR, M. and MEHLER, A. H. (1954). Synthesis of a metabolic product of histidine. *J. Amer. chem. Soc.*, **76**: 6205.

SHAPIRO, J., ALBERTS, H. W., WELCH, P. and METZ, J. (1965). Folate and vitamin B_{12} deficiency associated with lactation. *Brit. J. Haemat.*, **11**: 498–504.

SHEEHY, T. W., RUBINI, M. E., PEREZ-SANTIAGO, E., SANTINI, R., JR. and HADDOCK, J. (1961). Effect of "minute" and "titrated" amounts of folic acid on megaloblastic anemia of tropical sprue. *Blood*, **18**: 623–36.

SHEMIN, D., ABRAMSKY, T. and RUSSELL, C. S. (1954). The synthesis of protoporphyrin from delta-amino-levulinic acid in a cell-free extract. *J. Amer. chem. Soc.*, **76**: 1204–5.

SHIVE, W., ACKERMANN, W. W., GORDEN, M., GETZENDANER, M. E. and EAKIN, R. E. (1947). 5(4)-amino-4(5)-imidazolecarboxamide, a precursor of purines. *J. Amer. chem. Soc.*, **69**: 725–6.

SILVERMAN, M., KERESZTESY, J. C. and KOVAL, G. J. (1954). Isolatian of N-10-formyl-folic acid. *J. biol. Chem.*, **211**: 53–61.

SILVERMAN, M., LAW, L. W. and KAUFMAN, B. (1961). The distribution of folic acid activities in lines of leukemic cells of the mouse. *J. biol. Chem.*, **236**: 2530–3.

SIMPSON, R. E. and SCHWEIGERT, B. S. (1949). Folic acid metabolism studies. I. Occurrence of Blood Conjugases. *Arch. Biochem.*, **20**: 32–40.

SNELL, E. E. and MITCHELL, H. K. (1941). Purine and pyrimidine bases as growth substances for lactic acid bacteria. *Proc. Nat. Acad. Sci. U.S.*, **27**: 1–7.

SNELL, E. E. and PETERSEN, W. H. (1940). Growth factors for bacteria. X. Additional factors required by certain lactic acid bacteria. *J. Bact.*, **39**: 273–85.

SOLOMONS, E., LEE, S. L., WASSERMAN, M. and MALKIN, J. (1962). Association of anaemia in pregnancy and folic acid deficiency. *J. Obstet. Gynaec. Brit. Commw.*, **69**: 724–8.

SPRAY, G. H., FOURMAN, P. and WITTS, L. J. (1951). The excretion of small doses of folic acid. *Brit. med. J.*, **ii**: 202–5.

SPRAY, G. H. and WITTS, L. J. (1953a). The utilization of folic acid in anaemia and leukaemia. *Clin. Sci.*, **12**: 385–90.

SPRAY, G. H. and WITTS, L. J. (1953b). The utilization of folinic acid injected intravenously. *Clin. Sci.*, **12**: 391–7.

SPURLING, C. L., SACKS, M. S. and JIJI, R. M. (1964). Juvenile pernicious anemia. *New Eng. J. Med.*, **271**: 995–1003.

STOKES, J. L. (1944). Substitution of thymine for "folic acid" in the nutrition of lactic acid bacteria. *J. Bact.*, **48**: 201–9.

STOKSTAD, E. L. R. (1943). Some properties of a growth factor for Lactobacillus casei. *J. biol. Chem.*, **149**: 573–4.

STOKSTAD, E. L. R., FORDHAM, D. and DE GRUNIGEN, A. (1947). The inactivation of pteroylglutamic acid (liver *Lactobacillus casei* factor) by light. *J. biol. Chem.*, **167**: 877–8.

STOKSTAD, E. L. R. and MANNING, P. D. V. (1938). Evidence of a new growth factor required by chicks. *J. biol. Chem.*, **125**: 687–96.

STRELLING, M. K., BLACKLEDGE, G. D., GOODALL, H. B. and WALKER, C. H. M. (1966). Megaloblastic anaemia and whole-blood folate levels in premature infants. *Lancet*, **i**: 898–900.

SULLIVAN, L. W. and HERBERT, V. (1964). Suppression of hematopoiesis by *Ethanol. J. clin. Invest.*, **43**: 1048–62.

SUNDBERG, R. D., SCHAAR, F. and MAY, C. D. (1952). Experimental Nutritional megaloblastic anemia. II. Hematology. *Blood*, **7**: 1143–81.

SWENDSEID, M. E., BURTON, F. I. and BETHELL, F. H. (1943). Excretion of keto acids and hydroxyphenyl compounds in pernicious anemia. *Proc. Soc. exp. biol.*, **52**: 202–3.

SWENDSEID, M. E., SWANSON, A. L., MEYER, M. C. and BETHELL, F. H. (1952). The nutritional status of folic acid in persons with leukaemia and its possible relation to effects of aminopterin therapy. *Blood*, 7: 307–10.

TABOR, H. and RABINOWITZ, J. C. (1956). Intermediate steps in the formylation of tetrahydrofolic acid by formiminoglutamic acid in rabbit liver. *J. Amer. chem. Soc.*, 78: 5705–6.

TABOR, H., SILVERMAN, M., MEHLER, A. H., DAFT, F. S. and BAUER, H. (1953). L-Histidine conversion to a urinary glutamic acid derivative in folic-deficient rats. *J. Amer. chem. Soc.*, 75: 756–7.

TABOR, H. and WYNGARDEN, L. (1958). A method for the determination of formiminoglutamic acid in urine. *J. clin. Invest.*, 37: 824–828.

TABOR, H. and WYNGARDEN, L. (1959). The enzymatic formation of formiminotetrahydrofolic acid, 5,10-methenyltetrahydrofolic acid and 10-formyl-tetrahydrofolic acid in the metabolism of formiminoglutamic acid. *J. biol. Chem.*, 234: 1830–46.

TASKER, P. W. G. (1959). Concealed megaloblastic anaemia. *Trans. R. Soc. trop. Med. Hyg.*, 33: 291–4.

THIERSCH, J. B. (1952). Therapeutic abortions with a folic acid antagonist, 4-aminopteroyl-glutamic acid (4-amino-P.G.H.) administered by the oral route. *Amer. J. Obstet. Gyncae.*, 63: 1298–304.

THIRKETTLE, J. L., GOUGH, K. R. and READ, A. E. (1964). Diagnostic value of small oral doses of folic acid in megaloblastic anemia. *Brit. Med. J.*, i: 1286.

TOENNIES, G., FRANK, H. O. and GALLANT, D. L. (1956). Blood folic acid activity of normal humans, cancer patients, and non-cancer patients: with a few observations on animals. *Cancer*, 9: 1053–8.

TOENNIES, G. and PHILLIPS, P. M. (1959). Blood folic acid studies. V. Resolution of precursor and enzyme fractions of the blood folic acid system. *J. biol. Chem.*, 234: 2369–72.

TOPIE, J., LAPORTE, J., MONNIER, J., RIBET, A., BERNADET, and DAVERE, (1958). Anémie avec mégaloblastose médullaire au cours d'un traitement par la pyriméthamine (malocide). *Bull. mein Soc. Med. Hop. Paris*, 74: 902–6.

TRIER, A. S. (1961). Morphologic changes in human small intestinal mucosa induced by methotrexate. *Proc. Amer. Ass. Cancer Res.*, 3: 273.

TSCHESCHE, R. VON. (1947). Eine neue deutung des antibakteriellen wirkungsmechanismus der sulfonamide. *Z. Naturforsch*, 26: 10–11.

USDIN, E., PHILLIPS, P. M. and TOENNIES, G. (1956). Multiplicity of the folic acidactive factors of blood. *J. biol Chem.*, 221: 865–72.

USDIN, E. and PORATH, J. (1957). Separation of folic acid and derivatives by electrophoresis and anion exchange chromatography. *Arkiv. Kemi*, 11: 41–6.

VAN SCOTT, E. J. and REINERTSON, R. P. (1959). Morphologic and physiologic effects of chemotherapeutic agents in psoriasis. *J. invest. Derm.*, 33: 357–69.

VELEZ, H., GHITIS, J., PRADILLA, A. and VITALE, J. J. (1963). Megaloblastic anemia in Kwashiorkor. *Amer. J. clin. Nutr.*, 12: 54–65.

VELEZ, H., RESTREPO, A., BUSTAMENTE, J. and VITALE, J. J. (1965). Studies on folic acid requirements in adult man. *Amer. J. clin. Nutr.*, 16: 383–4.

VERWILGHEN, R., REYBROUCK, G., CALLENS, L. and CASEMANS, J. (1965). Anti-tuberculous drugs and sideroblastic anaemia. *Brit. J. Haemat.*, 11: 92–98.

VILTER, R. W., HORRIGAN, D., MUELLER, J. F., JARROLD, I., VILTER, C. F., HAWKINS, V. and SEAMAN, A. (1950). Studies on the relationships of vitamin B_{12}, folic acid, thymine, uracil and methyl group donors in persons with pernicious anaemia and related megaloblastic anemias. *Blood*, 5: 695–717.

VILTER, V. A., SPIES, T. D. and KOCH, M. B. (1945). Further studies on folic acid in the treatment of macrocytic anaemia. *Southern Med. J.*, 38: 781–5.

VILTER, V. A., VILTER, R. W. and SPIES, T. D. (1947). The treatment of pernicious and related anemias with synthetic folic acid. I. Observations on the maintenance of a normal hematologic status and on the occurrence of combined system disease at the end of one year. *J. lab. clin. Med.*, 32: 262–73.

VITALE, J. J., SETA, K., HELLERSTEIN, E. E. (1965). Folate deficiency secondary to iron depletion. *Fed. Proc.*, 24: 718.

VITALE, J. J., STREIFF, R. R. and HELLERSTEIN, E. E. (1965). Folate metabolism and iron deficiency. *Lancet*, ii: 393–4.

WALT, F., HOLMAN, S. and HENDRICKS, R. G. (1956). Megaloblastic anaemia of infancy in Kwashiorkor and other diseases. *Brit. med. J.*, i: 119–1203.

WATERS, A. H. and MOLLIN, D. L. (1961). Studies on the folic acid activity of human serum. *J. clin. Path.*, 14: 335–44.

WATERS, A. H. and MOLLIN, D. L. (1963). Observations on the metabolism of folic acid in pernicious anaemia. *Brit. J. Haemat.*, 9: 319–27.

WATSON-WILLIAMS, E. J. (1962). Folic acid deficiency in sickle-cell anaemia. *E. African Med. J.*, 39: 213–21.

WERKHEISER, W. C. (1961). Specific binding of 4-aminofolic acid analogues by folic acid reductase. *J. biol. Chem.*, 236: 888–893.

WILKINSON, J. F. and ISRAËLS, M. C. G. (1949). Pteroyl-polyglutamic acids in the treatment of pernicious anaemia. *Lancet*, ii: 689–91.

WILLIAMS, A. W. (1961). Light and electron microscope studies of the effect of 4-aminopteroylglutamic acid (aminoptern) on the mucous membrane of the small intestine of the rat. *Gut*, 2: 346–51.

WILLS, L. (1931). Treatment of "pernicious anaemia of pregnancy" and "tropical anaemia" with special reference to yeast extract as a curative agent. *Brit. med. J.*, i: 1059–64.

WILSON, H. E. and PITNEY, W. R. (1955). Serum concentrations of vitamin B_{12} in normal and nutritionally deficient monkeys. *J. lab. clin. Med.*, 45: 590–8.

WINSTEN, W. A. and EIGEN, E. (1950). Bioautographic studies with use of leuconstoc citrovorum 8081. *J. biol. Chem.*, 184: 155–61.

WOODS, D. D. (1940). The relation of p-aminobenzoic acid to the mechanism of the action of sulphanilamide. *Brit. J. exp. Path.*, 21: 74–90.

WOOLEY, D. E. and SPRINCE, H. (1945). The nature of some new dietary factors required by guinea pigs. *J. biol. Chem.*, 157: 447–53.

WRIGHT, L. D. and WELCH, A. D. (1943a). The metabolism of "folic acid". *Amer. J. med. Sci.*, 206: 128–129.

WRIGHT, L. D. and WELCH, A. D. (1943b). The production of folic acid by rat liver in vitro. *Science*, 98: 179–82.

YUNIS, A. A., ARIMURA, G. K., LUTCHER, C. L., BLASQUEZ, J. and HALLORAN, M. J. (1965). Biochemical lesion in dilantin induced erythroid aplasia. *J. clin. Invest.*, 44: 1114–5.

ZAKRZEWSKI, S. F. (1960). Purification and properties of folic acid reductase from chick liver. *J. biol. Chem.*, 235: 1776–9.

ZALUSKY, R. and HERBERT, V. (1961). Megaloblastic anemia in scurvy with response to 50 microgram of folic acid daily. *New Eng. J. Med.*, 265: 1033–8.

ZALUSKY, R., HERBERT, V. and CASTLE, W. B. (1962). Cyanocobalamin therapy, effect in folic acid deficiency. *Arch. int. Med.*, 109: 545–54.

CHAPTER 3

VITAMIN B₆*

VITAMIN B_6*

G. R. Lee, M.D.† and E. A. Deiss, M.D.

*The Department of Medicine,
University of Utah College of Medicine,
Salt Lake City, Utah*

HISTORY

In 1934 György reported his experience with rats fed a semi-synthetic diet supplemented with crystalline thiamine and riboflavin. These animals exhibited a reduced growth rate, and developed a characteristic inflammation of the paws, snout, and ears, which was later termed "acrodynia". The dermatitis could be prevented by adding to the diet an alcoholic extract of yeast. The name "vitamin B_6" was applied by György to the acrodynia-preventing component of the yeast extract.

Some four years later, Lepkovsky (1938), and almost simultaneously several other groups of investigators (Keresztesy and Stevens, 1938; György, 1938; Kuhn and Wendt, 1938; and Ichiba and Micchi, 1938) isolated crystalline substances with the properties of vitamin B_6. The chemical structure of the crystalline material was quickly established (Kuhn *et al.*, 1939; Stiller *et al.*, 1939), and its synthesis accomplished (Harris and Folkers, 1939). The name pyridoxine was proposed by György and Eckhardt (1939), and became generally accepted.

In 1942 Snell and his colleagues working with a microbiological assay system, was able to show that naturally occurring compounds other than pyridoxine had "vitamin B_6" activity. Later (Snell, 1944; Harris *et al.*, 1944) it was established that two compounds, pyridoxal and pyridoxamine, accounted for the vitamin activity not attributable to pyridoxine.

* This study was supported by a graduate training grant AM-5098, and a research grant AM-04489 from the National Institute of Arthritis and Metabolic Disease, National Institutes of Health, Bethesda, Maryland.
† Markle Scholar in Medical Science.

Between 1938 and 1945, a need for vitamin B_6 in the nutrition of many species was established. However, the role of the vitamin in human nutrition was not appreciated until 1950. In that year Snyderman and colleagues (1950) fed a vitamin B_6 deficient diet to two children with hydrocephalus. After 76 days, one child experienced a series of convulsions which disappeared after pyridoxine therapy. The other child developed hypochromic anemia after 130 days on the diet; treatment with pyridoxine resulted in reticulocytosis and the restoration of blood hemoglobin to normal levels.

Only one year later, the first spontaneously occurring cases of vitamin B_6 deficiency in humans were observed (Coursin, 1954; Molony and Parmelee, 1954). Between 1951 and 1953, a proportion of infants fed from birth with a commercial milk formula developed a convulsive disorder which responded to therapy with pyridoxine. The commercial formula was found to contain suboptimal amounts of vitamin B_6, and the addition of pyridoxine to the formula prevented the syndrome.

In the last 15 years it has become apparent that certain conditions may respond to pharmacological doses of pyridoxine, even though there is no evidence of vitamin B_6 deficiency. These conditions include pyridoxine-responsive anemia (Harris *et al.*, 1956), pyridoxine "dependency" (Hunt *et al.*, 1954) and cystathioninuria (Frimpter *et al.*, 1963).

CHEMICAL AND PHYSICAL PROPERTIES

The term "vitamin B_6" has no precise chemical meaning, since several compounds with different chemical structures have the biological properties of vitamin B_6. It is convenient to use the term in a biologic sense, however, as in referring to "vitamin B_6 deficiency". It is also convenient to refer to "vitamin B_6", or "the vitamin B_6 group", when discussing certain properties common to all members of the group. In discussing treatment or chemical actions, however, the more precise terms given below will be used.

Pyridoxine, pyridoxal, and pyridoxamine are derivatives of 2-methyl-3-hydroxy-5-hydroxymethyl pyridine (Stiller *et al.*, 1939; Snell, 1944; Harris *et al.*, 1944). The compounds differ from one another in the nature of the group occupying position 4. All three may occur in nature as derivatives formed by phosphorylation of the 5-hydroxymethyl group (Fig. 1) (McCormick *et al.*, 1961). The three compounds and their phosphorylated derivatives all have the biological properties of "vitamin B_6".

Pyridoxine hydrochloride may be crystallized from alcohol and acetone, in the form of white platelets which melt with slight decomposition at 204–206° (Stiller *et al.*, 1939; Keresztesy and Stevens, 1938). Pyridoxine is highly soluble in water. In acid solution, it is stable to heat and light. Pyridoxal and pyridoxamine are less stable to the effects of heat and light, especially in neutral and alkaline solutions (Cunningham and Snell, 1945).

Chemical, enzymatic and microbiological methods are available for the assay of vitamin B_6 activity (Storvick and Peters, 1964). These methods accurately measure the vitamin B_6 content of pure solutions; however, the determination of the vitamin B_6 content of biological materials is com-

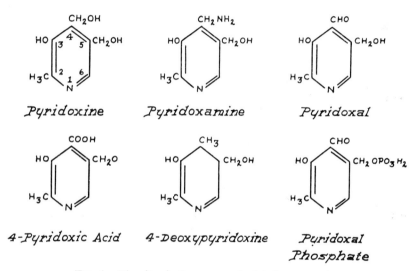

FIG. 1.   The vitamin B_6 group and related compounds.

plicated by the presence of phosphorylated forms and protein bound complexes. Complete extraction of a measurable form of the vitamin is therefore a prerequisite for a satisfactory assay method. As yet, no completely adequate extraction procedure has been described.

ABSORPTION, EXCRETION, AND METABOLIC FATE

All members of the vitamin B_6 group appear to be rapidly and quantitatively absorbed from the normal gastrointestinal tract (Scudi *et al.*, 1940a,b). There is some evidence that patients with adult celiac disease are deficient in the vitamin (Kowlessar *et al.*, 1964), an observation which implies that absorption may be defective in malabsorptive states (see p. 167).

The principal excretory product of vitamin B_6 is 4-pyridoxic acid (Huff and Perlzweig, 1944) (Fig. 1), a fluorescent compound that has no vitamin B_6 activity. It is formed from pyridoxal, through the action of a nonspecific aldehyde oxidase in the liver (Schwartz and Kjeldgaard, 1951).

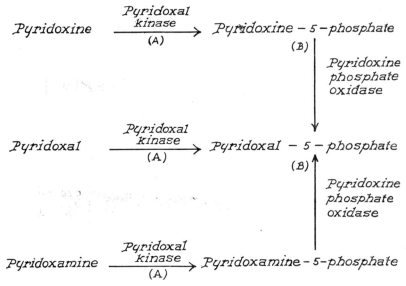

FIG. 2.   Metabolic pathways leading to the synthesis of pyridoxal-5-phosphate.

When a member of the vitamin B_6 group is administered to a human subject, most is excreted as 4-pyridoxic acid, regardless of the form given. However, increased excretion of active forms of the vitamin is observed as well. When pyridoxine is administered, there is increased excretion of all three members of the group. Ingestion of either pyridoxal or pyridoxamine leads to increased excretion of both of these compounds, but not of pyridoxine (Rabinowitz and Snell, 1949). Regardless of the form administered, not all of the administered material is accounted for, suggesting that there are additional excretory compounds or pathways as yet undiscovered.

The active coenzyme form of vitamin B_6 is pyridoxal-5-phosphate for most reactions; pyridoxamine-5-phosphate is active in transamination only. The fact that mammals are able to utilize all three members of the vitamin B_6 group with equal facility implies the existence of biochemical mechanisms that enable the organism to convert these compounds into the active coenzyme forms. For the most part, these conversions take place by means of two enzymatic reactions. The first of these is phosphorylation (Fig. 2A), a reaction catalysed by the enzyme pyridoxal kinase. This reaction requires the presence of adenosine triphosphate (ATP) as a source of phosphate. The form of the reaction is as follows:

$$\text{pyridoxal} + \text{ATP} \xrightarrow{\text{pyridoxal kinase}} \text{pyridoxal-5-phosphate} + \text{ADP}.$$

This reaction has been studied in bacteria, yeast, and mammalian tissues (Hurwitz, 1953, 1955; McCormack *et al.*, 1961). The enzyme is relatively non-specific, and will also bring about the phosphorylation of pyridoxamine, pyridoxine, and a number of synthetic pyridoxine analogs, including deoxypyridoxine.

The second important reaction is that catalysed by the enzyme pyridoxine phosphate oxidase (Wada and Snell, 1961) (Fig. 2B). This enzyme has the ability to convert either pyridoxine phosphate or pyridoxamine phosphate into pyridoxal phosphate. Flavin mononucleotide is an essential cofactor. Apparently it is the lack of this enzyme that makes it impossible for certain microorganisms to utilize pyridoxine or pyridoxamine for growth (Snell and Rannefeld, 1945).

In addition to these two major pathways, interconversion among the members of the vitamin B_6 group may be accomplished to a limited extent by several other reactions. These reactions, which are discussed fully in a review by Snell (1963), are of relatively little importance as far as a net conversion of pyridoxamine and pyridoxine to pyridoxal-5-phosphate is concerned.

THE BIOCHEMICAL ACTION OF PYRIDOXAL PHOSPHATE

Pyridoxal phosphate functions as a coenzyme in a wide variety of enzymatic reactions, almost all of which are concerned with the metabolism of amino acids. Several excellent reviews of the complex role of pyridoxal phosphate in mammalian biochemistry are available (Braunstein, 1960; Snell, 1958; Snell, 1961; Harris *et al.*, 1964).

The majority of the enzymatic reactions requiring pyridoxal phosphate as a cofactor can be made to take place non-enzymatically *in vitro* in the presence of either pyridoxal or pyridoxal phosphate (Longenecker and Snell, 1956). The use of these non-enzymatic reactions as chemical models

F*

has made it possible to identify the structural characteristics upon which the activity of pyridoxal phosphate depends. These characteristics include the heterocyclic pyridine ring, and the free formyl and phenolic groups in the configuration in which they exist in pyridoxal (Fig. 1). The phosphorylated 5-hydroxymethyl group is not essential in the non-enzymatic reactions, but is presumably important for binding with the apoenzyme (Metzler *et al.*, 1954).

The initial step in the reaction between pyridoxal and an amino acid is the formation of a Schiff base (Metzler *et al.*, 1954) (Fig. 3). In such a compound, the bonds about the alpha-carbon of the amino acid become labile. Most pyridoxal phosphate-catalysed reactions involve the groups

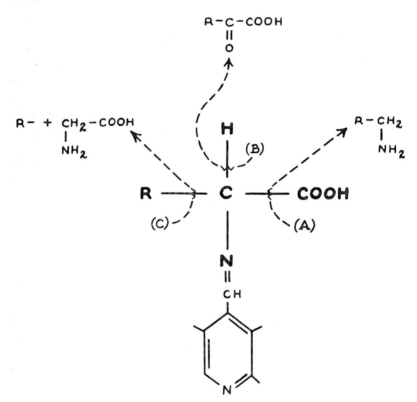

FIG. 3. Schiff base formed by an amino acid (bold face) and pyridoxal. The nature of the subsequent reaction depends upon the site at which cleavage of the labilized bonds takes place. If at "A", decarboxylation of the amino acid results: at "B", transamination; and at "C", rupture of the carbon chain.

attached by these bonds to the alpha-carbon. The apoenzyme confers substrate specificity and determines which of the groups about the alpha-carbon is to react. Because of this basic mechanism of action, most pyridoxal-requiring reactions will be one of three types (Snell, 1961) (Fig. 3A, B, and C).

One type of reaction (Fig. 3A) is decarboxylation:

$$\underset{\underset{NH_2}{|}}{R-CH-COOH} \longrightarrow R-CH_2-NH_2 + CO_2$$

Among the enzymes catalysing this type of reaction are those necessary for the synthesis of catecholamines (Holtz, 1959), 5-hydroxytryptamine (serotonin) (Holtz, 1959), histamine (Ganrot *et al.*, 1961), and γ-amino-butyric acid (Roberts and Frankel, 1950, 1951; Awapara *et al.*, 1950).

A second type of reaction (Fig. 3B) is transamination. This reaction is characterized by the formation of a keto acid from an amino acid of corresponding structure, with the simultaneous conversion of a second keto acid to the corresponding amino acid (Longenecker and Snell, 1956). This transfer of the amino group involves interconversion of pyridoxal phosphate and pyridoxamine phosphate; and, indeed, the transamination reaction appears to be the sum of two reactions:

(1) $\underset{\underset{NH_2}{|}}{R-CH-COOH}$ + enzyme-pyridoxal phosphate $\rightleftharpoons$

$\qquad \underset{\underset{O}{\|}}{R-C-COOH}$ + enzyme-pyridoxamine phosphate;

(2) $\underset{\underset{O}{\|}}{R'-C-COOH}$ + enzyme-pyridoxamine phosphate $\rightleftharpoons$

$\qquad \underset{\underset{NH_2}{|}}{R'-CH-COOH}$ + enzyme-pyridoxal phosphate;

$$R-CH-COOH + R'-C-COOH \rightleftharpoons R-C-COOH + R'-CH-COOH;$$
$$\quad\ |\qquad\qquad\quad \|\qquad\qquad\quad \|\qquad\qquad\quad |$$
$$\quad NH_2 \qquad\qquad\ O \qquad\qquad\quad O \qquad\qquad NH_2$$

The third type of reaction results from labilizing the bond between the α- and β-carbons (Fig. 3C). Reactions of this type are part of the catabolism of threonine and serine. The products are glycine and the residual aldehyde:

$$R-CH-CH-COOH \rightleftharpoons R-CHO + CH_2-COOH$$
$$\quad\ |\quad\ |\qquad\qquad\qquad\qquad\qquad\quad |$$
$$\quad OH\ NH_2 \qquad\qquad\qquad\qquad\qquad NH_2$$

In the case of serine, the formaldehyde formed is not free but is coupled with tetrahydrofolic acid to form N^{10}-hydroxymethyl-tetrahydrofolic acid, and thus becomes involved in purine and pyrimidine synthesis (Alexander and Greenberg, 1956). In some instances, the direction of the reaction illustrated above is predominantly from right to left. One such reaction is the synthesis of Δ-aminolevulinic acid from glycine and succinyl-coenzyme A, a pyridoxal phosphate-requiring reaction which is the initial step in the synthesis of heme (Kikuchi *et al.*, 1958).

Pyridoxal phosphate is a cofactor in a wide variety of other enzyme systems, including some amine oxidases (Yamada and Yasunubo, 1962), and amino acid dehydrases and desulfhydrases (Braunstein, 1960). Several enzymes involved in the metabolism of tryptophan require pyridoxal phosphate (Holtz and Palm, 1964) (see p. 167). Pyridoxal phosphate serves also as coenzyme in several reactions involving sulfur-containing amino acids, including both the synthesis and degradation of cystathionine (Binkley *et al.*, 1952).

Pyridoxal phosphate may be necessary for several reactions that do not seem to be related to amino acid metabolism. The compound has long been implicated in the metabolism of fatty acids, but its role remains undefined and is perhaps an indirect one (Mueller, 1964). It is also apparently involved in carbohydrate metabolism since it is a part of purified muscle *phosphorylase a* (Baranowski *et al.*, 1957), perhaps serving to stabilize the enzyme structurally (Illingworth *et al.*, 1958). A requirement for pyridoxal phosphate in normal oxalate metabolism appears probable in view of the hyperoxaluria which occurs in vitamin B_6 deficient animals, although the source of the excess oxalate remains unexplained (Runyan and Gershoff, 1965).

VITAMIN B$_6$ DEFICIENCY IN ANIMALS

Every species of animal tested has shown a need for vitamin B$_6$ in the diet. These include monkeys (McCall *et al.*, 1946), dogs (Fouts *et al.*, 1938), pigs (Wintrobe *et al.*, 1943), rats (György, 1934), mice (Schweigert *et al.*, 1946), hamsters (Schwartzman and Strauss, 1949), rabbits (Hove and Herndon, 1957), chickens (Jukes, 1939), ducks (Hegsted and Rao, 1945), turkeys (Bird *et al.*, 1943), and rainbow trout (McLaren *et al.*, 1947). The manifestations of vitamin B$_6$ deprivation vary somewhat from species to species, but for the most part the differences are in degree rather than in kind. The most regularly observed manifestations are anemia, neurological disturbances, and arrest of growth.

Anemia

Anemia was first noted in dogs (Fouts *et al.*, 1938), but it has also been observed in cats, pigs, and monkeys, as well as in chickens and ducks. In rats and other small animals, anemia is not always observed; however, an unusually prolonged existence on the deficient diet can result in anemia among surviving animals (Shen *et al.*, 1964). Even in the absence of anemia, impaired blood regeneration in response to phlebotomy is observed (Kornberg *et al.*, 1945).

A great deal of descriptive information is available concerning the anemia seen in swine. Since most of the pertinent observations in this species apply to other species as well, a description follows.

When 3–4-week-old pigs are fed a purified vitamin B$_6$ deficient diet, a decrease in the volume of packed red cells (VPRC) becomes apparent within 3–4 weeks. The VPRC declines progressively and is less than 20 ml/ 100 ml within 2–3 months. Values as low as 9 ml/100 ml have been observed. The anemia is hypochromic and microcytic; both the mean corpuscular volume (MCV) and the mean corpuscular hemoglobin concentration (MCHC) are reduced as compared with values in a control group. The hypochromia and microcytosis are also apparent on blood smear, and there is considerable aniso- and poikilocytosis. Erythrocytes containing Prussian blue positive inclusions are seen on smear. These cells, known as siderocytes, are still more numerous after splenectomy (Deiss *et al.*, 1966). The reticulocyte count is usually low and there is no evidence of increased blood destruction. The bone marrow is hyperplastic due to proliferation of normoblasts.

The anemia is accompanied by disturbed iron metabolism. A marked increase in serum iron may be detected early in the deficiency. Iron absorption is increased, and siderosis of the bone marrow, spleen, and liver may develop if the deficiency state is sufficiently prolonged. The plasma iron turnover is increased, and the rate of incorporation of iron into red cells is impaired (Bush *et al.*, 1956).

The concentration of free porphyrin in erythrocytes is markedly reduced in deficient animals as compared to controls. Furthermore, the reduction in porphyrin content may become apparent before the decrease in the VPRC (Cartwright and Wintrobe, 1948).

When vitamin B_6 is administered, there is a prompt reticulocytosis, a reduction in the serum iron, and a rapid increase in the VPRC and in erythrocyte porphyrins. After 20–30 days of therapy, the animal is hematologically normal. In early reports (Wintrobe *et al.*, 1943; McKibbin *et al.*, 1942), the response to pyridoxine was found to be incomplete; however, with present-day complete diets, total reversal of the deficiency is possible (Cartwright *et al.*, 1963).

Because the anemia was hypochromic and microcytic, impaired synthesis of hemoglobin was suspected. The finding of reduced free erythrocyte porphyrins suggested that the defect lay in the synthesis of the porphyrin prosthetic group of hemoglobin. In 1957, Schulman and Richert demonstrated that the synthesis of Δ-aminolevulinic acid (ALA), a precursor of porphyrins, was defective in vitamin B_6 deficient duck erythrocytes. It now appears well established that pyridoxal phosphate is an essential cofactor in this reaction and that the anemia results from impaired ALA synthesis.

Neurological manifestations

Vitamin B_6 deficiency is associated with a convulsive disorder in most species. In the pig, two types of seizures have been observed (Wintrobe *et al.*, 1943). One, a generalized convulsion with a tonic and a clonic phase followed by post-ictal confusion, stupor and ataxia, appears analogous to grand mal seizures in man. A second, milder variety of seizure consists of brief, jerky movements of the whole body, or a peculiar stiff-legged walk lasting only a few moments. Once seizures have been observed, the animal appears hyperirritable or "nervous", and seizures may sometimes be induced by a sudden noise or fright. Addition of pyridoxine to the diet completely prevents the seizures.

In rats, a similar hyperexcitable state is observed in association with "fits" in which the animal runs in circles, then becomes suddenly helpless and still, except for tonic and clonic muscle twitches. These episodes are often followed by coma or stupor (Chick *et al.*, 1940). The threshold for induction of seizures by electroshock is markedly reduced in such animals (Davenport and Davenport, 1948).

In chickens, three stages of neurologic abnormality may be observed: abnormal excitability; occasional uncontrolled, jerky, convulsive movements of body, legs and wings; and generalized seizures with post-ictal stupor (Lepkovsky and Kratzer, 1942).

Seizures are observed in most other species in which vitamin B$_6$ deficiency has been produced (Tower, 1956). In some, especially mice, monkeys, and cats, it is necessary to administer the antivitamin deoxypyridoxine in addition to the deficient diet before seizures occur.

In addition to convulsive disorders, other disturbances of the nervous system are seen, but with much less regularity. In general, these are related to degenerative changes in peripheral nerves. For example, in pigs after prolonged deficiency, an ataxia of the hind limbs develops, and histologic changes can be seen in the brachial and sciatic nerves, posterior roots and ganglia, and spinal cord. Similar manifestations have been noted in dogs, turkeys and calves (Tower, 1956).

Growth

In all species, growth of young animals is retarded as vitamin B$_6$ deficiency develops, and grown animals tend to lose weight. This is an early and striking finding in rats (Beaton *et al.*, 1954). The failure to gain weight is accompanied by loss of appetite, and a reduction of food intake. However, the reduced intake does not completely account for the effects on growth, since animals receiving isocaloric amounts of a control diet gain weight significantly faster than the deficient animals. These observations imply a failure to utilize the ingested food, and since vitamin B$_6$ is so intimately related to amino acid metabolism (see pp. 157–60), it would be reasonable to propose that defective protein synthesis accounts for the growth failure. However, carcass analyses show that the protein content of deficient animals is the same as that of controls; the difference in weight is accounted for by a difference in fat and water content. Thus, neither the loss of appetite nor the failure to grow is completely understood; however, it should be noted that this set of findings is common to many nutritional deficiencies, and is not a specific manifestation of vitamin B$_6$ lack.

Other manifestations

Dermatitis in the form of "rat acrodynia" was the first abnormality ascribed to vitamin B_6 deficiency, and served as a basis for early bio-assay methods. The characteristic symmetrical dermatitis involving the tail, paws, nose, mouth, and ears is produced after about 6–9 weeks of dietary deficiency in the rat. Similar skin lesions can also be produced in hamsters, rabbits, and, with the aid of deoxypyridoxine, in mice; however, a specific dermatitis is not characteristic of the deficiency in larger species.

Several observations suggest that pyridoxine deficiency is associated with defective immunological processes (Axelrod and Trakatellis, 1964). Production of circulating antibodies to common antigens is impaired in the deficient animal. Delayed hypersensitivity, in the form of the tuberculin reaction, or in homograft rejection, is also defective. Atrophy of various lymphoid tissues, including the spleen, thymus, and circulating lymphocytes, has been observed in several species.

In monkeys, lesions of arteries are seen which resemble human arteriosclerosis (Greenberg, 1964). Similar arterial lesions have been reported in dogs (Mushett and Emerson, 1957). In rats, although no such lesions are seen, hypertension has been reported (Olson, 1956).

Two other unusual manifestations are noted in monkeys: the incidence of dental caries is markedly increased, and there is a marked degree of liver damage varying from fatty infiltration to florid cirrhosis (Greenberg, 1964). Fatty infiltration of the liver has also been noted in pigs (Wintrobe *et al.*, 1943).

HUMAN REQUIREMENT FOR VITAMIN B_6

The minimum daily requirement for vitamin B_6 is not well established. This is due in part to the absence of a spontaneously occurring deficiency syndrome which might be studied, and in part to lack of agreement on a suitable test for vitamin B_6 deficiency. The test most commonly employed for this purpose is the so-called "tryptophan load test": the determination of certain tryptophan metabolites, especially xanthurenic acid, in the urine following the oral administration of tryptophan (Greenberg and Rinehart, 1948; Coursin, 1964b) (see p. 167, and Fig. 4). Other tests which have been used include the measurement of urinary 4-pyridoxic acid, both with and without prior oral administration of pyridoxine (Wachstein and Gudaitis, 1953; Sarett, 1951), urinary *N*-methyl nicotinamide after a tryptophan load (Schweigert and Pearson, 1947), plasma and leukocyte vitamin levels (Coursin and Brown, 1961; Boxer *et al.*, 1957), trans-aminases in plasma, erythrocytes, and leukocytes (Raica and Sauberlich, 1964; Cheney *et al.*, 1965), urinary taurine (Swan *et al.*, 1964), and blood urea following an alanine test load (Hawkins *et al.*, 1946). Unfortunately, none of these procedures is entirely satisfactory, because of technical difficulties in measuring the compounds in some instances, because of lack of sensitivity in some, and because most are not specific for vitamin B_6 deficiency.

The experimental determination of the requirement in the adult male has been the subject of a series of studies by the U.S. Army (Baker *et al.*, 1964; Sauberlich, 1964). Both natural and purified diets deficient in vitamin B_6 were fed to healthy young adult males, a variety of biochemical and clinical parameters were followed, and the effect of pyridoxine supplementation was observed. In these subjects, the minimum pyridoxine supplement necessary to prevent all manifestations of deficiency varied with the amount of protein intake; the daily requirement was 1.25 mg and 1.5 mg, respectively, for diets providing 30 and 100 gm of protein per day.

The National Academy of Sciences–National Research Council suggested that 1.5–2.0 mg daily in the adult, and 400 mcg in infants, represent adequate allowances (Food and Nutrition Board, 1964). Actual dietary intake of vitamin B_6 in the United States, however, was estimated to range from 1.1 to 3.6 mg per day in "adequate" diets, and from 0.7 to 1.4 mg per day in "poor" diets (Mangay Chung *et al.*, 1961). If these various estimates are correct, it would appear that, for a substantial portion of the population of the United States, vitamin B_6 intake is marginal.

VITAMIN B_6 AND HUMAN DISEASE

Deficiency of vitamin B₆

Clinically recognizable deficiency of vitamin B_6 has rarely been reported in man. This is due in part to the wide distribution of the vitamin in foods of both plant and animal origin. Muscle, liver, kidney, and many seeds and grains are excellent sources, but comparatively low concentrations are present in milk (Snell and Keevil, 1954). Pyridoxal and pyridoxamine predominate in foods from animal sources; whereas plant materials yield primarily pyridoxine (Rabinowitz and Snell, 1948).

In the adult human, attempts to produce clinical evidence of vitamin B_6

deficiency by means of experimental diets have been mostly unsuccessful. In contrast, biochemical abnormalities due to vitamin B_6 deficiency have been produced easily.

Convincing evidence that vitamin B_6 is an essential nutrient for man was presented in 1950 by Synderman, Carretero, and Holt. Two mentally defective infants were fed a diet deficient in vitamin B_6. Weight gain ceased, 4-pyridoxic acid vanished from the urine, and conversion of tryptophan to N-methylnicotinamide was subnormal. One infant developed convulsions after 76 days; hypochromic microcytic anemia was observed in the other after 130 days. Treatment with pyridoxine corrected all of these abnormalities.

In a study in normal adult males (Sauberlich, 1964), convulsions occurred in one subject during the seventh week of a vitamin B_6 deficient diet. Electroencephalographic abnormalities were observed in other subjects, as early as 21 days after the study was begun. Following pyridoxine administration, the electroencephalogram returned to normal in all subjects.

Cases thought to represent spontaneously occurring instances of deficiency of vitamin B_6 were reported shortly after pyridoxine was synthesized. Four patients with multiple nutritional deficiencies were described in whom weakness, irritability, difficulty in walking and abdominal pain persisted following treatment with thiamine, nicotinic acid, and riboflavin (Spies *et al.*, 1939). Dramatic relief of symptoms was observed within hours of administration of pyridoxine, and the symptoms were therefore ascribed to vitamin B_6 deficiency. It is difficult to explain the manifestations exhibited by these patients in terms of present knowledge of vitamin B_6 functions.

In 1951 a synthetic milk preparation, the pyridoxine content of which was 60 mcg per liter, was marketed in the United States as an infant-feeding formula. During the next two years, an outbreak of vitamin B_6 deficiency occurred among infants who were fed from birth exclusively with this product (Nelson, 1956; Snyderman, 1955; Hunt, 1957; Molony and Parmelee, 1954; Coursin, 1954; May, 1954). The manifestations of the disorder, which consisted of hyperirritability and convulsions, responded promptly to the administration of pyridoxine. Similar symptoms, also controlled by pyridoxine, have been observed in breast-fed infants, presumably as a result of the low vitamin B_6 content of the mother's breast milk (Bessey *et al.*, 1957). Apart from these cases in infants, instances of symptomatic vitamin B_6 deficiency have seldom been reported (Theron *et al.*, 1961; Lerner *et al.*, 1958; Leevy *et al.*, 1965).

Malabsorption. Failure to absorb vitamin B$_6$ normally might be expected to produce manifestations of deficiency, particularly if dietary intake were marginal. The tryptophan load test was abnormal in several adults with celiac disease (Kowlessar *et al.*, 1964). In these patients the test returned nearly to normal following parenteral administration of 180 mg of pyridoxine. Anemia was observed in another patient with celiac disease in whom the tryptophan load test also was abnormal. The anemia resembled that seen in experimental vitamin B$_6$ deficiency in that hypochromia of the erythrocytes was present, reticuloendothelial iron was increased in the bone marrow, and ringed sideroblasts were prominent. These abnormalities disappeared after treatment with gluten-free diet and the anemia was ascribed to malabsorption of vitamin B$_6$ (Dawson *et al.*, 1964).

Alteration in tryptophan metabolism without other evidence of vitamin B$_6$ deficiency

Xanthurenic acid was first detected in the urine of vitamin B$_6$ deficient animals in 1942 (Fouts and Lepkovsky; Lepkovsky and Nielsen). After oral administration of tryptophan, Greenberg *et al.* (1949) observed increased xanthurenic acid excretion in humans fed a vitamin B$_6$ deficient diet. The tryptophan load test is based upon these observations, and has become the most frequently used test for the diagnosis of vitamin B$_6$ deficiency.

Pyridoxal phosphate is a necessary cofactor for several enzymes involved in the metabolism of tryptophan (Fig. 4). As might be anticipated, in vitamin B$_6$ deficiency states, metabolic products of tryptophan in addition to xanthurenic acid have been demonstrated in the urine. It has been suggested that the enzymes differ in their sensitivity to a decreased supply of pyridoxal phosphate. The tryptophan metabolite present in greatest quantity in the urine would therefore depend in part on the severity of the vitamin B$_6$ deficiency (Coursin, 1964b).

Abnormal tryptophan metabolism unrelated to vitamin B$_6$ deficiency has been demonstrated in thiamine and in riboflavin deficiency (Porter *et al.*, 1948), and also, rarely, in patients with thyrotoxicosis (Wachstein and Lobel, 1956; Wohl *et al.*, 1960), malignancies (Wachstein and Lobel, 1956; Crepaldi and Parpajola, 1964; Perissinotto *et al.*, 1964), diabetes mellitus (Oka and Leppanen, 1963; Rosen *et al.*, 1955), porphyria (Price *et al.*, 1959), rheumatoid arthritis (Flinn *et al.*, 1964; McKusick *et al.*, 1964), scleroderma (Price *et al.*, 1957), epilepsy (Hagberg *et al.*, 1964),

and various psychoses (Price *et al.*, 1959). In the reported cases, there were
no identifiable symptoms referable to vitamin B_6 deficiency, and treatment
with pyridoxine produced no symptomatic change. In some instances
excretion of tryptophan metabolites became more nearly normal following
treatment with large amounts of pyridoxine; a completely normal pattern
after such treatment was rarely seen, however. The significance of these
observations is not known, but the view that these patients are vitamin B_6
deficient is not justified by the presently available data.

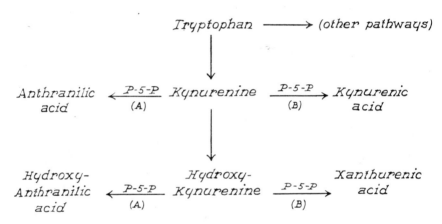

FIG. 4. The origin of urinary tryptophan metabolites measured in the
tryptophan load test. Tryptophan is converted first to kynurenine by
means of the tryptophan pyrrolase reaction. The kynureninase reaction
(A) is very sensitive to deficiency of pyridoxal-5-phosphate; consequently,
increased amounts of kynurenine, hydroxykynurenine, kynurenic acid
and xanthurenic acid appear in the urine of vitamin B_6 deficient animals
following the administration of a tryptophan load. The transaminase
reaction (B) may also become impaired if deficiency of P-5-P is severe.
Thus, the relative proportions of the four compounds may vary with the
degree of deficiency.

In contrast to the low incidence of apparent abnormalities of tryptophan
metabolism in the above diseases is the high frequency with which such
abnormalities were observed in pregnancy (Wachstein and Gudaitis,
1952, 1953a). Increased excretion of xanthurenic acid after an oral tryptophan load was found in the majority of pregnant women, beginning in the
12th week of pregnancy (Wachstein and Gudaitis, 1952). However,
abnormal tryptophan metabolism did not develop if a daily 10 mg supple-

ment of pyridoxine was given; a smaller supplement was incompletely effective (Wachstein and Gudaitis, 1953a). Significant improvement in the metabolism of tryptophan was observed within 30 min of a single 2.5 mg dose of pyridoxine (Wachstein and Gudaitis, 1953a). Urinary 4-pyridoxic acid was normal in pregnant women, but the increase following oral pyridoxine administration was subnormal, suggesting greater pyridoxine retention (Wachstein and Gudaitis, 1953b). Blood levels of pyridoxal phosphate and pyridoxamine phosphate were subnormal during the last trimester (Coursin and Brown, 1961). These observations suggest that mild deficiency of vitamin B$_6$ may occur in pregnancy, presumably because of an increased requirement. If so, there is no evidence of an increase in morbidity or mortality of either mother or fetus as a result of this deficiency (Hillman *et al.*, 1963). Adequately controlled evaluation (Hesseltine, 1946) failed to support early claims of the value of pyridoxine therapy for nausea and vomiting of pregnancy and for hyperemesis gravidarum.

Abnormal tryptophan load tests and reduced plasma pyridoxal phosphate and transaminase levels have been observed in elderly subjects. These observations have been cited as evidence for a high incidence of subclinical vitamin B$_6$ deficiency in this age group (Ranke *et al.*, 1960; Hamfelt, 1964). The observed metabolic abnormalities were readily correctable by a supplement of pyridoxine. The data were interpreted as indicating a greater requirement for vitamin B$_6$ in this age group, but the adequacy of the subjects' diets was not investigated.

An interesting explanation for the abnormal tryptophan metabolism observed in these various conditions has recently been offered (Altman and Greengard, 1966). *Tryptophan pyrrolase* is the enzyme governing the amount of tryptophan that is converted to kynurenine. It has been demonstrated in rats that an increase in the amount of hepatic tryptophan pyrrolase can be induced by increasing the concentration of its substrate, or by a variety of maneuvers which increase adrenal cortical secretion. In a group of nutritionally normal patients with a variety of diseases, it was shown that the amount of kynurenine excreted in the urine following oral administration of tryptophan could be correlated directly with hepatic tryptophan pyrrolase activity. Following administration of cortisol, both tryptophan pyrrolase and urinary kynurenine strikingly increased. Tryptophan pyrrolase therefore appears to be inducible in man as well as in the rat. The kynureninuria seen in patients with diseases not associated with vitamin B$_6$ deficiency might be due to production of kynurenine in an amount which exceeds the capacity of the pyridoxal-requiring enzymes to catalyse it. Thus, neither diminished activity of these enzymes nor deficiency of vitamin B_6 need be postulated to explain abnormal results of the tryptophan load test.

Metabolic inhibitors

In addition to these spontaneously occurring disorders, symptoms or chemical signs of vitamin B_6 deficiency may be produced by a number of substances which interfere with normal functions of the vitamin.

The most thoroughly studied of these compounds is 4-deoxypyridoxine. This antimetabolite differs from pyridoxine in that a methyl rather than a hydroxymethyl group occupies the critical 4-position (Fig. 1). Deoxypyridoxine is phosphorylated by pyridoxal kinase, thus competitively inhibiting phosphorylation of pyridoxine and pyridoxal (Hurwitz, 1959, 1960); the 4-deoxypyridoxine-5-phosphate thus formed in turn competes with pyridoxal-5-phosphate for binding sites on the several apoenzymes (Hurwitz, 1959, 1960; Umbreit and Waddell, 1949).

Vilter and his associates (1953) administered deoxypyridoxine to 50 adults. Two-thirds developed signs which disappeared following pyridoxine therapy. The most frequently observed sign was a seborrhea-like skin lesion occurring most commonly at the nasolabial fold. Glossitis developed in some of the subjects, and cheilosis and stomatitis were present in a few. Three patients developed a symmetrical peripheral neuropathy, characterized by hyperesthesia and paresthesias of the feet and legs. Absolute lymphopenia was observed in most. Mild normocytic normochromic anemia was observed in a few patients, but no reticulocytosis followed pyrixodine therapy. Convulsions were not observed in these patients.

Several medically important therapeutic agents react directly with pyridoxal to inactivate the vitamin. The most important of these is isonicotinylhydrazide (INH), the compound of greatest usefulness in the treatment of tuberculosis. This compound, along with other hydrazides of similar structure, reacts with the carbonyl oxygen of pyridoxal to form the hydrazone, which is a potent inhibitor of pyridoxal kinase but which does not have vitamin B_6 activity (McCormick *et al.*, 1961).

Some individuals who receive INH develop a peripheral neuropathy, involving both sensory and motor nerves (Biehl and Vilter, 1954a, 1954b; Pegum, 1952; Jones and Jones, 1953). The occurrence of this phenomenon is dose-related (Biehl and Vilter, 1954a). It is frequent only when doses greater than about 5 mg per kg per day are employed, and is rarely observed at the more usually employed therapeutic levels. The neuropathy is preventable by simultaneous administration of pyridoxine (Biehl and Vilter, 1954a, 1954b; Ross, 1958; Carlson *et al.*, 1956); once developed, however, this complication is not always reversible by pyridoxine therapy, unless the administration of INH is discontinued (Biehl and Vilter, 1954a). Certain other toxic symptoms produced by INH, such as confusion, psychosis, and convulsions, are not regularly prevented by simultaneous use of pyridoxine (Ross, 1958) and may not be due to the anti-vitamin B_6 effect of INH.

In addition to its neurologic effects, INH therapy has coincided with the development of anemia in a few reported instances (Bowman, 1961; McCurdy, 1963; Redleaf, 1962; Kohn *et al.*, 1963; McCurdy and Donohue, 1966). The syndrome in these patients resembled that seen in experimental vitamin B_6 deficiency in animals, in that marrow iron stores were increased, transferrin was saturated, and a response to treatment with pyridoxine was observed. However, in some patients the response to therapy was incomplete (McCurdy and Donohue, 1966).

A second drug employed in the treatment of tuberculosis, cycloserine, apparently inactivates pyridoxal by binding directly with it (Roze and Straminger, 1963). Cycloserine produces toxic signs of central nervous system origin, such as convulsions, and the simultaneous administration of pyridoxine is said to have prevented the occurrence of these complications (Epstein *et al.*, 1959). Sideroblastic anemia has been reported in patients receiving cycloserine, but the relationship of the anemia to possible disturbances in vitamin B_6 function was not studied (Verwilghen *et al.*, 1965).

Still another drug that inactivates pyridoxal is penicillamine (Kuchinskas *et al.*, 1957; duVigneaud *et al.*, 1957), a compound useful in the therapy of Wilson's disease because of its ability to chelate copper (Aposhian, 1961). In studies *in vitro*, both the D- and L-isomers of penicillamine inactivated free pyridoxal phosphate, but only the L-form inhibited pyridoxal-enzyme complexes (Ueda *et al.*, 1960). Presumably because of this difference, L-penicillamine is very much more toxic (Aposhian and Aposhian, 1959), and it produces signs of vitamin B_6 deficiency in animals (Wilson and duVigneaud, 1950; Kuchinskas and duVigneaud, 1957). For this reason, only D-penicillamine is used therapeutically (Aposhian, 1961). Even with this isomer, however, the tryptophan load test has been observed to be abnormal (Jaffe *et al.*, 1964; Asatoor, 1964), and to return to normal following pyridoxine supplementation (Jaffe *et al.*, 1964). The occurrence of abnormal tryptophan load tests among patients treated with D-penicillamine is inconstant, however, and may be dose-related (Gibbs and Walshe, 1966).

The pyridoxine-responsive disorders

Three clinical disorders have been described in which pyridoxine appears to be effective when administered in pharmacologic doses. The disorders may be referred to as "pyridoxine-responsive" rather than "pyridoxine-deficient", since in most cases evidence of deficiency is lacking. Scriver (1966) has used the term "pyridoxine-dependency" in referring to all of these syndromes. We have limited the use of this term to its original application, the convulsive disorder of children to be described below.

Pyridoxine-responsive anemia. The spontaneous occurrence of anemia responding to pyridoxine therapy was first observed in 1956 by Harris and his co-workers. By 1964, Horrigan and Harris had accumulated data on 72 patients with "pyridoxine-responsive anemia". Data on 41 of these patients had appeared in published reports, and the remainder were gleaned from personal communications to the authors.

Pyridoxine-responsive anemia was observed primarily in males; less than 20% of the recorded patients were females. In several instances the anemia was probably present from birth; however, there was a significant incidence in all decades and the oldest reported patient was 87 years of age.

In about one-third of the reported cases, there were indications of similar diseases in other family members, especially siblings. The male predominance suggested a sex-linked heredity pattern, and, indeed, members of the families reported as "sex-linked anemia" by Rundles and Falls (1946) have responded to pyridoxine (Bishop and Bethell, 1959). In other families, however, an autosomal hereditary pattern was suggested (Cotton and Harris, 1962).

The patient characteristically sought medical attention because of symptoms of slowly progressive anemia. Other symptoms of vitamin B_6 deficiency were conspicuous by their absence. None of the patients had noted convulsions, nor were skin lesions reported. Furthermore, in the great majority of cases, the dietary history was normal.

Physical examination revealed the signs of anemia. The only other physical findings of note were enlargement of the liver and spleen, present in about half of the patients.

Usually the degree of anemia was severe; in over half the cases, the blood hemoglobin concentration was less than 7.0 gms/100 ml. The anemia was usually hypochromic and microcytic. A hypochromic population of cells almost invariably was observed on blood smear, and in most cases the mean corpuscular hemoglobin concentration was subnormal. Microcytosis was less regularly present, but the mean corpuscular volume was subnormal in over 60 % of the patients. Additional morphological findings included marked aniso- and poikilocytosis, and, occasionally, significant numbers of target cells. Siderocytes, erythrocytes with iron-containing granules, were often prominent, especially in splenectomized patients (Raab *et al.*, 1961). There was no characteristic disturbance of leukocytes; in some cases leukopenia was observed; in others, leukocytosis. The platelets were usually unremarkable.

The bone marrow was cellular, and usually normoblastic with a decreased myeloid–erythroid cell ratio. In a small proportion of the reported cases, the marrow was megaloblastic. Iron stains demonstrated marked increases in reticulum-cell hemosiderin as well as in sideroblasts. In many cases, so called "ringed" sideroblasts, which are said to indicate mitochondrial iron-loading, were observed.

Evidence of iron overload was present in virtually all cases. The serum iron was increased and the serum transferrin was more than 80 % saturated. Evidence of siderosis of the liver was present in a large majority of biopsies. Marrow iron findings have been mentioned above. In some cases, the degree of iron overloading was such that a diagnosis of hemochromatosis was suggested. Indeed, diabetes mellitus or a diabetic glucose tolerance curve was noted in nearly half the cases in which the finding was sought. In addition, fibrosis accompanied marked siderosis in two-thirds of reported liver biopsies, providing a histologic basis for a diagnosis of pigmentary cirrhosis.

Studies with ^{51}Cr labeled red cells indicated that erythrocyte survival was either normal or only slightly reduced. Studies with ^{59}Fe revealed that the plasma iron turnover rate was increased and that erythrocyte iron incorporation was reduced. Early uptake of ^{59}Fe by the liver was observed by means of *in vivo* surface counting. These kinetic data are consistent with "ineffective erythropoiesis", i.e., the production of a population of nonviable erythrocytes.

Abnormal excretion of tryptophan metabolites following a loading dose was noted in about half of the cases in which the test was done.

The above features make up a distinctive clinical picture, which resembles in many ways that seen in the vitamin B$_6$ deficient animal. However, it must be noted that a response to pyridoxine cannot be predicted by the presence of such a picture. Cases with identical findings, but lacking the response to vitamin B$_6$ therapy, have been described under several different names, including "sideroachrestic anemia" (Heilmeyer, 1958) and "sideroblastic anemia" (Mollin, 1965).

The response to pyridoxine therapy was variable and incomplete. There was usually a rise in reticulocyte count with a peak about 7–10 days after therapy began. In only about half of the cases did the blood hemoglobin concentration return to normal, and even in these the morphological abnormalities persisted. In the remaining cases, there was a rise in hemoglobin concentration, but to less than normal values. On withdrawal of therapy, relapse was usually rapid, with a fall in hemoglobin levels having been noted within 2–16 weeks.

The minimum effective dose of pyridoxine was rarely determined. Ordinarily large doses, up to 100 or 200 mg per day, were administered. In one case (Horrigan and Harris, 1964), the minimum dose necessary to maintain remission was established as 20 mg intramuscularly twice a week, or 50 mg by mouth daily. In a few cases, responses to as little as 2.5–5 mg per day were noted; whereas in others requirement of a dose as large as 100 mg per day was established.

In most instances in which therapy has been interrupted and relapse has occurred, the patient responded again to the reinstitution of pyridoxine treatment. In some, however, the patient became refractory to therapy. It is interesting that in two patients in whom this refractory state developed, the free erythrocyte porphyrins increased during therapy even though the blood hemoglobin did not rise (Bottomley, 1965). A similar, but even more dramatic, rise in erythrocyte porphyrins during pyridoxine therapy was observed in a case of "sideroachrestic anemia" who had never responded to pyridoxine therapy with a reticulocytosis or rise in hemoglobin (Lee *et al.*, 1966).

A number of other agents were administered to these patients, and occasional responses were observed. These agents included liver extract (Horrigan, 1961), plasma (Erslev *et al.*, 1960), tryptophan (Horrigan, 1961) and androgens (Gardner and Nathan, 1962). Folic acid was effective in certain cases in which the anemia was megaloblastic (Horrigan and Harris, 1964).

Pyridoxine dependency. In 1954, Hunt *et al.* described an infant in whom convulsions developed on the first day of life. The seizures persisted despite barbiturate therapy but ceased within 15–30 min after the intramuscular administration of a multivitamin preparation. It was subsequently demonstrated that the seizures could be prevented by the oral administration of 2 mg of pyridoxine daily, but that failure to supply the vitamin precipitated a recurrence. Mental retardation had been progressive from birth and was not corrected by therapy. Ten years later

(Coursin, 1964b), daily pyridoxine supplementation was still necessary and mental development was not improved.

Since the first case, there have been a number of similar reports (Garty *et al.*, 1962; Scriver, 1960; Scriver and Hutchison, 1963; Waldinger and Berg, 1963). The term "pyridoxine dependency" has been applied to this disorder. It is distinguished from the occasional occurrence of pyridoxine deficient convulsions in children by the earlier age of onset, the occasional familial incidence, the association with mental retardation, the continuous need for unusually high doses of pyridoxine and the prompt relapse when therapy is interrupted. As in the original report, the tryptophan load test has usually been normal. Prompt institution of pyridoxine therapy has resulted in normal mental development in addition to seizure control (Waldinger and Berg, 1963).

Cystathioninuria. Markedly excessive urinary excretion of the amino acid cystathionine has been reported in six patients (Harris *et al.*, 1959; Frimpter *et al.*, 1963, 1965; Berlow and Efron, 1964, 1966; Shaw *et al.*, 1967; and Perry *et al.*, 1967). Four of the patients were mentally retarded, but other clinical findings were quite variable, and not clearly related to the cystathioninuria. Additional metabolic abnormalities were observed in three patients; one had acromegaly; another, nephrogenic diabetes insipidus; and another, phenylketonuria. Two patients had congenital anomalies: bilateral talipes calcaneovalgus in one, persistence of first gill-cleft remnants in the other. Miscellaneous findings included epilepsy in one patient, thrombocytopenia in one, and anemia in another.

Lesser degrees of cystathioninuria were observed in relatives of 2 of the 6 cases. The hereditary pattern was consistent with autosomal transmission of the trait.

Pyridoxine had been administered to 5 of the patients. In all, a marked reduction in cystathionine excretion was observed. In general, no other clinical improvement was evident. An exception was the patient of Perry *et al.* (1967) whose severe anemia proved to be pyridoxine responsive. The mental deficiency was not improved in any of the subjects. It has been suggested that earlier diagnosis and treatment might prevent mental impairment, but there are no data to support this suggestion.

"Xanthurenic aciduria". A fourth possible pyridoxine responsive disorder has been described by Knapp (1962). He has detected abnormal tryptophan load tests in 43 of 74 individuals in 9 kindreds. The observed

abnormalities, which consisted of xanthurenic aciduria or kynureninuria or both, disappeared after oral administration of pyridoxine in a dose of 100 mg. Many of the subjects had no clinical abnormalities, but there was a high incidence of allergic manifestations such as urticaria and asthma.

The presence of an hereditary deficiency of the enzyme kynureninase was suggested, but no enzyme assays were performed. Problems of interpretation of abnormal tryptophan load tests have been discussed on pp. 167–70. These considerations are particularly important in this instance, since Knapp administered relatively high doses of tryptophan (10 g), which may induce apparent abnormalities in normal subjects (Coon, 1966). For these reasons, it is not at all clear that a clinical entity has been defined by the above observations or, if so, what enzyme system is disturbed.

Pathogenesis of the pyridoxine responsive disorders

The pathogenesis of the pyridoxine responsive disorders remains unknown. However, a number of observations suggest that hereditary or acquired defects in pyridoxal phosphate dependent enzymes may be responsible.

An hereditary incidence of all three disorders has been noted: all three conditions have been described in siblings. In the case of pyridoxine-responsive anemia, a sex-linked hereditary pattern has been noted in several families. In many instances, inherited disorders may be related to the lack of a specific enzyme.

In some cases, pyridoxine responsive anemia appears to be acquired late in life, rather than inherited. Acquired defects in an enzyme system or systems might be postulated under these circumstances; for example, the presence of enzyme inhibitors must be considered.

Evidence will be summarized below suggesting that one pyrodixal-phosphate-dependent enzyme system is defective in each of the pyrodixine-responsive disorders. In the case of pyridoxine responsive anemia, the affected enzyme appears to the *ALA synthetase;* in that of cystathioninuria, *cystathionase*; and in that of pyridoxine dependency, *glutamic acid decarboxylase.*

Pyridoxine responsive anemia. ALA synthetase catalyses the formation of Δ-aminolevulinic acid (ALA) from succinyl coenzyme A and glycine, a reaction that requires pyridoxal phosphate as a cofactor (Schulman and Richert, 1957). ALA is an essential precursor to heme, the prosthetic group of hemoglobin (Fig. 5). A number of defects present in patients with pyridoxine responsive anemia could be explained by defective heme synthesis, including the hypochromia of the erythrocytes, the decreased erythrocyte porphyrins and the disturbances in iron metabolism. The latter occur because, in the absence of protoporphyrin, iron cannot be incorporated into the hemoglobin molecule; it consequently accumulates in mitochondria, leading to the formation of ringed sideroblasts and siderocytes. Iron which is not utilized also accumulates in serum, resulting in an elevated plasma iron level.

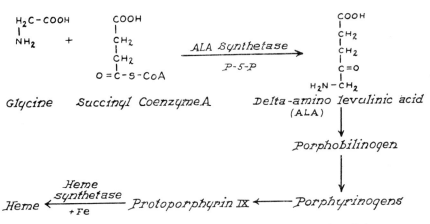

FIG. 5. The biosynthesis of heme. Pyridoxal-5-phosphate (P-5-P) is a co-factor in the synthesis of delta-amino levulinic acid (ALA).

Direct assays of ALA synthetase are very difficult to carry out in human hematopoietic tissues. In two patients with pyridoxine responsive anemia (Labbe, 1964; Vogler and Mingioli, 1965), *in vitro* heme synthesis by bone marrow cells or reticulocytes in the presence of ^{14}C-labeled glycine or ALA was studied. Synthesis from ALA proceeded normally, but synthesis from glycine was impaired, findings which are consistent with defective ALA synthesis.

There are a few observations *in vivo* that may be cited as evidence for defective ALA synthesis in pyridoxine responsive anemia. In patients with this disorder, the free erythrocyte porphyrin is usually reduced, and increases to normal levels on therapy, a response which is similar to that of the deficient animal. This observation suggests that a defect in the synthesis of protoporphyrin has been overcome by the therapy. Perhaps even more interesting is the observation that the free porphyrins may rise strikingly with pyridoxine therapy when the blood hemoglobin concentration remains unchanged (Bottomley, 1965; Lee *et al.*, 1966), a phenomenon that is not observed in normal individuals. In the patients in which such a response has been seen, a block at the step in which iron combines with protoporphyrin has been postulated. This second block enables one to detect the *in vivo* effect of pyridoxine therapy on porphyrin synthesis.

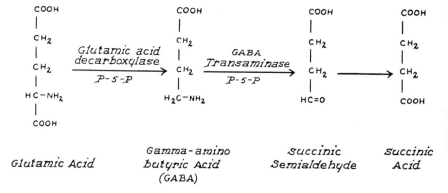

FIG. 6.   The metabolism of γ-amino butyric acid (GABA). Pyridoxal-5-phosphate is a co-factor in both the synthesis and utilization of GABA.

Pyridoxine dependency. In this disorder, a malfunction of the enzyme glutamic acid decarboxylase (GAD) has been suggested (Scriver, 1960). This enzyme, present only in nervous tissue, is essential for the synthesis of γ-aminobutyric acid (GABA) (Fig. 6). GABA is a substrate for oxidative energy metabolism of the brain, and is, in addition, a neuro-depressant; a physiologic role as a feedback inhibitor in neuronal function has been proposed (Roberts *et al.*, 1964).

No assays for GAD or GABA have been performed in pyridoxine-dependent children, because of obvious difficulties in obtaining the appropriate tissues. An *in vivo* study which bears on the matter is that of Sokoloff *et al.* (1959). These investigators measured the oxygen consumption of the brain in a child with pyridoxine dependency. Oxygen consumption dropped markedly when pyridoxine therapy was interrupted and during the seizures that followed. When pyridoxine therapy was re-instituted, oxygen consumption increased. This type of response is the reverse of that seen when seizures are induced by electroshock or metrazol, is similar to that seen with seizures due to hypoglycemia, and implies the lack of a substrate essential to cerebral oxidative metabolism. The authors suggested that GABA might be the deficient substrate.

In vitamin B$_6$ deficient animals, GAD activity is decreased and may be restored to normal by the addition of pyridoxal phosphate (Roberts *et al.*, 1951). Administration of large amounts of GABA resulted in the temporary alleviation of seizures in deficient animals (Roberts *et al.*, 1958), and in a pyridoxine dependent child (Marie, 1960). Large doses are necessary because of a significant blood-brain barrier to GABA.

Despite these observations, there is lack of agreement on the role of GAD or GABA in this syndrome, and in the seizures of vitamin B$_6$ deficiency (Holtz and Palm, 1964; Roberts, 1964).

Cystathioninuria. This disease is presumed to be a consequence of the hereditary lack of cystathionase. This enzyme catalyses one step in the catabolism of methionine, namely, the degradation of cystathionine to cysteine and homoserine (Matsuo and Greenberg, 1958) (Fig. 7). Frimpter (1965) assayed the activity of this enzyme in liver tissue obtained at biopsy from two patients with cystathioninuria and found it to be markedly decreased as compared with normal. Finkelstein *et al.* (1965) confirmed this observation with hepatic tissue from another patient.

Alternate hypotheses. Another way in which a pyridoxine responsive disorder could come about would be through a disturbance in the metabolic pathways leading to pyridoxal phosphate formation (p. 156). Deficiencies in pyridoxine phosphate oxidase or in pyridoxal kinase could lead to cellular deficiency of pyridoxal phosphate despite an adequate supply of dietary vitamin B$_6$. Almost no data are available regarding the activity of these enzymes in human disorders. As was noted by Snell (1964), a defect in pyridoxine phosphate oxidase should result in a disorder that would be responsive to pyridoxal but not pyridoxine. A deficiency in pyridoxal kinase, on the other hand, might lead to a disorder more responsive to phosphorylated vitamin B$_6$ derivatives than to their non-phosphorylated counterparts.

Such responses have not been reported in human disease syndromes, but few studies have been done. In at least one case of pyridoxine responsive anemia (Raab *et al.*, 1961), no additional effects were noted when either pyridoxal or pyridoxamine were added to the regimen. It should be noted that microbiological models for the above syndromes exist. Certain lactobacilli, for example, lack pyridoxine phosphate oxidase and cannot utilize pyridoxine for growth, others lack pyridoxal kinase and require phosphorylated vitamin B_6 derivatives.

Still another mechanism that might produce an increased need for pyridoxine would be excessive excretion of the vitamin. Such an abnormality might result from increased hepatic aldehyde oxidase activity, from

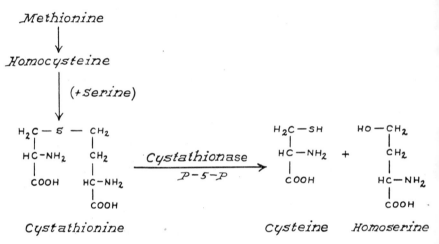

FIG. 7.   The metabolism of cystathionine. Pyridoxal-5-phosphate (P-5-P)
is a co-factor for the enzyme cystathionase.

a renal defect or from deficient tissue binding of vitamin B_6. Some early observations in pyridoxine dependency in infants suggested an abnormal excretory pattern of vitamin B_6 metabolites (Coursin, 1960; Scriver, 1960). Excretion of active forms of the vitamin was higher in relation to 4-pyridoxic acid excretion than was the case in normal infants. More recent investigations in 5 patients disclosed no differences in the excretory pattern (Scriver and Cullen, 1965).

Some investigators have cited the occasionally observed abnormalities in the tryptophan load test as evidence for disordered vitamin B_6 metabolism, or for cellular vitamin B_6 lack in patients with pyridoxine responsive anemia. It should be noted that an abnormal tryptophan load test cannot at present be considered to be specific for abnormal vitamin B_6

metabolism, since abnormalities in the test have been described in a wide variety of diseases in which other evidence for abnormal vitamin B_6 function was lacking (see p. 170).

Mode of action of pyridoxine

If one accepts the thesis that the pyridoxine responsive disorders represent enzymatic defects, how might the effect of pyridoxine be explained? Certainly, it is unusual for the administration of a coenzyme to increase the activity of an enzyme system when the enzyme itself is defective.

Non-enzymatic effects of pyridoxal phosphate. Reference has previously been made to the observations which established that pyridoxal phosphate could accomplish chemically and non-enzymatically any of the reactions which occur in association with an enzyme (pp. 157–58). Whether this property of pyridoxal has any relation to its pharmacological effects remains uncertain, however, since unphysiological conditions of pH and temperature are usually necessary before these reactions can be made to work non-enzymatically.

Defective coenzyme-apoenzyme binding. Scriver (1960) has suggested that the nature of the defect in the apoenzyme system in pyridoxine dependency is such that an increased amount of pyridoxal phosphate is required for normal enzymatic activity. An example of this kind of defect might be an amino-acid substitution involving the coenzyme binding site of the apoenzyme and resulting in decreased affinity of enzyme for coenzyme. Possibly such a defect could be overcome by increasing co-enzyme concentration.

A similar mechanism has been proposed to explain cystathioninuria (Frimpter, 1965), and some experimental data were presented in support of the thesis. Cystathionase activity was found to be decreased in tissue obtained at liver biopsy from two patients with cystathioninuria. Furthermore, the *in vitro* addition of pyridoxal phosphate corrected the defect. On the other hand, Finkelstein *et al.* (1965), using different assay conditions, was able to confirm the enzyme defect, but not its correction by added pyridoxal phosphate.

Chelation of toxic substances. Another possible mode of action of pyridoxine is the removal of inhibition of an enzyme system by chelation

G

of an inhibitory substance. Such a theory was proposed by Bishop and Bethell (1959), as an explanation for pyridoxine responsive anemia. They suggested that ALA synthetase was inhibited by the excessive amount of intracellular iron present, and that pyridoxine was effective because it chelated the toxic iron. Some biochemical support for such an effect of iron was noted by Brown (1958), who found that heme synthesis could be inhibited *in vitro* by excessive amounts of added iron. A strong point against this attractive hypothesis was made by Horrigan and Harris (1964) who removed their patient's excessive iron load by phlebotomy over a long period of time. After removal of the iron the patient was still anemic and the anemia was still responsive to pyridoxine.

DOSAGE AND TOXICITY

Pyridoxine hydrochloride is the form of vitamin B_6 that is ordinarily employed for therapeutic use. For most purposes, the oral route of administration is entirely satisfactory. However, parenteral preparations are also available and may be used in patients with malabsorption, or in situations in which a rapid response is desirable, for example, in the treatment of convulsions in infants.

No toxic effects of pyridoxine have been described in man. When enormous doses have been employed, convulsions and other neurologic symptoms have been produced in several species of laboratory animals. The median lethal dose for orally administered pyridoxine was 5.5 gm/kg in rats (Unna, 1954).

Because of the lack of toxicity and the low cost of pyridoxine, little effort has been made to determine the minimal effective dose in the various pyridoxine responsive disorders. It is probable that the quantities used were often greatly in excess of needs. As much as 200 mg per day have been used for the therapy of pyridoxine dependency in infants or of pyridoxine responsive anemia. Under some circumstances, the distinction between vitamin deficiency and a pyridoxine "responsive" disorder can be made by a more conservative approach to therapy. For example, a 10-day trial of 2–5 mg of pyridoxine per day should result in relief of symptoms due to deficiency. On the other hand, there are no known contraindications to very large doses whenever the clinical situation warrants their use.

When pyridoxine is administered with agents such as INH (Biehl and

Vilter, 1954a; Carlson *et al.*, 1956) or cycloserine (Epstein *et al.*, 1959), 40 mg per day has been adequate to prevent neurologic complication. A need for pyridoxine supplementation in patients receiving D-penicillamine has not been established. Gibbs and Walshe (1966) have suggested, however, that a pyridoxine supplement may be warranted in such patients during periods of rapid growth, or if they become pregnant, or if their dose of D-penicillamine is as much as 40 mg/kg per day.

In most of the conditions in which abnormalities in tryptophan metabolism, correctable with pyridoxine therapy, have been described, no clinical benefit from such therapy was reported.

REFERENCES

(a) BOOKS, REVIEWS, AND MONOGRAPHS

AXELROD, A. E. and TRAKATELLIS, A. C. (1964). Relationship of pyridoxine to immunological phenomena. *Vitam. Horm.*, 22: 591–608.
BRAUNSTEIN, A. E. (1960). Pyridoxal phosphate. In: *The Vitamins*, 2nd ed., vol. 2, pp. 113–84. BOYER, P. D., LARDY, H. and MYRBACK, K. (Ed.). Academic Press, New York.
COURSIN, D. B. (1964a). Vitamin B$_6$ metabolism in infants and children. *Vitam. Horm.* 22: 756–86.
EFRON, M. (1965). Aminoaciduria. *New Engl. J. Med.*, 272: 1058–67, 1107–13.
GREENBERG, L. D. (1964). Arteriosclerotic, dental and hepatic lesions in pyridoxine deficient monkeys. *Vitam. Horm.*, 22: 677–94.
HARRIS, J. W. and HORRIGAN, D. L. (1964). Pyridoxine-responsive anemia—prototype and variations on the theme. *Vitam. Horm.*, 22: 722–55.
HARRIS, R. S., WOOL, I. G. and LORRAINE, J. A. (Eds.) (1964). International Symposium on Vitamin B$_6$ in honor of Professor Paul György. *Vitam. Horm.*, 22: 359–885.
HOLTZ, P. (1959). Role of L-dopa decarboxylase in the biosynthesis of catecholamines in nervous tissue and the adrenal medulla. *Pharmacol. Rev.*, 11: 317–29.
HOLTZ, P. and PALM, D. (1964). Pharmacological aspects of vitamin B$_6$. *Pharmacol. Rev.*, 16: 113–78.
HORRIGAN, D. L. and HARRIS, J. W. (1964). Pyridoxine-responsive anemia: analysis of 62 cases. *Adv. Int. Med.*, 12: 103–74.
ROBERTS, E., WEIN, J., SIMONSEN, D. G. (1964). Gamma-aminobutyric acid (gamma ABA), vitamin B$_6$ and neuronal function—A speculative synthesis. *Vitam. Horm.*, 22: 504–60.
SAUBERLICH, H. E. (1964). Human requirements for vitamin B$_6$. *Vitam. Horm.*, 22: 807–23.
SNELL, E. E. (1958). Chemical structure in relation to biological activities of Vitamin B$_6$. *Vitam. Horm.*, 16: 78–125.
SNELL, E. E. (1961). The role of vitamin B$_6$ in catalysis of reactions of amino acids. In: *The Mechanism of Action of Water-Soluble Vitamins*, pp. 18–31. DEREUCK, A. V. S. and O'CONNOR, M. (Ed.). Little, Brown, Boston.

SNELL, E. E. (1963). Some enzymatic transformations of vitamin B_6 and their inhibition. In: *Proc. 5th Int. Congr. Biochem*, vol. IV, pp. 268–77. DESUIELLE, P. A. E. (Ed.). MacMillan, New York.
SNELL, E. E. (1964). Some notes on the metabolism of vitamin B_6. *Vitam. Horm.*, **22**: 485–94.
SNELL, E. E. and KEEVIL, C. S., JR. (1954). Pyridoxine and related compounds. IX. Occurrence in foods. In: *The Vitamins*, vol. 3, pp. 255–63. SEBRELL, W. H., JR. and HARRIS, R. S. (Ed.). Academic Press, New York.
STORVICK, C. A. and PETERS, J. M. (1964). Methods for the determination of vitamin B_6 in biological materials. *Vitam. Horm.*, **22**: 833–54.
TOWER, D. B. (1956). Neurochemical aspects of pyridoxine metabolism and function. *Amer. J. clin. Nutr.*, **4**: 329–45.
UNNA, K. R. (1954). Pyridoxine and related compounds. XI. Pharmacology. In: *The Vitamins*, vol. 3, pp. 290–3. SEBRELL, W. H., JR. and HARRIS, R. S. (Ed.). Academic Press, New York.

(b) ORIGINAL PAPERS

ALEXANDER, N. and GREENBERG, D. M. (1956). Studies on the purification and properties of the serine-forming enzyme system. *J. biol. Chem.*, **220**: 775–85.
APOSHIAN, H. V. (1961). Biochemical and pharmacological properties of the metal-binding agent penicillamine. *Fed. Proc.*, **20**: Suppl. 10, 185–88.
APOSHIAN, H. V. and APOSHIAN, M. M. (1959). N-acetyl-DL-penicillamine, a new oral protective agent against the lethal effects of mercuric chloride. *J. Pharmacol. exp., Ther.*, **126**: 131–35.
ASATOOR, A. M. (1964). Pyridoxine deficiency in the rat produced by D-penicillamine. *Nature, Lond.*, **203**: 1382–83.
AWAPARA, J., LANDAU, A. J., FUERST, R. and SEALE, B. (1950). Free gamma-aminobutyric acid in brain. *J. biol. Chem.*, **187**: 35–9.
BAKER, E. M., CANHAM, J. E., NUNES, W. T., SAUBERLICH, H. E. and McDOWELL, M. E. (1964). Vitamin B_6 requirement for adult man. *Amer. J. clin. Nutr.*, **15**: 59–66.
BARANOWSKI, T., ILLINGWORTH, B., BROWN, D. H. and CORI, C. F. (1957). The isolation of pyridoxal-5-phosphate from crystalline muscle phosphorylase. *Biochim. biophys. Acta (Amst.)*, **25**: 16–21.
BEATON, J. R., BEARE, J. L., BEATON, G. H., CALDWELL, E. F., OZAWA, G. and McHENRY, E. W. (1954). Studies on vitamin B_6. V. Chronological sequence of biological defects in the vitamin B_6 deprived rat. *J. biol. Chem.*, **207**: 385–91.
BERLOW, S. and EFRON, M. (1964). *Studies in cystathioninuria*. Presented at Meeting of Midwest Society for Pediatrics Research, Winnipeg. October 13, 1964. Quoted in: EFRON, M. (1965).
BESSEY, O. A., ADAM, D. J. D. and HANSEN, A. E. (1957). Intake of vitamin B_6 and infantile convulsions: A first approximation of requirements in infants. *Pediatrics*, **20**: 33–44.
BIEHL, J. P. and VILTER, R. W. (1954a). Effects of isoniazid on pyridoxine metabolism. *J. Amer. med. Ass.*, **156**: 1549–52.
BIEHL, J. P. and VILTER, R. W. (1954b). Effect of isoniazid on vitamin B_6 metabolism; Its possible significance in producing isoniazid neuritis. *Proc. Soc. exp. Biol., N.Y.*, **85**: 389–92.
BINKLEY, F., CHRISTENSEN, G. M. and JENSEN, W. N. (1952). Pyridoxine and the transfer of sulfur. *J. biol. Chem.*, **194**: 109–13.

BIRD, F. H., KRATZER, F. H., ASMUNDSEN, V. S. and LEPKOVSKY, S. (1943). Pyridoxine deficiency in turkeys. *Proc. Soc. exp. Biol., N.Y.*, **52**: 44–5.

BISHOP, R. C. and BETHELL, F. H. (1959). Hereditary hypochromic anemia with transfusion hemosiderosis treated with pyridoxine. *New. Engl. J. Med.*, **261**: 486–9.

BOTTOMLEY, S. S. (1965). Observations on free erythrocyte protoporphyrin in sideroachrestic anemia. *Clin. Chim. Acta*, **12**: 542–5.

BOWMAN, W. D., JR. (1961). Abnormal ("ringed") sideroblasts in various hematologic and non-hematologic disorders. *Blood*, **18**: 662–71.

BOXER, G. E., PRUSS, M. D. and GOODHEART, R. S. (1957). Pyridoxal-5-phosphoric acid in whole blood and isolated leukocytes of man and animals. *J. Nutr.*, **63**: 623–36.

BROWN, E. G. (1958). Evidence of involvement of ferrous iron in the biosynthesis of delta-aminolevulinic acid by chicken erythrocyte preparations. *Nature, Lond.*, **182**: 313–15.

BUSH, J. A., JENSEN, W. N., ASHENBRUCKER, H., CARTWRIGHT, G. E. and WINTROBE, M. M. (1956). The kinetics of iron metabolism in swine with various experimentally induced anemias. *J. Exp. Med.*, **103**: 161–71.

CARLSON, H. B., ANTHONY, E. M., RUSSELL, W. F., JR. and MIDDLEBROOK, G. (1956). Prophylaxis of isoniazed neuropathy with pyridoxine. *New Engl. J. Med.*, **255**: 118–22.

CARTWRIGHT, G. E., KURTH, D. and WINTROBE, M. M. (1963). Hematologic response of pyridoxine deficient swine to pyridoxine. *Proc. Soc. exp. Biol., N.Y.*, **114**: 7–9.

CARTWRIGHT, G. E. and WINTROBE, M. M. (1948). Studies on free erythrocyte protoporphyrin, plasma copper, and plasma iron in normal and in pyridoxine deficient swine. *J. biol. Chem.*, **172**: 557–65.

CHEN, S. C., WONG, P. Y. C. and OGURO, M. (1964). Experimental production of pyridoxine deficiency in rats. *Blood*, **23**: 679–87.

CHENEY, M. C., CURRY, D. M. and BEATON, G. H. (1965). Blood transaminase activity in vitamin B₆ deficiency: Specificity and sensitivity. *Canad. J. Physiol. Pharmacol.*, **43**: 579–89.

CHICK, H., ELSADR, M. M. and WORDEN, A. M. (1940). Occurrence of fits of an epileptiform nature in rats maintained for long periods on a diet deprived of vitamin B₆. *Biochem. J.*, **34**: 595–600.

COTTON, H. B. and HARRIS, J. W. (1962). Familial pyridoxine-responsive anemia. *J. clin. Invest.*, **41**: 1352.

COURSIN, D. B. (1954). Convulsive seizures in infants with pyridoxine deficient diet. *J. Amer. med. Assoc.*, **154**: 406–8.

COURSIN, D. B. (1960). Seizures in vitamin B₆ deficiency. In: *Inhibition of the Nervous System and Gamma Amino Butyric Acid*, pp. 294–301. ROBERTS, E. (Ed.), Pergamon Press, London.

COURSIN, D. B. (1964b). Recommendations for standardization of the tryptophan load test. *Amer. J. clin. Nutr.*, **14**: 56–61.

COURSIN, D. B. and BROWN, V. C. (1961). Changes in vitamin B₆ during pregnancy. *Amer. J. Obstet. Gynec.*, **51**: 82–6.

CREPALDI, G. and PARPAJOLA, A. (1964). Excretion of tryptophan metabolites in different forms of haemoblastosis. *Clin. chim. Acta*, **9**: 106–17.

CUNNINGHAM, E. and SNELL, E. E. (1945). The vitamin B₆ group. VI. The comparative stability of pyridoxine, pyridoxamine and pyrodoxal. *J. biol. Chem.*, **158**: 491–5.

DAVENPORT, V. D. and DAVENPORT, H. W. (1948). Brain excitability in pyridoxine deficient rats. *J. Nutr.*, **36**: 263–75.

DAWSON, A. M., HOLDSWORTH, C. D. and PITCHER, C. S. (1964). Sideroblastic anaemia in adult coeliac disease. *Gut*, **5**: 304–8.

186 *Hematopoietic Agents*

DEISS, A., KURTH, D., CARTWRIGHT, G. E. and WINTROBE, M. M. (1966). Experimental production of siderocytes. *J. clin. Invest.*, **45**: 353–64.
EPSTEIN, I. G., NAIR, K. G., MULINOS, M. G. and HABER, A. (1959). Pyridoxine and its relation to cycloserine neurotoxicity. A pharmacological and clinical study. *Antibiot. Ann.*, pp. 472–81.
ERSLEV, A. J., LEAR, A. A. and CASTLE, W. B. (1960). Pyridoxine responsive anemia. *New Engl. J. Med.*, **262**: 1209–14.
FLINN, J. H., PRICE, J. M., YESS, N. and BROWN, R. R. (1964). Excretion of tryptophan metabolites by patients with rheumatoid arthritis. *Arthr. and Rheum.*, **7**: 201–10.
FOOD AND NUTRITION BOARD (1964). *Recommended dietary allowances.* National Acad. Sci. National Res. Council Publ. 1146.
FOUTS, P. J., HELMER, O. M., LEPKOVSKY, S. and JUKES, T. H. (1938). Production of microcytic hypochromic anemia in puppies on synthetic diet deficient in rat antidermatitis factor (vitamin B_6). *J. Nutr.*, **16**: 197–207.
FOUTS, P. J. and LEPKOVSKY, S. (1942). A green pigment producing compound in urine of pyridoxine-deficient dogs. *Proc. Soc. exp. Biol., N.Y.*, **50**: 221–2.
FRIMPTER, G. W. (1965). Cystathioninuria: nature of the defect. *Science*, **149**: 1095.
FRIMPTER, G. W., HAYMOVITZ, A. and HORWITH, M. (1963). Cystathioninuria. *New Engl. J. Med.*, **268**: 333–9.
GANROT, P. O., ROSENGREN, A. M. and ROSENGREN, E. (1961). On the presence of different histidine decarboxylating enzymes in mammalian tissues. *Experientia, Basel*, **17**: 263–4.
GARDNER, F. H. and NATHAN, D. S. (1962). Hypochromic anemia and hemochromatosis. Response to combined testosterone, pyridoxine and liver extract therapy. *Amer. J. med. Sci.*, **243**: 447–57.
GARTY, R., YONIS, Z., BRAHAM, J. and STEINITZ, K. (1962). Pyridoxine-dependent convulsions in an infant. *Arch. Dis. Childh.*, **37**: 21–4.
GIBBS, K. and WALSHE, J. M. (1966). Penicillamine and pyridoxine requirements in man. *Lancet*, **1**: 175–9.
GREENBERG, L. D., BOHR, D. F., McGRATH, H. and RINEHART, J. F. (1949). Xanthurenic acid excretion in the human subject on a pyridoxine deficient diet. *Arch. Biochem.*, **21**: 237–9.
GREENBERG, L. D. and RINEHART, J. F. (1948). Xanthurenic acid excretion in pyridoxine deficient Rhesus monkeys. *Fed. Proc.*, **7**: 157.
GYÖRGY, P. (1934). Vitamin B_2 and the pellagra like dermatitis in rats. *Nature, Lond.*, **133**: 498–9.
GYÖRGY, P. (1938). Crystalline vitamin B_6. *J. Amer. chem. Soc.*, **60**: 983–4.
GYÖRGY, P. and ECKHARDT, R. E. (1939). Vitamin B_6 and skin lesions in rats. *Nature, Lond.*, **144**: 512.
HAGBERG, B., HAMFELT, A. and HANSSON, O. (1964). Epileptic children with disturbed tryptophan metabolism treated with vitamin B_6. *Lancet*, **1**: 145.
HAMFELT, A. (1964). Age variation in vitamin B_6 metabolism in man. *Clin. chim. Acta*, **10**: 48–54.
HARRIS, H., PENROSE, L. S. and THOMAS, D. H. H. (1959). Cystathioninuria. *Ann. hum. Genet.*, **23**: 442–53.
HARRIS, J. W., WHITTINGTON, R. M., WEISMAN, R. and HORRIGAN, D. L. (1956). Pyridoxine responsive anemia in the human adult. *Proc. Soc. exp. Biol., N.Y.*, **91**: 427–32.
HARRIS, S. A. and FOLKERS, K. (1939). Synthesis of vitamin B_6. *J. Amer. chem. Soc.*, **61**: 1245–7.
HARRIS, S. A., HEYL, D. and FOLKERS, D. (1944). The vitamin B_6 group. II. The structure and synthesis of pyridoxamine and pyridoxal. *J. Amer. chem. Soc.*, **66**: 2088–92.

HAWKINS, W. W., MACFARLAND, M. C. and McHENRY, E. W. (1946). Nitrogen metabolism in pyridoxine deficiency. *J. biol. Chem.*, **166**: 223–9.

HEGSTED, D. M. and RAO, M. N. (1945) Nutritional Studies with the Duck. II. Pyridoxine deficiency. *J. Nutr.*, **30**: 367–74.

HEILMEYER, L. (1958). Anemies sideroachrestiques. *Sang.*, **29**: 465–75.

HESSELTINE, H. C. (1946). Pyridoxine Failure in Nausea and Vomiting of Pregnancy. *Amer. J. Obstet. Gynec.*, **51**: 82–6.

HILLMAN, R. W., CABAUD, P. G., NILSSON, D. E., ARPIN, P. D. and TUFANA, R. J. (1963). Pyridoxine supplementation during pregnancy. Clinical and laboratory observations. *Amer. J. clin. Nutr.*, **12**: 427–30.

HORRIGAN, D. L. (1961). Unidentified erythropoietic substance in liver. *Blood*, **18**: 535–42.

HOVE, E. L. and HERNDON, J. F. (1957). Vitamin B$_6$ deficiency in rabbits. *J. Nutr.*, **61**: 127–36.

HUFF, J. W. and PERLZWEIG, W. A. (1944). A product of oxidative metabolism of pyridoxine, 2-methyl-3-hydroxy-4-carboxy-5-hydroxy-methylpyridine-4-pyridoxic acid. *J. biol. Chem.*, **155**: 345–55.

HUNT, A. D. (1957). Abnormally high pyridoxine requirement. Summary of evidence suggesting relation between this finding and clinical pyridoxine "deficiency". *Amer. J. clin. Nutr.*, **5**: 561–5.

HUNT, A. D., JR., STOKES, J., JR., McCRORY, W. W. and STROUD, H. H. (1954). Pyridoxine dependency: A report of a case of intractable convulsions in an infant controlled by pyridoxine. *Pediatrics*, **13**: 140–5.

HURWITZ, J. (1952). The enzymic phosphorylation of vitamin B$_6$ derivatives and their effects on tyrosine decarboxylase. *Biochim. biophys. Acta*, **9**: 496–8.

HURWITZ, J. (1953). The enzymatic phosphorylation of pyridoxal. *J. biol. Chem.*, **205**: 935–47.

HURWITZ, J. (1955). Enzymatic phosphorylation of vitamin B$_6$ analogues and their effect on tyrosine decarboxylase. *J. biol. Chem.*, **217**: 513–25.

ICHIBA, A. and MICCHI, K. (1938). Crystalline vitamine B$_6$. *Scient. Papers Inst. phys. chem. Res., Tokyo*, **34**: 623–6.

ILLINGWORTH, B. I., JANSZ, H. S., BROWN, D. H. and CORI, C. F. (1958). Observations on the function of pyridoxal-5-phosphate in phosphorylase. *Proc. Nat. Acad. Sci., Washington*, **44**: 1180–91.

JAFFE, I. A., ALTMAN, K. and MERRYMAN, P. (1964). The anti-pyridoxine effect of penicillamine in man. *J. clin. Invest.*, **43**: 1869–73.

JONES, W. A. and JONES, G. P. (1953). Peripheral neuropathy due to isoniazid. *Lancet*, **1**: 1073–4.

JUKES, T. H. (1939). Vitamin B$_6$ deficiency in chicks. *Proc. Soc. exp. Biol., N.Y.*, **42**: 180–2.

KERESZTESY, J. C. and STEVENS, J. R. (1938). Crystalline vitamin B$_6$. *Proc. Soc. exp. Biol., N.Y.*, **38**: 64–5.

KIKUCHI, G., KUMAR, A., TALMEGE, P. and SHEMIN, D. (1958). The enzymatic synthesis of delta-aminolevulinic acid. *J. biol. Chem.*, **233**: 1214–9.

KOHN, R., HEILMEYER, L. and CLOTTEN, R. (1963). Pyridoxine-responsive sideroachrestic anaemia in the course of isoniazid treatment. *Germ. med. Mth.*, **8**: 103–7.

KORNBERG, A., TABOR, H. and SEBRELL, W. H. (1945). Blood regeneration in pyridoxine-deficient rats. *Amer. J. Physiol.*, **143**: 434–9.

KOWLESSAR, O. D., HAEFNER, L. J. and BENSON, G. D. (1964). Abnormal tryptophan metabolism in patients with adult celiac disease with evidence for deficiency of vitamin B$_6$. *J. clin. Invest.*, **43**: 894–903.

KUCHINSKAS, E. J., HORRATH, A. and DUVIGNEAUD, V. (1957). The anti-vitamin B$_6$ action of L-penicillamine. *Arch. Biochem.*, **68**: 69–75.

KUCHINSKAS, E. J. and DUVIGNEAUD, V. (1957). An increased vitamin B_6 requirement in the rat on a diet containing L-penicillamine. *Arch. Biochem.*, **66**: 1–9.

KUHN, R. and WENDT, G. (1938). The adermin (vitamin B_6) isolated from rice paste and yeast. *Berichte deutsch. chem. Gesellschrift.*, **71**: 1118.

KUHN, R., WESTPHAL, K., WENDT, G. and WESTPHAL, O. (1939). Synthesis of adermine. *Naturwissenschrift*, **27**: 469–70.

LABBE, R. (1964). Quoted in HORRIGAN and HARRIS (1964).

LEE, G. R., CARTWRIGHT, G. E. and WINTROBE, M. M. (1966). The response of free erythrocyte protoporphyrin to pyridoxine therapy in a patient with sideroachrestic (sideroblastic) anemia. *Blood*, **27**: 557–67.

LEEVY, C. M., BAKER, H., TEN HOVE, W., FRANK, O. and CHERRICK, G. R. (1965). B-complex vitamins in liver disease of the alcoholic. *Amer. J. clin. Nutr.*, **16**: 339–46.

LEPKOVSKY, S. (1938). Crystalline Factor I. *Science*, **87**: 169–70.

LEPKOVSKY, S. and KRATZER, F. H. (1942). Pyridoxine deficiency in chicks. *J. Nutr.*, **24**: 515–21.

LEPKOVSKY, S. and NIELSEN, E. (1942). A green pigment-producing compound in the urine of pyridoxine-deficient rats. *J. biol. Chem.*, **144**: 135–8.

LEPKOVSKY, S., ROBAZ, E. and HAAGEN-SMIT, A. J. (1943). Xanthurenic acid and its role in the tryptophane metabolism of pyridoxine-deficient rats. *J. biol. Chem.*, **149**: 195–201.

LERNER, A. M., DECARLI, L. M. and DAVIDSON, C. S. (1958). The association of pyridoxine deficiency and convulsions in alcoholism. *J. lab. clin. Med.*, **52**: 920–1.

LEWIS, W. C., CALDEN, G., THURSTON, J. R. and GILSON, W. E. (1957). Psychiatric and neurological reactions to cycloserine in the treatment of tuberculosis. *Dis. Chest*, **32**: 172–82.

LONGENECKER, J. B. and SNELL, E. E. (1956). On the mechanism and optical specificity of transaminase reactions. *Proc. Nat. Acad. Sci., Wash.*, **42**: 221–7.

MANGAY CHUNG, A. S., PEARSON, W. N., DARBY, W. S., MILLER, O. N. and GOLDSMITH, G. A. (1961). Folic acid, vitamin B_6, pantothenic acid and vitamin B_{12} in human dietaries. *Amer. J. clin. Nutr.*, **9**: 573–82.

MARIE, J. (1960). Personal communication, cited in SCRIVER (1960).

MATSUO, Y. and GREENBERG, D. M. (1958). A crystalline enzyme that cleaves homoserine and cystathionine. *J. biol. Chem.*, **230**: 561–71.

MAY, C. D. (1954). Vitamin B_6 in human nutrition: A critique and an object lesson. *Pediatrics*, **14**: 269–79.

McCALL, K. B., WAISMAN, H. A., ELVEHJEM, C. A. and JONES, E. S. (1946). Study of pyridoxine and pantothenic acid deficiencies in the monkey (*Macaca mulatta*). *J. Nutr.*, **31**: 685–97.

McCORMICK, D. B., GREGORY, M. E. and SNELL, E. E. (1961). Pyridoxal phosphokinases. I. Assay, distribution, purification and properties. *J. biol. Chem.*, **236**: 2076–84.

McCORMICK, D. B. and SNELL, E. E. (1961). Pyridoxal phosphokinase. II. Effects of inhibitors. *J. biol. Chem.*, **236**: 2085–8.

McCURDY, D. C. (1963). INH conditioned pyridoxine responsive anemia. *Clin. Res.*, **11**: 59.

McCURDY, P. R. and DONOHOE, R. F. (1966). Pyridoxine-responsive anemia conditioned by isonicotinic acid hydrazide. *Blood*, **27**: 352–62.

McKIBBIN, J. M., SCHAEFER, A. E., FROST, D. V. and ELVEHJEM, C. A. (1942). Studies on anemia in dogs due to pyridoxine deficiency. *J. biol. Chem.*, **142**: 77–84.

McKUSICK, A. B., SHERWIN, R. W., JONES, L. G. and HSU, J. M. (1964). Urinary excretion of pyridoxine and 4-pyridoxic acid in rheumatoid arthritis. *Arthr. Rheum.*, **7**: 636–53.

MCLAREN, B. A., KELLER, E., O'DONNEL, D. J. and ELVEHJEM, C. A. (1947). The nutrition of rainbow trout. I. Studies of vitamin requirements. *Arch. Biochem.*, **15**: 169–78.

METZLER, D. H., IKAWA, M. and SNELL, E. E. (1954). A general mechanism for vitamin B$_6$-catalyzed reactions. *J. Amer. Chem. Soc.*, **76**: 648–52.

MOLLIN, D. L. (1965). Sideroblasts and sideroblastic anemia. *Brit. J. Haemat.*, **11**: 41–51.

MOLONEY, C. J. and PARMELEE, A. H. (1954). Convulsions in young infants as a result of pyridoxine (vitamin B$_6$) deficiency. *J. Amer. Med. Assoc.*, **154**: 405–6.

MUELLER, J. F. (1964). Vitamin B$_6$ in fat metabolism. *Vitam. Horm.*, **22**: 787–96.

MUSHETT, C. W. and EMERSON, G. (1957). Arteriosclerosis in pyridoxine deficient monkeys and dogs. *Fed. Proc.*, **16**: 367.

NELSON, E. H. (1956). Association of Vitamin B$_6$ deficiency with convulsions in infants. *Publ. Hlth Rep., Wash.*, **71**: 445–8.

OKA, M. and LEPPANEN, V. V. E. (1963). Metabolism of tryptophan in diabetes mellitus. *Acta med. Scand.*, **173**: 361–4.

OLSON, N. (1956). Discussion of: RINEHART, J. F. and GREENBERG, L. D. Vitamin B$_6$ deficiency in the rhesus monkey with particular reference to the occurrence of atherosclerosis, dental caries and hepatic cirrhosis. *Amer. J. Clin. Nutr.*, **4**: 327–8.

PEGUM, J. S. (1952). Nicotinic acid and burning feet. *Lancet*, **2**: 536.

PERISSINOTTO, B., BENASSI, C. A. and ALLEGRI, G. (1964). Urinary excretion of tryptophan metabolites in patients with renal pelvis and parenchyma tumours. *Urol. int., Basel*, **17**: 175–82.

PORTER, C. C., CLARK, I. and SILBER, R. H. (1948). The effect of B vitamin deficiencies on tryptophan metabolism in the rat. *Arch. Biochem.*, **18**: 339–43.

PRICE, J. M., BROWN, R. R. and PETERS, H. A. (1959). Tryptophan metabolism in porphyria, schizophrenia, and a variety of neurologic and psychiatric diseases. *Neurology, Minneap.*, **9**: 456–68.

PRICE, J. M., BROWN, R. R., RUKAVINA, J. G., MENDELSON, C. and JOHNSON, S. A. M. (1957). Scleroderma (acrosclerosis). II. Tryptophan metabolism before and during treatment by chelation (EDTA). *J. invest. Derm.*, **29**: 289–98.

RAAB, S. O., HAUT, A., CARTWRIGHT, G. E. and WINTROBE, M. M. (1961). Pyridoxine responsive anemia. *Blood*, **18**: 285–302.

RABINOWITZ, J. C. and SNELL, E. E. (1948). The vitamin B$_6$ group. XIV. Distribution of pyridoxal, pyridoxamine, and pyridoxine in some natural products. *J. biol. Chem.*, **176**: 1157–67.

RABINOWITZ, J. C. and SNELL, E. E. (1949). Vitamin B$_6$ group. XV. Urinary excretion of pyridoxal, pyridoxamine, pyridoxine, and 4-pyridoxic acid in human subjects. *Proc. Soc. exp. Biol., N.Y.*, **70**: 235–40.

RAICA, N., JR. and SAUBERLICH, H. E. (1964). Blood cell transaminase activity in human B$_6$ deficiency. *Amer. J. clin. Nutr.*, **15**: 67–72.

RANKE, E., TAUBER, S. A., HORONICK, A., RANKE, B., GOODHART, R. S. and CHOW, B. F. (1960). Vitamin B$_6$ deficiency in the aged. *J. Geront.*, **15**: 41–4.

REDLEAF, P. D. (1962). Pyridoxine-responsive anemia in a patient receiving isoniazid. *Dis. Chest.*, **42**: 222–6.

ROBERTS, E. and FRANKEL, S. (1950). Gamma-aminobutyric acid in brain: its formation from glutamic acid. *J. biol. Chem.*, **187**: 55–63.

ROBERTS, E. and FRANKEL, S. (1951). Glutamic acid decarboxylase in brain. *J. biol. Chem.*, **188**: 789–95.

ROBERTS, E., ROTHSTEIN, M. and BAXTER, C. F. (1958). Some metabolic aspects of gamma-aminobutyric acid. *Proc. Soc. exp. Biol., N.Y.*, **97**: 796–802.

ROBERTS, E., YOUNGER, F. and FRANKEL, S. (1951). Influence of dietary pyridoxine on glutamic decarboxylase activity of brain. *J. biol. Chem.*, **191**: 277–85.

ROSEN, D. A., MAEGWYN-DAVIES, G. D., BECKER, B., STONE, H. H. and FRIEDENWALD, J. S. (1955). Xanthurenic acid excretion studies on diabetics with and without retinopathy. *Proc. Soc. exp. Biol., N.Y.*, **88**: 321–3.

ROSS, R. R. (1958). Use of pyridoxine hydrochloride to prevent isoniazid toxicity. *J. Amer. Med. Assoc.*, **168**: 273–5.

ROZE, V. and STRAMINGER, J. L. (1963). The non-enzymatic reaction between D-cycloserine and pyridoxal phosphate. *Fed. Proc.*, **22**: 423.

RUNDLES, R. W. and FALLS, H. F. (1946). Hereditary (? sex-linked) anemia. *Amer. J. Med. Sci.*, **211**: 641–58.

RUNYAN, T. J. and GERSHOFF, S. N. (1965). The effect of vitamin B_6 deficiency in rats on the metabolism of oxalic acid precursors. *J. biol. Chem.*, **240**: 1889–92.

SARETT, H. P. (1951). A study of the measurement of 4-pyridoxic acid in urine. *J. biol. Chem.*, **189**: 769–77.

SCHULMAN, M. P. and RICHERT, D. A. (1957). Heme synthesis in vitamin B_6 and pantothenic acid deficiencies. *J. biol. Chem.*, **226**: 181–9.

SCHWARTZ, R. and KJELDGAARD, N. O. (1951). The enzymatic oxidation of pyridoxal by liver aldehyde oxidase. *Biochem. J.*, **48**: 333–7.

SCHWARTZMAN, G. and STRAUSS, L. (1949). Vitamin B_6 deficiency in the Syrian hamster. *J. Nutr.*, **38**: 131–53.

SCHWEIGERT, B. S. and PEARSON, P. B. (1947). Effect of vitamin B_6 deficiency on the ability of rats and mice to convert tryptophane to N′-methylnicotinamide and nicotinic acid. *J. biol. Chem.*, **168**: 555–67.

SCHWEIGERT, B. S., SAUBERLICH, H. E., ELVEHJEM, C. A. and BAUMANN, C. A. (1946). Dietary protein and the vitamin B_6 content of mouse tissue. *J. biol. Chem.*, **165**: 187–96.

SCRIVER, C. R. (1960). Vitamin B_6-dependency and infantile convulsions. *Pediatrics*, **26**: 62–74.

SCRIVER, C. R. and CULLEN, A. M. (1965). Urinary vitamin B_6 and 4-pyridoxic acid in health and in vitamin B_6 dependency. *Pediatrics*, **36**: 14–20.

SCRIVER, C. R. and HUTCHISON, J. H. (1963). The vitamin B_6 deficiency syndrome in human infancy: biochemical and clinical observations. *Pediatrics*, **31**: 240–50.

SCUDI, J. V., KOONES, H. F. and KERESZTESY, J. C. (1940). Urinary excretion of vitamin B_6 in the rat. *Proc. Soc. exp. Biol., N.Y.*, **43**: 118–22.

SCUDI, J. V., UNNA, K. and ANTOPOL, W. (1940). A study of the urinary excretion of vitamin B_6 by a colorimetric method. *J. biol. Chem.*, **135**: 371–6.

SHEN, S. S. WONG, P. Y. C. and OGURO, N. (1964). Experimental production of pyridoxine deficiency anaemia in rats. *Blood*, **23**: 678–87.

SNELL, E. E. (1944). The vitamin B_6 group. I. Formation of additional members from pyridoxine and evidence concerning their structure. *J. Amer. Chem. Soc.*, **66**: 2082–8.

SNELL, E. E., GIURARD, B. M. and WILLIAMS, R. J. (1942). Occurrence in natural products of a physiologically active metabolite of pyridoxine. *J. biol. Chem.*, **143**: 519–30.

SNELL, E. E. and RANNEFELD, A. N. (1945). The vitamin B_6 group. III. The vitamin activity of pyridoxal and pyridoxamine for various organisms. *J. biol. Chem.*, **157**: 475–89.

SNYDERMAN, S. E. (1955). Vitamin B_6 in infant nutrition. *Merck Rep.*, **64**: 3–6.

SNYDERMAN, S. E., CARRETERO, R. and HOLT, L. E. (1950). Pyridoxine deficiency in the human being. *Fed. Proc.*, **9**: 371–2.

SOKOLOFF, L., LASSEN, N. A., MCKHANN, G. M. and TOWER, D. B. (1959). Effects of pyridoxine withdrawal on cerebral circulation and metabolism in a pyridoxine dependent child. *Nature, Lond.*, **183**: 751–3.

SPIES, T. D., BEAN, W. B. and ASHE, W. F. (1939). A note on the use of vitamin B$_6$ in human nutrition. *J. Amer. Med. Assoc.*, **112**: 2414–5.

STILLER, E. T., KERESZTESY, J. C., STEVENS, J. R. and FOLKERS, H. (1939). The structure of vitamin B$_6$. *J. Amer. Chem. Soc.*, **61**: 1237–45.

SWAN, P., WENTWORTH, J. and LINKSWILER, H. (1964). Vitamin B$_6$ depletion in man: urinary taurine and sulfate excretion and nitrogen balance. *J. Nutr.*, **84**: 220–8.

THERON, J. J. PRETORIUS, P. J., WOLF, H. and JOUBERT, C. P. (1961). The state of pyridoxine nutrition in patients with kwashiorkor. *J. Pediat.*, **59**: 439–50.

UEDA, K., AKEDO, H. and SUDA, M. (1960). Intestinal absorption of amino acids. IV. Participation of pyridoxal phosphate in the active transfer of L-amino acids through the intestinal wall. *J. Biochem., Tokyo*, **48**: 584–92.

UMBREIT, W. W. and WADDELL, J. G. (1949). Mode of action of deoxypyridoxine. *Proc. Soc. exp. Biol., N.Y.*, **70**: 293–9.

VERWILGHEN, R., REYBROUCK, G., CALLENS, L. and COSEMAUS, J. (1965). Antituberculosis drugs and sideroblastic anaemia. *Brit. J. Haemat.*, **11**: 92–8.

DUVIGNEAUD, V., KUCHINSKAS, E. J. and HORVATH, A. (1957). L-penicillamine and rat liver transaminase activity. *Arch. Biochem.*, **69**: 130–7.

VILTER, R. W., MUELLER, J. F., GLAZER, H. S., JARROLD, T., ABRAHAM, J., THOMPSON, C. and HAWKINS, V. R. (1953). The effect of vitamin B$_6$ deficiency induced by desoxypyridoxine in human beings. *J. lab. clin. Med.*, **42**: 335–57.

VOGLER, W. R. and MINGIOLI, E. S. (1965). Heme synthesis in pyridoxine responsive anemia. *New Engl. J. Med.*, **273**: 347–53.

WACHSTEIN, M. and GUDAITIS, A. (1952). Disturbance of vitamin B$_6$ metabolism in pregnancy. *J. lab. clin. Med.*, **40**: 550–7.

WACHSTEIN, M. and GUDAITIS, A. (1953a). Disturbance of vitamin B$_6$ metabolism in pregnancy. II. The influence of various amounts of pyridoxine hydrochloride upon the abnormal tryptophan load test in pregnant women. *J. lab. clin. Med.*, **42**: 98–107.

WACHSTEIN, M. and GUDAITIS, A. (1953b). Disturbance of vitamin B$_6$ metabolism in pregnancy. III. Abnormal vitamin B$_6$ load test. *Amer. J. Obstet. Gynec.*, **66**: 1207–13.

WACHSTEIN, M. and LOBEL, S. (1955). Abnormal tryptophan metabolism in various diseases particularly hyperthyroidism and its relation to vitamin B$_6$. *Fed. Proc.*, **14**: 422.

WACHSTEIN, M. and LOBEL, S. (1956). The relation between tryptophane metabolism and vitamin B$_6$ in various diseases as studied by paper chromatography. *Amer. J. Clin. Path.*, **26**: 910–25.

WADA, H. and SNELL, E. E. (1961). The enzymatic oxidation of pyridoxine and pyridoxamine phosphates. *J. biol. Chem.*, **236**: 2089–95.

WALDINGER, C. and BERG, R. B. (1963). Signs of pyridoxine dependency manifest at birth in siblings. *Pediatrics*, **32**: 161–8.

WILSON, J. E. and DUVIGNEAUD, V. (1950). Inhibition of the growth of the rat by L-penicillamine and its prevention by aminoethanol and related compounds. *J. biol. Chem.*, **184**: 63–70.

WINTROBE, M. M., FOLLIS, R. H., JR., MILLER, M. H., STEIN, H. J., ALCAYAGA, R., HUMPHREYS, S., SUKSTA, A. and CARTWRIGHT, G. E. (1943). Pyridoxine deficiency in swine; with particular reference to anemia, epileptiform convulsions, and fatty liver. *Bull. Johns Hopk. Hosp.*, **72**: 1–25.

WOHL, M. G., LEVY, H. A., SZUTKA, A. and MALDIA, G. (1960). Pyridoxine deficiency in hyperthyroidism. *Proc. Soc. exp. Biol., N.Y.*, **105**: 523–7.

SUPPLEMENTARY BIBLIOGRAPHY

YAMADA, H. and YASUNOBU, K. T. (1962). The nature of the prosthetic groups of plasma amine oxidase. *Biochem. biophys. Res. Commun.*, **8**: 387–90.

ALTMAN, K. and GREENGARD, O. (1966). Correlation of kynurenine excretion with liver tryptophan pyrrolase levels in disease and after hydrocortisone induction. *J. clin. Invest.*, **45**: 1527–34.

BERLOW, S. and EFRON, M. (1966). Studies in cystathioninemia. *Amer. J. Dis. Child.*, **112**: 135–42.

COON, W. W. (1966). The tryptophan load and pyridoxine deficiency. *Amer. J. Clin. Path.*, **46**: 345–8.

FINKELSTEIN, J. D., MUDD, S. H., IRREVERRE, F. and LASTER, L. (1966). Deficiencies of cystathionase and homoserine dehydratase activities in cystathioninuria. *Proc. Nat. Acad. Sci.*, **55**: 865–72.

KNAPP, A. (1962). Genetische Factoren beim Tryptophanstoffwechsel des Menschen. In: *Protides of the biological fluids, Proceedings of the 9th Colloquium*. PEETERS, H. (Ed.). Elsevier, N.Y.

PERRY, T. L., ROBINSON, G. C., TEASDALE, J. M. and HANSEN, S. (1967). Cystathioninuria, nephrogenic diabetes insipidus and anemia. *New Engl. J. Med.*, **276**: 721–5.

SCRIVER, C. R. (1967). Vitamin B_6 deficiency and dependency in man. *Amer. J. Dis. Child.*, **113**: 109–14.

SHAW, K. N. F., LIEBERMANN, E., KOCH, R. and DONNELL, G. N. (1967). Cystathioninuria. *Amer. J. Dis. Child.*, **113**: 119–28.

CHAPTER 4

IRON

J. C. Dreyfus

Université de Paris, Institut de Pathologie Moléculaire,
Groupe I.N.S.E.R.M., Paris, France

IRON is essential to hematopoiesis, for it is a constituent element of hemo-globin. Lack of iron, whatever its origin, thus leads to anemia. An excess of iron may be found in diseases that do not necessarily affect the blood. Very large doses of iron produce harmful effects due to the pharmacological action of iron. This means that, from the therapeutic point of view, iron metabolism involves three problems: the treatment of deficiency, of chronic overload, and of poisoning.

HISTORY

The presence of iron in the tissues has been recognized for more than two centuries: in 1713 Lemmery and Geoffroy demonstrated the metal in tissues. Its presence in hemoglobin was observed in the 19th century, and in 1867 Hoppe-Seyler crystallized hemoglobin. The discovery of cyto-chromes by MacMunn in 1886 was not generally accepted until the publi-cation of Keilin's work in 1925. This date marks the beginning of the modern era.

The presence of iron in serum was discovered in 1925 by Fontès and Thivolle; plasma-transport protein in 1945 by Holmberg and Laurell; and storage protein in 1936 by Laufberger.

The therapeutic value of iron has been known since early antiquity. There have been legends and empirical observations on the subject for more than 3000 years (see Beutler *et al.*, 1963). Paracelsus (1493–1541) introduced iron into medical practice. Lange, and later Sydenham (1624–89), used it against chlorosis. Blaud (1832) was the first to lay down rules for its use. At the beginning of the 20th century iron therapy fell out of favor, but when the need for iron in the synthesis of hemoglobin had been demonstrated (Heath *et al.*, 1932), and still more after studies with radioactive iron pioneered by Hahn in 1939, iron assumed a definitive and important place in therapeutics.

I. BIOLOGICAL COMPOUNDS OF IRON

Iron is on the dividing line between bulk and the trace elements. The adult human body contains no more than about 5 g of it. Yet its presence in all organisms and in all cells, its inclusion in several of the most important constituents of living matter, and our relatively wide knowledge of its biochemistry and physiology give it a special position.

Iron is never found in the mineral state, but always in organic combination. It is usually combined with proteins, but it may or may not be included in particular prosthetic groups.

Of all biochemically active metals, iron is the most versatile; it may be found in a wide variety of biological molecules. However, none of the functions of iron is strictly specific to it, and some people regard its peculiar importance as an accident of evolution.

The following properties of iron account for its usefulness in biological systems (see Dreyfus and Schapira, 1958):

(1) Iron in solution provides a concentration of positive charges. By distorting dipoles, this charge weakens covalent bonds and facilitates their breakage.

(2) The covalent bonds of iron are directed towards the six angles of an octahedron, thus orientating the molecules that enter into combination with it.

(3) Iron can exist in two stable oxidation states, Fe^{2+} and Fe^{3+}, and also in several unstable oxidation states. Iron complexes are intermediates in electron-transfer reactions.

The valency structure of iron complexes is such that iron can exist as divalent Fe^{2+}, or as trivalent Fe^{3+}. Furthermore, the bonding may be either ionic or covalent. In the ionic form, the orbitals of the 3d sub-shell are occupied by unpaired electrons—5 in Fe^{3+} and 4 in Fe^{2+}. In the covalent form, each orbital receives an additional electron from a donor. Only one unpaired electron remains to Fe^{3+}, and none to Fe^{2+}, which in this case forms diamagnetic complexes. Measurement of the magnetic moment allows the number of unpaired electrons to be determined. There is still controversy over the question why certain compounds always assume the covalent form, while others are variable or predominantly ionic.

Eichhorn (1960) has attempted to provide an explanation based on the existence of compounds with high field-intensity, of which the electrons remain in the same orbital, and compounds with low field-intensity of which the electrons do not so remain.

High field-intensity proteins are typified by cytochrome *c*. This molecule acts as a transmitter of electrons, and there is no change in the configuration about the iron atom in the course of transmission. Thus the molecule has the electronic configuration, which confers the maximum of stability upon it: cytochrome *c* has a single unpaired electron in the oxidized state, and is diamagnetic in the reduced state.

This constitution differs from that of other known heminic proteins, hemoglobin as well as enzymes (peroxidases and catalases). In these compounds only five iron bonds are permanent, the sixth being reserved for the substrate, or, in the case of hemoglobin, for oxygen. All these molecules are low field-intensity compounds in the absence of substrate (or oxygen). The sixth position is occupied by water; the iron is in the ionic state, and strongly paramagnetic. When the substrate or oxygen is bound, a high field-intensity complex is formed, and the bonds become covalent.

Iron-containing compounds may be divided into two main categories, according to whether the iron is or is not in the form of heminic compounds. Table 1 shows the distribution of the most important of them in man.

TABLE 1. IRON IN THE HUMAN BODY

Form	Amount, g
Hemoglobin	3.00
Cytochromes, catalase, siderophilin	0.01
Ferritin + hemosiderin	0.70
Muscular iron:	
myoglobin	0.15
non-hemin iron	0.50

A. HEMINIC COMPOUNDS

These are by far the better known. Their iron is combined with a porphyrin—protoporphyrin in hemoglobin, myoglobin, catalase, peroxidases, and cytochrome *b*. In a modified form this compound, known as hem when the iron is divalent, and as hematin when it is trivalent, also provides the prosthetic groups of cytochromes c and a_3. A much less common form is the "*Spirographis* hemin", found in chlorocruorines and cytochrome a.

The protoporphyrin ring is composed of four pyrrole rings joined by methylene bridges to form a ring of 16 carbon atoms and 4 nitrogen atoms, lying in one plane, and stabilized by conjugate double bonds. Naturally-occurring protoporphyrin has 3 kinds of substituent groups: 4 methyl, 2 vinyl, and 2 propionic groups. Since it corresponds with type III etioporphyrin the methyl groups occupy positions 1, 3, 5, and 8. In Fischer's nomenclature of compounds with 3 substituents, it is given the number IX: the vinyl groups are at 2 and 4, and the propionic at 6 and 7.

The iron lies at the centre of the molecule, and is bound to the four nitrogen atoms in the plane of the ring, leaving free two coordinate valencies, of which one is for the protein. Hem or hematin can be found at all levels of life: hematin is an essential growth factor for *H. influenzae* and certain flagellates (Lwoff, 1943).

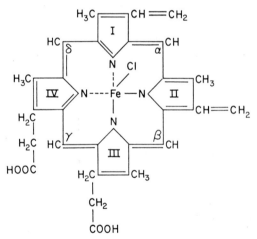

FIG. 1. The structure of hematin.

The bonds between iron and porphyrin are very firm, in hematin even more than in hem; they are unaffected by reagents for ionized iron. Before iron can be estimated in these compounds, it must first be converted to an inorganic form.

Hem gives a broad absorption band in the visible part of the spectrum with maxima at 550 and 575×10^{-6} mm. It also gives the very intense absorption band, common to all porphyrin derivatives, between 400 and 420×10^{-6} mm (Soret's band). However, it has lost the characteristic red fluorescence of the porphyrins.

The combination of hem, or hematin, with proteins produces some of the most important compounds in biochemistry.

Hemoglobins and myoglobin

In hemoglobin, iron is in the divalent state. The hem is combined with a molecule of a specific globin. There are four hem groups in a molecule of hemoglobin, whereas myoglobin contains only one. Hemoglobin contains 0.34% of iron.

State of iron in hemoglobin (Pauling and Coryell, 1936). In the isolated prosthetic group, hem or hematin, iron is combined with porphyrin by ionic bonds; hem and hematin are in effect paramagnetic. Hematin has 5 unpaired electrons in the outer 3d orbital, as in ferric ions; hem, a ferrous compound, has only 4.

Of all the nitrogenous compounds of hem, only reduced hemoglobin is paramagnetic. Its magnetic moment of 5 Bohr magnetons approaches that of ferrous ions.

On the other hand, its compounds with oxygen and carbon monoxide are diamagnetic, which shows that iron completely loses its ionic character in these compounds, and that the binding of oxygen or CO to the sixth coordinate bond of the iron changes the nature of the bonds between iron and porphyrin.

In methemoglobin, where the iron is trivalent and has lost the power of combining reversibly with oxygen, paramagnetism returns: in the acid or neutral state it has five unpaired electrons. In an alkaline medium only three unpaired electrons remain.

Type of bond between iron and protein

Of the two valences of iron that are not combined with porphyrin, one is reserved for binding oxygen and the other provides the bond between the prosthetic group and the globin. The last few years have seen considerable progress in two directions. Firstly, the sequence of all the amino acids in human hemoglobin (141 in the α chain, 146 in the β chain) has been elucidated (Braunitzer *et al.*, 1961; Konigsberg *et al.*, 1961). Secondly, the remarkable work of Kendrew (1962) on myoglobin, and of Perutz (1962, 1964) on hemoglobin, has revealed the tertiary structure of the chains and the spatial relationship of the amino acids. Thus hem is known to be inserted in a crevice in the outer surface of the globin; so the four hem groups are at some distance from each other, which only makes the interaction of hem with hem when oxygen is bound even more of a mystery. The iron atom is linked to a histidine residue in the chain, and more loosely to a second, "distal" histidine. With certain mutations of the chain, where one of these histidines is replaced by another amino acid, the hemglobin is rendered unstable, and readily converted to methemoglobin.These are the M hemoglobins (of which several are already known) which are the basis of the methemoglobinemias (Gerald *et al.*, 1957).

Figs 2 and 3 show the structure of horse hemoglobin according to Kendrew *et al.* (1962), and the sequence of amino acids in the α and β chains of human hemoglobin.

Cytochromes (Nicholls, 1963; Paleus and Paul, 1963)

Numerous kinds of cytochromes have been described in recent years. They still conform to the conventional description of three classes: cytochromes, a (or a_3), b, and c each with a different kind of prosthetic group. In the cytochromes, of which the function is the transmission of electrons, iron changes reversibly from divalent to trivalent form, while remaining, as explained above, bonded by covalent linkage.

The three types of cytochrome differ according to the structure of their prosthetic groups.

(1) The hematin of the b cytochromes is protohematin, identical with that of methemoglobin, retaining the vinyl groups at positions 2 and 4.

(2) In cytochrome c the vinyl groups are saturated, each forming a thio-ester linkage with a cysteine residue of the protein.

(3) The a cytochromes form a more varied group: in the a type hematins one of the lateral chains undergoes oxidation or is saturated. In most cases a methyl group is oxidized to formyl. In cytochrome a_2, one of the pyrrole rings appears to be saturated, giving a chlorhemin structure.

The properties of the various cytochromes cannot be discussed in detail in an article on iron, but certain aspects of comparative biochemistry need consideration.

(1) Now that the amino acid sequences of numerous c-cytochromes from animals and microorganisms are known (Margoliash *et al.*, 1961) it is possible to say which sequences are probably essential—because

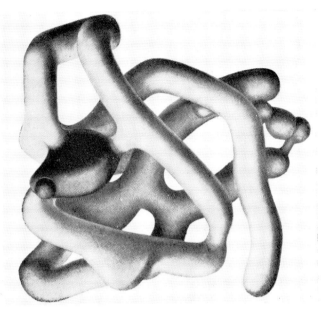

Fig. 2. The shape of the molecule of myoglobin.

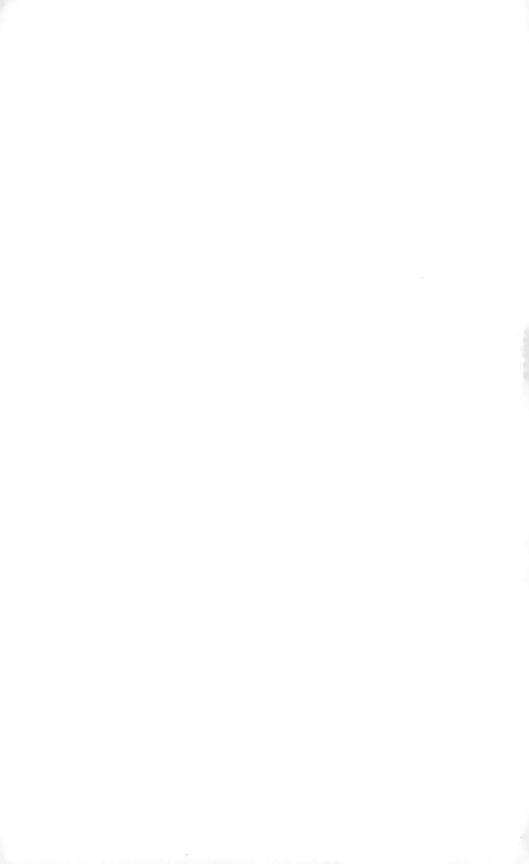

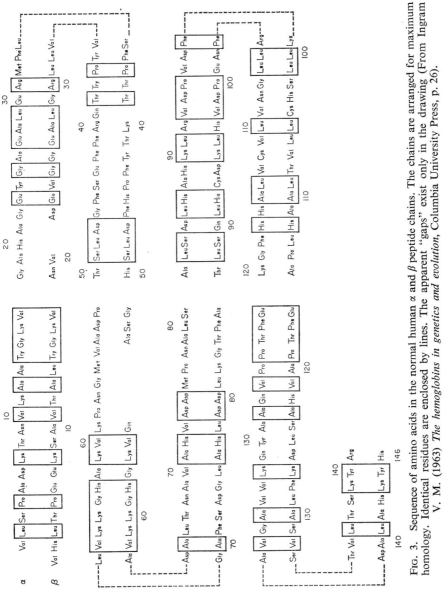

FIG. 3. Sequence of amino acids in the normal human α and β peptide chains. The chains are arranged for maximum homology. Identical residues are enclosed by lines. The apparent "gaps" exist only in the drawing (From Ingram V. M. (1963) *The hemoglobins in genetics and evolution*, Columbia University Press, p. 26).

present in organisms of every level—and which have been modified in the course of evolution.

(2) The evolution of cytochromes, both chemical and physical, probably reflects adaptation to differing biological conditions. The cytochrome system reflects the respiratory needs of the cell: if these are small, cytochromes may be found either in low concentration or with low specific activity.

(3) Lastly, though the chemical function of all cytochromes is the transfer of electrons, they do not necessarily all form part of the respiratory chain. Those of the chloroplasts take part in photosynthetic reactions, and others are concerned with the reduction of sulfates or nitrates.

(4) Recently the sequence of one cytochrome b, calf liver cytochrome b_5, has been elucidated (Ozols and Strittmatter, 1967). It shows striking homologies with hemoglobin and myoglobin, while cytochrome c does not.

Finally, a cytochrome called P 450, which plays a prominent part in terminal oxidations associated with the endoplasmic reticular membranes of liver and other tissues has been described (Symposium of electron transport system in Microsomes, 1965) and extensively studied (Lu *et al.*, 1969).

Catalases and peroxidases

Catalases and peroxidases are enzymes acting on peroxides, of which the most important is hydrogen peroxide, to liberate oxygen. This oxygen is molecular in the case of catalase, whereas peroxidases liberate atomic oxygen in the presence of an acceptor. The distinction between the two is in fact somewhat arbitrary. The iron in these enzymes is always in the trivalent state.

1. *Catalases.* (See Nicholls and Schonbaum, 1963). These are proteins containing four molecules of hematin; their molecular weight is about 240,000. A catalase (from ox liver) was first crystallized in 1937. Their physiological function is still under discussion. Catalases are found in all organisms excepting certain bacteria. In mammals the highest levels are found in liver and erythrocytes. The function usually attributed to them is protection against peroxides formed during oxidation. Two sets of findings cast doubt on this theory.

Firstly, the enzyme does not protect hemoglobin against slowly generated peroxides, and bacteria are not protected by catalase against the action of a glucose-notatin system.

Secondly, the strongest argument is from cases of acatalasemia in man that have been reported in Japan (Nishimura *et al.*, 1959), and in Switzerland (Aebi *et al.*, 1963). Their erythrocytes contain no catalase, yet have a normal life-span. In higher organisms catalase may be a "fossil enzyme". The same probably cannot be said further down the evolutionary scale: in certain microorganisms (*Rhodospirillum*) catalase can be induced by culture under aerobic conditions (Clayton, 1960). For the present, only biochemistry, not physiology, is likely to explain the function of this enzyme.

2. *Peroxidases.* (See Paul, 1963). The peroxidases are enzymes capable of releasing atomic oxygen from a peroxide in the presence of an acceptor. They do not form a homogeneous group. Some are not heminic compounds but flavoproteins (streptococcal peroxidases and glutathione peroxidase). It should also be mentioned that some proteins with no enzymatic properties of their own are able to activate the peroxidase-like properties of other proteins. The standard example is the haptoglobin of Polonovski and Jayle (1939).

The heminic peroxidases may have protohematin as their prosthetic group. The best known instance is horse-radish peroxidase, crystallized by Theorell in 1942. Peroxidases of the same type have been found in other plants. They contain one molecule of hematin (and thus one atom of iron) for a molecular weight of about 40,000.

Heminic peroxidases have also been found in microorganisms (various cytochrome-*c*-peroxidases in yeast, *Pseudomonas fluorescens* and hematin-dependant bacterial mutants).

In animals, two interesting peroxidases have recently been described in which hematin, instead of being firmly bound to protein, is readily detached (e.g. by passage over an ion-exchange material), and behaves more like a coenzyme than a prosthetic group. These are tryptophan pyrrolase, an inducible enzyme found in liver (Feigelson and Greengard, 1961; Knox and Mehler, 1951) and in a mutant of *Pseudomonas*, which seems, however, to be an oxygenase rather than a peroxidase (Hayaishi, 1963); and a peroxidase found in the submaxillary gland of the rat which catalyses the iodination of tyrosine or other substrates (Serif and Kirkwood, 1958).

The heminic peroxidases do not all contain protohematin. Verdoperoxidases are known in which the prosthetic group is so firmly bound to the protein that it cannot yet be removed intact, but it is probably verdohematin. The most fully studied are myeloperoxidase in leucocytes (Agner, 1958) and lactoperoxidase in milk (Polis and Shmuckler, 1953).

B. NON-HEMINIC COMPOUNDS

The only common factor of these very numerous and wide-spread compounds is negative. They are much less well known than the heminic compounds; often they are peculiar to categories of organisms, and not ubiquitous like cytochromes.

Siderochromes

This is a group of compounds isolated during the past fifteen years from cultures of microorganisms. The siderochromes give a broad absorption band at $420–440 \times 10^{-6}$ mm.

In 1947 Reynolds, Schatz, and Waksman made the discovery of grisein, an antibiotic, followed by that of a similar derivative, albamycin. These

TABLE 2. SIDERAMINES AND SIDEROMYCINS ISOLATED TO DATE
(FROM PRELOG, 1964)

	Siderochromes	
	Sideramines	Sideromycins
Ferrichrome	Ferrioxamine A	Grisein
Coprogen	Ferrioxamine B	Albomycin
Terregens factor	Ferrioxamine C	
	Ferrioxamine D_1	Ferrimycin A_1
	Ferrioxamine D_2	Ferrimycin A_2
	Ferrioxamine E	Ferrimycin B
	Ferrioxamine F	ETH 22765
	Ferrioxamine G	
	Ferrichrysin	LA 5352
	Ferricrocin	LA 5937
	Ferrirhodin	
	Ferrirubin	

antibiotics belong to the group of sideromycins. Since 1952 a number of growth factors called sideramines have been described. A whole series of compounds, the ferrioxamines, have recently been isolated.

Table 2 shows the list according to Prelog (1964) of the siderochromes that have so far been isolated, divided into sideramines (growth factors), and sideromycins (antibiotics), which are mutually antagonistic.

Constitution. The constitution has been worked out after isolation of various compounds by methods similar to those used for the cobalamines, based on extraction with a phenol–chloroform mixture followed by chromatography, electrophoresis, and counter-current separation. The formulae of several sideramines have been established by Swiss research groups. The structure differs in the ferrichromes of fungi, which contain trihydroxamic acids in the form of cyclohexapeptides, and in the ferri-oxamines, of which the hydroxamic acids have a straight configuration.

As examples the formulae of a sideramine, of ferrioxamine B, and of what is known of that of a sideromycin, ferrimycin A, are shown in Fig. 4.

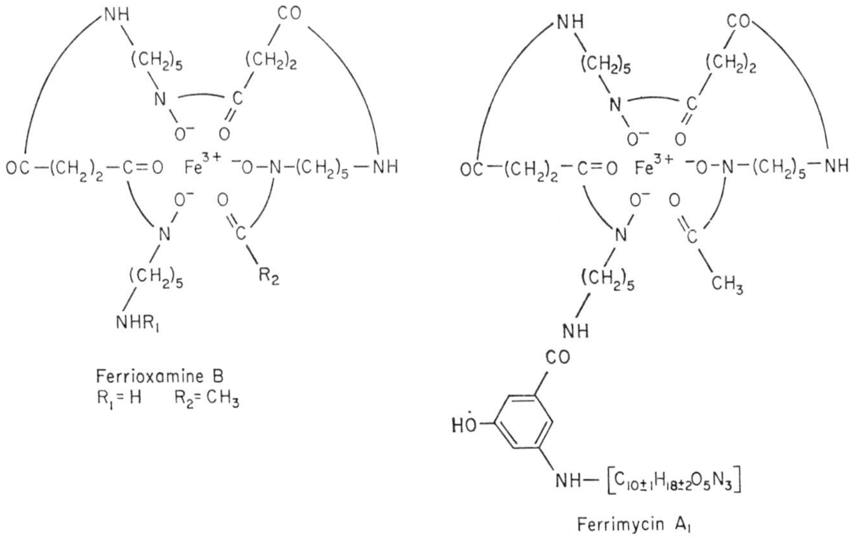

Ferrioxamine B
$R_1 = H$ $R_2 = CH_3$

Ferrimycin A_1

FIG. 4. Structure of ferrioxamine B and ferrimycin A_1.

Although this last is not yet completely known it can easily be seen that ferrimycin is a derivative of ferrioxamine B. It is therefore not surprising that even under relatively mild conditions a transformation of the anti-biotic to sideramine can take place

Biological function of sideramines. The activity of sideramines as growth factors can be shown directly in certain organisms such as *Arthrobacter terrogenes* or *Microbacterium lacticum*.

In some cases sideramines can replace hemin in hemin-dependent organisms. It is probable that sideramines promote the incorporation of iron in porphyrins. In the presence of sideromycins this reaction does not take place, and sideramines can no longer replace hemin.

Desferrioxamine

If iron is removed from ferrioxamines, desferrioxamines are obtained; they have considerable and highly selective ability to chelate iron.

Because of their high specificity and their lack of toxicity, the desferrioxamines, especially desferrioxamine D, find a therapeutic use in the treatment of iron excess in the body, whether chronic (hemochromatosis and hemosiderosis) or acute (poisoning by iron salts) (Schwarzenbach *et al.*, 1963).

Siderophilin (transferrin) and conalbumin

Siderophilin and conalbumin are proteins with the property of binding a fixed proportion of iron. Chemically they are closely related, though their biological functions are very different. Siderophilin is the vehicle for iron in the serum; conalbumin is a protein from egg white.

The presence of iron in the serum was discovered in 1925 by Fontès and Thivolle. The analytical properties of siderophilin were reported by Holmberg and Laurell (1945), and by Schade and Caroline (1946). It was first crystallized in 1947 by Surgenor, Koechlin, and Strong.

Siderophilin can be prepared in the pure state from plasma or from Cohn's fraction IV. It is a protein, colourless in the absence of metals, pink in the presence of iron, and yellow in the presence of copper. Under electrophoresis it migrates like a β_1 globulin. The molecular weight is about 90,000 (83,000 according to the latest estimate), and it can bind two atoms of iron. Thus it differs both from ferritin and hemoglobin: unlike ferritin, the protein can bind a clearly defined number of iron atoms; unlike hemoglobin, the protein in the natural state may or may not contain iron.

Type of bond between iron and siderophilin

In the neutral state iron is very firmly bound to siderophilin: the stability constant is very high (10^{29}), and is exceeded only by that of desferrioxamine. When the pH falls dissociation takes place, and in the usual method of estimating serum iron the first step is the release of iron by acid. The bonds are also split by reduction. The exact nature of the groups that attach the iron to the protein are not known with certainty. It is likely that CO_3H^- ions and one or more tyrosine molecules are involved. *In vitro*, the protein can also bind copper and zinc. *In vivo*, siderophilin is exclusively a vehicle for iron.

In the plasma, iron is bound to siderophilin, which is normally only one-third saturated. Normal adult human plasma contains about 0.3 g of siderophilin per 100 ml, which is capable of binding 350 mcg of iron, but contains only 140 mcg. Its physiological function will be further discussed when the metabolism of iron is considered. It may be mentioned that a fair number of mutants of siderophilin have been found in man; these mutants are genetically transmitted, and like haptoglobin, siderophilin forms one of the genetic "serum groups" (Bearn and Parker, 1963; Smithies, 1957). A similar polymorphism has been found in rhesus monkeys and chimpanzees.

The physicochemical properties of conalbumin (Fraenkel–Conrat and Feeney, 1950) are very similar to those of siderophilin. It was the first to be isolated, and the first to be studied. It has been suggested that conalbumin is identical with the iron-transport protein in the serum of birds. Finally, a lactosiderophilin with similar properties, isolated from milk, has been described, and recently a lactoferrin in white blood cells (Masson *et al.*, 1969).

Ferroxidase

It has been shown by Curzon (1960) that oxidase activity of plasma is enhanced by ferrous ions. This activity is due to the copper protein, ceruloplasmin. Osaki and Waalas (1966, 1967) demonstrated that ferrous ion not only is an activator, but also a privileged substrate of the enzyme, which functions in oxidizing ion to the ferric state. They therefore called this enzyme ferroxidase (ferro: O_2, oxidoreductase, E.C.1.12.3). Its exact role in iron metabolism is not yet known, but may be important.

Non-heminic iron-containing enzymes

Ferredoxin

Ferredoxin is an enzyme discovered by San Pietro and Lang in 1958. It is essential to certain electron-transfer reactions, and takes part especially in the separation of photosynthetic reactions in light and in darkness (Singer and Kearney, 1963). Ferredoxin is reduced by a chloroplast pigment in the light, and reoxidized by NADP in the dark. Its redox potential is -0.432, which makes it one of the most readily oxidized electron carriers. It appears to be necessary for nitrogen fixation by micro-organisms such as *Clostridium pasterianum*, and it takes part in photosynthesis (Arnon, 1965). The structure of ferredoxin has now been fully established. It appears to have a molecular weight of about 12,000, and to contain 10 atoms of iron—nearly 5%. Its aminoacid sequence has been completely worked out for spinach ferrodoxin and is made of 97 aminoacids (Matsubara *et al.*, 1967).

Other non-heminic iron-containing enzymes

The following enzymes appear to contain iron, or at least to require its presence for their activity: Aconitase (Dickman and Cloutier, 1951) catalyses the interconversion of citric, isocitric, and aconitic acids. Its iron is divalent.

Phenol oxygenases catalyse the opening of the ring in the presence of molecular oxygen. They require the presence of iron, though none has yet been demonstrated in the naturally occurring molecule. One example is pyrocatechase, which converts catechol to *cis,cis*muconic acid (Hayaishi, 1963).

With a whole group of flavine-containing enzymes iron is not the only coenzyme. The most studied is succinate dehydrogenase (Massey, 1958). As in other non-heminic iron compounds, the iron is less firmly bound than in the heminic proteins, and can be removed simply by deproteinization. To the absorption bands of flavine (460 and 345×10^{-6} mm) the presence of iron adds a band at 420×10^{-6} mm, which must not be mistaken for a Soret band. With a molecular weight of about 200,000, the molecule contains four atoms of iron, and one of flavine (flavine dinucleotide linked to a hexapeptide). The functional relationship between the two coenzymes and their respective roles have not yet been established.

Other flavine-containing dehydrogenases (Singer, 1963) also contain iron; these enzymes are bound to mitochondria, and are involved in respiratory oxidation-reduction chains. The best known are choline dehydrogenase, extracted from hepatic mitochondria, which in its present state of purity contains four atoms of iron and one of flavine for a molecular weight of 850,000 of protein; and α-glycerophosphate dehydrogenase from mitochondria (Ringler, 1961), which differs from that from cytoplasm discovered by Meyerhof in 1919. It appears to contain one atom of iron for a molecular weight of 35,000. The iron content of mitochondrial dehydrogenase is fairly high: sixteen atoms (and one of flavine) for a protein molecular weight of 10^6.

Lastly, certain nitrate reductases (e.g. of *E. coli*, but not of *Neurospora crassa*) contain iron and also molybdenum (Nason, 1963).

Ferritin and hemosiderin

These two proteins are the means of iron storage in higher animals. As early as 1894 Schmiedeberg recognized that iron was bound to a protein which he called ferratin. Laufberger in 1937 was the first to isolate and crystallize a protein containing over 20% of iron, which he called ferritin. Knowledge of it was quickly increased by the work of Granick (1946). In recent years it has been widely studied—chemically, biologically, and by electron microscopy. Whereas ferritin is a well defined protein, the nature of hemosiderin is still under discussion.

Properties of ferritin

Ferritin is a protein composed of micelles containing iron, and a protein, apoferritin, which may be prepared from ferritin by reduction followed by dialysis.

Colorless apoferritin has a molecular weight of 480,000 (Rothen, 1944). It crystallizes in the presence of cadmium sulphate under the same conditions and in the same form as ferritin. Electrochromatography of its tryptic hydrolysate shows that it is composed of identical subunits, of which there appear to be 20 (Saddi *et al.*, 1961), which would give each a molecular weight around 25,000.

Condition of iron in ferritin

If the maximum iron content is accepted as 24%, the molecular weight of saturated ferritin comes to 800,000. But all degrees of iron saturation are possible. The iron is in the form of a complex, in micelles surrounded by a shell of protein, the nature of which is still uncertain. A composition of the type $(FeOOH)_8$ $(FeO:PO_3H_2)$ has been suggested; theoretically this would give 57% of iron in the micelle, which is very close to the actual percentage.

The magnetic properties of the iron in ferritin are singular (Michaelis, 1947): three unpaired and two paired electrons, giving four covalent and two ionic bonds. This intermediate type is found only in ferritin (and hemosiderin) and in alkaline methemoglobin. The iron may be bound to SH groups in the protein (Mazur *et al.*, 1950). Under the electron microscope, the micelles in ferritin can be clearly seen in the form of tetrads or six-grained structures (Bessis and Breton-Gorius, 1959; Richter, 1958; Haggis, 1965). Inferences drawn from the X-ray pattern and from the decomposition into sub-units have led P. Harrison (1964) to believe that the protein consists of 20 sub-units at the extremities of a pentagonal dodecahedron; and if micelles occupy their interstices they must be in the form of solid icosahedrons, with a diameter of 70 Å. Figure 5 shows a model of an apoferritin molecule.

The presence of ferritin or a similar pigment is not peculiar to vertebrates. It has been reported in a worm, *Arenicola marina* and in molluscs and plants.

Hemosiderin (Cook, 1929; Shoden and Sturgeon, 1960)

The nature of hemosiderin is much more difficult to establish than that of ferritin, and there are considerable differences of opinion about it. The difficulty lies with the protein moiety of the molecule. Unlike ferritin, hemosiderin is virtually insoluble in water, and very difficult to extract. Two distinguishing features have been suggested: one physicochemical—insolubility; and the other histochemical—the Perls reaction to prussian blue, said to be given only by hemosiderin. But it can no longer be accepted that this reaction is negative with ferritin. The picture has changed as a result of electron-microscope studies (Farrant, 1954; Richter, 1958; Bessis and Breton-Gorius, 1959) which show no difference in the appearance of the two proteins; these workers consider that hemosiderin is no more than a slightly modified ferritin. The biological relationship between the two proteins will be considered later.

Non-heminic iron in muscle (Dreyfus, 1950; Schapira and Dreyfus, 1948)

Of the various non-heminic forms of iron the greatest amount, apart from the ferritin-hemosiderin system, is in muscle. Since the quantity is not reduced in anemia its function cannot be storage. Apart from small amounts of flavoferroproteins its chemical nature is unknown. The usual media for extracting iron dissolve only a part of it; thus muscle contains

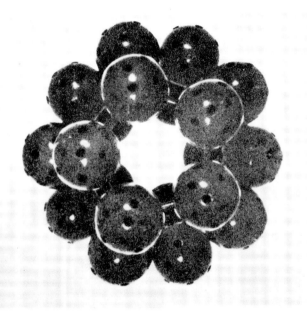

FIG. 5. Model of supposed quaternary structure of apoferritin (From Harrison, 1964).

a proportion of "concealed" iron, perhaps bound to the contractile proteins, myosin and actin. The level of iron in muscle may change in muscular disease; the most striking change is seen with experimental muscular atrophy, which causes a considerable increase.

II. IRON METABOLISM

This account is based on the metabolism of iron in mammals, especially in man, which has had by far the most study.

The metabolism of iron differs fundamentally from that of the principal cations of the body: it is balanced not by the excretion of excess but by the actual amount absorbed; absorption is thus the determining phase. Iron is a precious metal to the organism, which tends to retain and not eliminate it (McCance and Widdowson, 1937). Iron metabolism may be considered in the following five stages: absorption, transport, utilization storage, and excretion. The whole of this metabolism is centred on hematopoiesis, for, of the 5 g of iron contained in the adult human body, hemoglobin represents 70%. Iron is probably directly involved in the biosynthesis of hemoglobin in the bone marrow (Karibian and London, 1965; Waxman and Rabinowitz, 1965; Gribble and Schwartz, 1965; Grayzel *et al.*, 1966).

A. ABSORPTION

The whole of the metabolism is governed by the first stage.

1. *Factors determining the amount absorbed* (Elvehjem, 1935; Bannerman, 1965)

Absorption depends on several factors: dose, valency, degree of ionization:

(a) The absolute quantity absorbed increases with the dose, but the percentage falls (Brock and Hunter, 1937).

(b) In most animals and in man, ferrous ions are much better absorbed than are ferric ions (Lintzel, 1931; Bergeim and Kirch, 1949). Heminic iron, until recently thought to be unavailable, is in fact almost as well absorbed as inorganic iron (Hallberg and Solvell, 1960; Callender, 1957, 1964).

(c) Solution and ionization are promoted by gastric acidity. But not all authors agree that free hydrochloric acid is essential, and absorption in achlorhydric subjects is variable (Moore and Dubach, 1956).

These various factors are easily controlled when iron salts are given. The absorption of iron from the diet is complicated by the entry of further variables:

(a) The form of iron depends on the type of food: vegetables contain only non-heminic iron, but meat contains both heminic and non-heminic forms.

(b) Reducing agents promote absorption. The best known is ascorbic acid.

(c) Other compounds, however, act as inhibitors. The most effective appear to be phosphates, which lead to the formation of insoluble compounds, and above all phytin (calcium inositol hexaphoshate).

2. *Methods of investigating digestive absorption of iron*

The earliest technique to be used was evaluation of the therapeutic effect of iron preparations in animals or iron-deficient patients. It can be accepted—but only in very broad terms—that in cases of iron deficiency the whole of the absorbed iron is used for hematopoiesis. This far from exact method has been brought up to date by the use of radioactive iron.

In practice, assessment of iron balance is the only accurate method. The quantity absorbed is derived from the quantities in the diet and in the excreta.

This method is extremely laborious, but is practicable with the help of radioactive iron. A direct method can now be used: radioactive iron is ingested, and, after an interval of 4–6 days (according to the species)

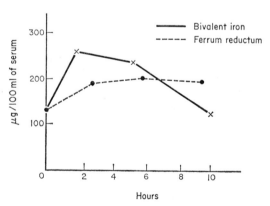

FIG. 6.   Iron tolerance curve.

to ensure intestinal elimination of iron, the total body radiation is measured. This technique can be applied to small animals in numerous laboratories; its use has recently been extended to man, but it is available in only a few specialized laboratories. A simpler means of estimating absorption, used in clinical practice, depends on induced hypersideremia. The serum iron is estimated before taking a dose of iron, and again 2, 4, and 6 hr after. From the results a graph of induced hypersideremia is drawn (iron tolerance curve). Usually the peak level gives a fair indication of the degree of absorption. But in practice there are two types of result: greatly increased sideremia always indicates much absorption; but a flat curve may indicate either deficient absorption or masking of absorption by loss of iron from the plasma to the tissues. The test has therefore to be interpreted with caution.

3. *Physiopathological variations*

Generally speaking, the principal factor in the regulation of absorption in the normal subject is the body's need for iron. Absorption increases with need, as in children, in girls, and above all during pregnancy and lactation. The daily requirement is about 1 mg in men, 2 mg in adolescents and women, and 3 mg during pregnancy (Moore, 1960). Among pathological states, iron deficiency produces the greatest increase, as shown by the graph of induced hypersideremia. But with endogenous excess of iron (idiopathic hemochromatosis) absorption is likewise increased.

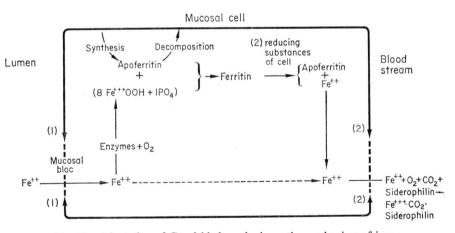

Fig. 7. Adaptation of Granick's hypothesis on the mechanism of iron absorption.

4. Mechanism of absorption

The principal site of iron absorption is the upper part of the small intestine—duodenum and proximal jejunum (Arrowsmith and Minnich, 1941). Most of the iron is then carried in the venous blood to the liver; a small part enters the lymphatics. The mechanism is still not clear. The one coherent theory to explain it was advanced by Granick in 1946. This supposes that there is a gradient of redox potential across the intestinal mucosa. Ferrous iron is first converted to ferric, and then combined with apoferritin to give ferritin. It is again reduced at the opposite pole of the cell, and released into the plasma to be taken up by siderophilin. Excessive dietary iron is held back in an intestinal store as ferritin.

This theory of a refractory state or mucosal block involves several obscurities. It has been severely criticized, but has not been supplanted. Nevertheless, W. H. Crosby (1953) has suggested a possible mechanism: iron is absorbed by the intestinal mucosa; part of it enters the blood, but the excess is retained; the intestinal mucosal cells, however, are short-lived, and after one or two days they desquamate into the intestinal lumen, taking with them the iron which they have retained.

New vistas on the mechanism of iron absorption have been put forward by Davis *et al.* (1966, 1967). They described a gastric protein, which they called gastroferrin, and which is able to chelate iron in a manner analogous to that of transferrin. During iron-deficiency anemia the amount of iron-binding protein increases (Luke *et al.*, 1967), while it decreases in hemochromatosis (Davis *et al.*, 1966). It is still too early to evaluate the importance of this new protein in iron absorption. If confirmed, the authors' work might be the first clue towards an understanding of mechanism of iron absorption (Morgan *et al.*, 1970).

B. TRANSPORT

1. Mechanism

Iron is transported in the plasma in the manner first shown by Fontès and Thivolle in 1925. It is bound to a β_1-globulin, siderophilin or transferrin (Holmberg and Laurell, 1945). This is confirmed by the following experiment: radioactive ^{59}Fe is injected into an animal, or added *in vitro* to human or animal plasma. The plasma is subjected to paper electrophoresis, and then to autoradiography. Only the band corresponding with β_1-globulins is radioactive.

Siderophilin is only partly saturated with iron. The serum levels of iron and free siderophilin allow three parameters subject to physiopathological variation to be defined:

(a) The serum iron (S.I.) corresponds with the siderophilin already saturated with iron; it can be measured directly.

(b) The unsaturated iron binding capacity (U.I.B.C.) corresponds with the unsaturated siderophilin.

(c) The total iron binding capacity (T.I.B.C.) corresponds with the total siderophilin. It is the sum of the S.I. and the U.I.B.C.

(d) The coefficient of saturation (C.S.), representing the proportion of siderophilin in the plasma that is in fact saturated, is calculated from these data. It is given by the formula (S.I.)/(T.I.B.C.) = C.S. Siderophilin normally forms 4% of the total plasma proteins, i.e. about 300 mg per 100 ml. Expressed as iron its normal value (T.I.B.C.) in either sex is 340 $\pm$ 40 mcg per 100 ml of plasma. The coefficient of saturation is about 40% in men (S.I. = 135 $\pm$ 55 mcg) and 35% in women (S.I. = 120 $\pm$ 60 mcg). In view of the considerable variation, an individual serum iron level cannot be considered abnormal unless it differs widely from the mean (below 80 mcg or above 190 mcg in a man; below 70 mcg or above 180 mcg in a woman).

In animals the serum iron level is of the same order as in man or rather higher (about 200 mcg per 100 ml in the rat and the rabbit).

2. Pathophysiological variation

As we have seen, sideremia is on the average lower in women than in men. This difference appears at puberty. At birth the S.I. is high, and the T.I.B.C. is low. During the first two years of life the position is reversed; the S.I. falls, and the T.I.B.C. and U.I.B.C. rise. Afterwards there is a change in the opposite direction until the adult values are reached. During pregnancy and lactation the relative deficiency is reflected in lowered S.I. and raised T.I.B.C.

TABLE 3. NORMAL VALUES AND PHYSIOLOGICAL VARIATIONS

	Serum Iron	U.I.B.C.	T.I.B.C.	S.C.
Man	135 $\pm$ 55	205	340 $\pm$ 40	40 $\pm$ 20
Woman	120 $\pm$ 60	220	340 $\pm$ 40	35 $\pm$ 15
New-born	170 $\pm$ 40	90	260 $\pm$ 20	65 $\pm$ 10
Infant under 2 years	95 $\pm$ 30	295	390 $\pm$ 40	24 $\pm$ 10
Pregnant woman (end of pregnancy)	80 $\pm$ 30	365	445 $\pm$ 40	17 $\pm$ 10

The given numbers are mean values, expressed in mcg iron per 100 ml of serum $\pm$ 2σ (σ = standard deviation)

H

In pathological states the estimation of serum iron and siderophilin gives valuable information. The most important changes can be classified as follows.

(a) In iron-deficiency anemia, whether due to inadequate intake or to loss by bleeding, there is a fall of serum iron with desaturation of siderophilin, of which the elements are:

> (i) lowered S.I.;
> (ii) raised total siderophilin (T.I.B.C.);
> (iii) fall of C.S., sometimes below 10%.

(b) In anemia with hemolysis (hemolytic anemia, pernicious anemia) there are, during episodes of hemolysis:

> (i) raised S.I.;
> (ii) lowered T.I.B.C.;
> (iii) raised C.S.

Between episodes of hemolysis, and in treated subjects, the S.I. and C.S are instead often lowered.

(c) Infectious jaundice gives a similar picture:

> (i) raised S.I.;
> (ii) normal or slightly lowered T.I.B.C.;
> (iii) raised C.S.;

whereas obstructive jaundice causes no change.

(d) These changes reach a maximum in hemochromatosis and hemosiderosis:

> (i) very high S.I.;
> (ii) low T.I.B.C.;
> (iii) high C.S., often reaching unity and signifying total saturation of siderophilin.

(e) In infections there are:

> (i) low S.I.;
> (ii) low T.I.B.C.;
> (iii) normal or slightly lowered C.S.

This is the one time when the changes in serum iron and siderophilin are not in opposite directions.

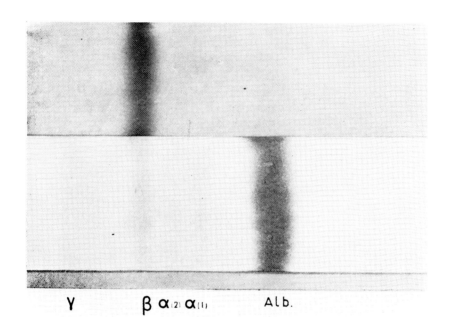

γ   β α$_{(2)}$ α$_{(1)}$ Alb.

FIG. 8.   Electrophoresis of serum proteins (bottom) and autoradiography (top) showing fixation of iron on β-globulins. (By courtesy of Dr. Paoletti).

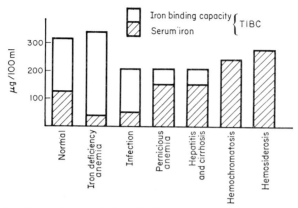

Fig. 9. Serum iron and iron-binding capacity (total iron-binding capacity) in normal subjects and in various pathological conditions.

Figure 9 shows the pathological variations in serum iron and siderophilin.

(S.C. = saturation coefficient)

3. *Mode of action of siderophilin*

Three main questions arise:

(a) What part does siderophilin play in absorption? The above tables show that the level of iron in the serum is nearly always inversely related to that of siderophilin. A raised T.I.B.C. nearly always coincides with increased absorption. Yet it has not been possible to show a causal relationship between the two phenomena.

(b) Does siderophilin accompany iron into the organs or not? The half-life of iron in the plasma averages, as will be shown, 100 min. That of siderophilin is several days. It is certain that siderophilin releases iron to the tissues without itself crossing the vascular barrier, and that it is solely a means of transport in the plasma (Laurell, 1951).

(c) Is siderophilin directly concerned in hematopoiesis? It appears (Katz and Jandl, 1964) that the iron-siderophilin complex attaches itself specifically to the surface of the erythroblast, allowing iron to be incorporated into the cell. A pathological finding shows the importance of siderophilin-transferrin: a case is known of atransferrinemia; this patient has a severe and intractable anemia (Heilmeyer *et al.*, 1961, 1964). In another case, atypical transferrin was found with a very high serum iron (Westerhausen *et al.*, 1969).

C. EXCRETION

It is generally accepted that the body is unable to rid itself of iron (McCance and Widdowson, 1937). Urinary and intestinal excretion are both minimal. However, the accepted view is called in question from time to time; a point of discussion is the amount of iron in sweat, hair, nails, and desquamated cells (Mitchell and Hamilton, 1949; Finch, 1965). The special case of iron in desquamated intestinal cells has been mentioned above, but here the metal may be said not to have been really absorbed. Total estimation is the best method: a labeled dose of iron is injected, and if possible the total radioactivity, or otherwise the level of labeled iron in the blood, is followed for several years, and from it the amount excreted is derived. The appropriate iron isotope for this purpose is ^{55}Fe, since its half-life is 3 years.

TABLE 4. DAILY EXCRETION OF IRON
(IN μMCG PER 24 HR)

Urine	100–200
Bile	10
Feces	300
Sweat	100

Cell desquamation
    nails
    hair
	200–1000

The total excretion by an adult man may be put at about 1 mg (according to Finch, 600 mcg) in 24 hr, and this is the amount to be replaced by absorption from the 10–20 mg provided by an average diet. Menstrual loss brings the average requirement of a woman to 2 mg per day, and pregnancy or lactation raise it to 3 mg.

D. STORAGE

Most of the iron absorbed is used in hematopoiesis. Part of it, normally 20–25%, is used in the renewal of other iron compounds or for replenishing stores.

Stores of iron are maintained in the liver, spleen, and bone marrow, in the form of ferritin (Hahn *et al.*, 1943). If radioactive iron is injected into an animal, ferritin taken from it in the next few hours is radioactive (Loftfield and Harris, 1956). In the presence of radioactive iron, sections of liver synthesize labeled ferritin. *In vitro* synthesis of this kind seems possible even in a cell-free system (Saddi and Von der Decken, 1964, 1965; Yu Fu Li and Fineberg, 1965). It has been shown that not only is the administered iron incorporated into ferritin but that the synthesis of ferritin is stimulated to the exclusion of any other liver protein molecule (Saddi, personal communication). This "induced" synthesis of a protein can be shown even more strikingly, and in this respect ferritin is an exceptionally interesting example. In the young rat there are virtually no reserves of ferritin or apoferritin in the liver. However, one need only inject a fairly large dose of iron (e.g. as the saccharate) for the protein to appear in the liver. Injection of iron thus serves not only to load the specific storage protein, apoferritin, but also to promote the biosynthesis of the protein itself. Ferritin behaves as an "adaptive" protein. However, iron does not act only in stimulating the synthesis of the protein, since actinomycin does not prevent the increase in synthesis.

1. *Evaluation of storage*

This may be done in various ways:

(a) The standard procedure is to estimate the iron in the tissues, which in man may be done by puncture-biopsy of the liver. Examination is usually confined to a histochemical test (Perls or Turnbull reaction). Investigation of bone-marrow smears or sections, or of iron granules in bone-marrow normoblasts (sideroblasts) have been suggested (Grunberg, 1941; Mouriquand, 1958).

(b) After injecting a tracer dose of radioactive iron, it is possible to measure the amount of radioactive iron taken up by the liver and spleen with a scintillation counter.

2. *Pathophysiological variation*

At birth there is considerable storage in the liver, which is increased in the first days by physiological hemolysis. In the early months these stores are depleted, and in the following years are replenished only very slowly. In women the stores are generally scanty, and they are further reduced during pregnancy. Women are also far more liable than men to iron deficiency. This difference between the sexes is not found in all animal species.

In pathological states one may find:

(a) Reduction or even total disappearance of stores in iron deficiency, whether due to inadequate intake, to digestive disorders (which prevent absorption), or to bleeding.

(b) Increased storage in various syndromes: severe hemolytic anemias, and especially primary or secondary hemochromatosis. This increase leads to accumulation of ferritin, and later of hemosiderin, in the paren-chymatous cells of the liver and spleen, and sometimes in the cells of the reticuloendothelial tissues. Hemosiderin, which is insoluble, is easily detected histochemically.

E. UTILIZATION

Most of the iron taken into the plasma is needed for the synthesis of hemoglobin. A 70–kg adult has about 900 g of hemoglobin, containing 3 g of iron. The average life-span of a red cell is about 120 days. The hemo-globin broken down and resynthesized every day thus amounts to 900/120 g, i.e. 7.5 g, involving 25 mg of iron. The origin of this 25 mg of iron, greatly exceeding the dietary 1 mg, and the mechanism whereby the cor-puscular iron is replaced, may perhaps be explained by studies of the kinetics of erythrocytic iron (Huff *et al.*, 1951; Finch, 1959; Pollycove, 1961, 1964; Wasserman *et al.*, 1952). This is done by means of radioactive iron, ^{59}Fe. If a tracer dose of ^{59}Fe is injected intravenously, it leaves the plasma; the rate at which it leaves follows an exponential curve, and may be taken as an indication of the movement of iron across the vascular barier. The biological "period" of radioactive iron (the time in which radioactivity is reduced by half) is of the order of from 90 min to 2 hr. The whole of the plasma iron is replaced about eight times in 24 hr. Since the total plasma iron amounts to some 4 mg (3 l of plasma with 130 mcg per 100 ml), the amount of iron replaced in 24 hr is around 30 mg. Of this 30 mg, about 25 mg (80%) is used for the synthesis of hemoglobin, and so goes to the bone marrow.

If it is accepted that 80% of the plasma iron goes to the bone marrow, the replacement of plasma iron is a measure of the activity of the whole marrow. This is normally well below its maximum; it can be increased at least five-fold (recovery from iron-deficiency anemia, hemolytic anemias, polycythemia). It can also be greatly diminished (aplastic anemias, depression of hematopoiesis after irradiation, antihematopoietic drugs, massive transfusion).

Effective erythropoietic activity, culminating in the release of red cells into the circulation, is evaluated from the amount of radioactive iron taken up by the red cells. This is assessed by measuring the radioactivity of the circulating red cells for some days after the injection. Given the blood volume, the proportion of injected iron incorporated in the red cells can be calculated. This coefficient of utilization is normally $75 \pm 5\%$. The rest is allocated almost entirely to storage, and it is clear that in most cases the condition of the stores determines the value of the coefficient.

If there are no reserves, utilization increases and may reach 100%.

When the stores are increased, the coefficient of utilization falls, even if hematopoiesis is normal (hemochromatosis).

The study of iron kinetics of erythrocytes is often very complex, and may involve drawing conclusions from doubtful premises, but it gives some interesting results. It helps to distinguish certain pathological conditions:

(a) *Hyperfunction* of bone marrow, for instance in hemolytic anemia, where the activity of the marrow may be multiplied by six. The anemia results from the fact that even this intense activity is not enough to compensate for destruction when the rate of destruction is more than 5–7 times the normal.

(b) *Hypofunction* of marrow may be relative (medullary fibrosis); the marrow cannot then increase production to balance even moderate destruction. Or it may be absolute and lead to aplastic anemia.

(c) *Dysfunction* of marrow may also be seen (pernicious anemia, thalassemia). The turnover of iron in the highly active marrow is rapid, but hematopoiesis is ineffective, and only an inadequate number of red cells reach the circulation.

The biosynthesis of hemoglobin certainly originates with the plasma iron. But it must be added that investigations by electron microscopy (Bessis and Breton-Gorius, 1961) suggest that iron from destroyed red cells is directly resumed and absorbed by erythropoietic cells.

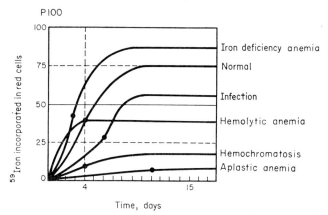

FIG. 10. Utilisation of radioactive iron by the red cells in normal subjects and in various pathological conditions.

F. REGULATION OF IRON METABOLISM

The fine adjustment of iron metabolism is under the control of the endocrine glands and the autonomic nervous system (Schaeffer, 1964). One of the most obvious effects of this control is the diurnal rhythm of sideremia, which has to be borne in mind when studying variations in serum iron (Hemmeler, 1944). This attains its maximum in the morning, and falls progressively throughout the day. The endocrine glands certainly have an effect, and a complex one. There are differences between men and women in the levels both of hemoglobin and of serum iron (Widdowson and McCance, 1948). This difference is apparently not due to menstrual loss, for it is found in young women after castration (Vahlquist, 1950). It is probably due to a hypersideremic effect of male sex hormones. Incidentally, such differences are by no means the rule among animal species. The pituitary, adrenal, and thyroid hormones also have effects, which vary according to species. But in almost every case corticotrophin and cortisone appear to depress sideremia.

III. IRON AND NUTRITION

The available information on the amount of iron in the diet is far from complete. The average intake probably lies between 10 and 30 mg (W.H.O., 1958). Table 5 shows the changes in iron intake in the United States between 1936 and 1955. It is complemented by Table 6, which shows the iron content of different drinks (MacDonald, 1963).

TABLE 5. IRON IN CITY DIETS, U.S.A. IN A WEEK IN SPRING. (AVERAGE IN MG PER PERSON PER DAY FROM FOOD USED AT HOME)

	All households	Income thirds		
		Lowest	Middle	Highest
1936	11.8	10.2	11.8	14.0
1942	13.6	12.8	13.5	13.8
1948	15.9	15.6	15.8	16.2
1955	17.0	16.4	17.0	17.6

Household Food Consumption Survey. U.S. Dept. of Agriculture, Rep. No. 16, 1955. (1955 Survey based on approx. 6000 housekeeping households of 1 or more persons, about 3000 of which were urban).

TABLE 6. IRON CONTENT OF VARIOUS ALCOHOLIC BEVERAGES. (FROM MACDONALD, (1963)).

U.S. beer	0.1 mg/l
Gin, whiskey, bourbon, scotch	0.6 mg/l
U.S. (New York) wine	2.3 mg/l
U.S. (California) wine	2.6 mg/l
3 U.S. wines popular with Boston alchoholics	4.4 mg/l
44 French wines, red and white, sold in Boston	6.2 mg/l
Cider and wine from Rennes, France	10–16 mg/l

These figures may be compared with the requirements, which vary with the physiological conditions, shown in table 7.

The amount of iron needed in the diet is thus about ten times the physiological requirement. For a long time the only way to find out whether food provided satisfactory digestive absorption was to assess the iron which could be extracted from it. This result was compared with its efficacy in curing anemia in rats. These results agreed fairly well, but they were difficult to extrapolate to man.

TABLE 7. ESTIMATED IRON REQUIREMENT (IN MG/DAY)

	Urine, sweat, feces	Menses	Pregnancy	Growth	Total
Men and post-meno-pausal women	0.5–1				0.5–1
Menstruating women	0.5–1	0.5–1			1 –2
Pregnant women	0.5–1		1–2		1.5–2.5
Children (average)	? 0.5			0.6	1
Girls (age 12–15)	0.5–1	0.5–1		0.6	1 –2.5

Table 8 shows the total and available quantities of iron in a number of foods (Sunderman and Boerner, 1949).

In the past few years radioactive iron has been used to assess the intestinal absorption of iron. Two methods are available. For the first, which is the more precise but the harder to carry out, radioactive food is prepared (eggs laid by radioactive hens, vegetables grown on soil enriched with labeled iron, radioactive hemoglobin etc.). For the second, radioactive iron is added to the food-stuff. Figure 11 (after Moore, 1964) shows

H*

TABLE 8. FOODS AND THEIR IRON CONTENT (FROM SUNDERMAN AND BOERNER, 1949)

Foods of low iron content (0–0.99 mg/100 g)	mg/100 g	Foods of moderate iron content (1.0–4.99 mg/100 g)	mg/100 g	Foods of high iron content (5.0–18.2 mg/100 g)	mg/100 g
Buttermilk	0.07	Mayonaise	1.0	Egg yolk, fresh	7.2
Chocolate milk	0.07	Eggs, whole, fresh	2.7	Eggs, whole, dried*	8.7
Dry skimmed milk	0.58	Chuck roast	2.8	Corned beef, dried or chipped*	5.1
Dry whole milk	0.58	Corned beef, canned	4.0	Liver, fresh	12.1
Evaporated milk	0.17			Heart, fresh	6.2
Fresh skimmed	0.07	Hamburger	2.4	Liver sausage	5.4
Fresh whole milk	0.07	Loin steaks	2.5	Tongue, fresh	6.9
Cream	0.06	Round steaks	2.9	Oysters	7.1
Ice cream	0.10	Stewing meat	2.4	Beans, dry seed, common or kidney*	10.3
Cheddar cheese	0.57	Lamb	2.7	Beans, lima, dry seed*	7.5
Cottage cheese	0.46	Ham	2.3	Peas, spread*	6.0
Cream cheese	0.17	Pork chop	2.5	Soya-beans, whole, mature*	8.0
Bacon	0.8	Pork link sausage	1.6	Peaches, dried (sulfered)*	6.9
Butter	0.2	Veal	2.9	Oatmeal*	5.2
French dressing	0.1	Baloney	2.2	Bouillon cubes*	9.2
Lard & other shortening	0	Frankfurter	2.3	Wheat-germ	8.1
Oleomargarine	0.2	Hash	1.3	Yeast, brewers	18.2
Salad & cooking oil	0	Chicken	1.9		
Cod	0.9	Turkey	3.8		
Asparagus, fresh	0.9	Salmon	1.3		
Cabbage, fresh	0.5	Sardines	1.8		
Carrots, fresh	0.8	Shrimp	2.0		
Celery, fresh	0.5	Tuna	1.7		
Corn, fresh	0.5	Beans, canned	3.4		
Cucumbers, fresh	0.3	Almonds	4.4		
Eggplant, fresh	0.4	Peanut butter	1.9		
Lettuce	0.5	Peanuts, roasted	1.9		
Okra	0.7	Pecans	2.4		
Onions, mature	0.5	Walnuts, english	2.1		
Parsnip	0.7	Beans, lima, green	2.3		
Peppers, green, fresh	0.4	Beet greens	3.2		
Potatoes, white	0.7	Beets	1.0		
Rutabegas, fresh	0.4	Broccoli	1.3		
Squash, fresh	0.4	Brussel sprouts	1.3		
Squash, winter	0.6	Cauliflower	1.1		
Sweet potatoes	0.7	Chard	4.0		
Tomatoes	0.6	Dandelion greens	3.1		
Turnips	0.5	Kale	2.2		
Canned corn	0.5	Lettuce	1.1		
Canned sauerkraut	0.5	Mustard greens	2.9		
Tomato catsup	0.8	Peas, green	1.9		
Tomato juice	0.4	Radishes	1.0		

Foods of low iron content (0–0.99 mg/100 g)	mg/ 100 g	Foods of moderate iron content (1.0–4.99 mg/100 g)	mg/ 100 g	Foods of high iron content (5.0–18.2 mg/100 g)	mg/ 100 g
Tomatoes, canned	0.6	Spinach	3.0		
Asparagus, pureed	0.7	Turnip greens	2.4		
Apples, fresh	0.3	Lima beans	1.7		
Apricots, fresh	0.5	Peas, green, canned	1.8		
Avocado	0.6	Spinach, canned	1.6		
Banana	0.6	Tomato puree	1.1		
Blueberries	0.8	Beets, puree	1.8		
Strawberries	0.8	Beans, green, puree	1.0		
Other berries	0.9	Carrots, puree	1.0		
Cantaloupe	0.4	Greens, mixed, pureed	1.4		
Grapefruit	0.3				
Grapes	0.6	Peas, puree	1.8		
Lemon	0.1	Spinach, puree	1.0		
Orange	0.4	Vegetable soup	1.0		
Peach	0.6	Plums, canned	1.1		
Pear	0.3	Apricots, dried	4.9		
Pineapple	0.3	Prunes, dried (un-sulfered)	3.9		
Plums	0.5	Fruits (apricots & apples, strained)	1.3		
Rhubarb	0.5	Pears & pineapple, strained	1.3		
Tangerines	0.4	Prunes, strained	3.4		
Watermelon	0.2	Cornmeal, whole-grain	2.7		
Applesauce, canned	0.2	Wheat flour, enriched	2.9		
Apricots, canned	0.3	Whole-wheat flour	3.8		
Cherries, canned	0.3	Whole-wheat bread	2.6		
Cranberry sauce	0.3	Crackers	1.5		
Grapefruit juice	0.4	Cornflakes	1.0		
Orange juice	0.4	Farina, enriched	1.3		
Pineapple juice	0.5	Wheat flakes, puffed	3.7		
Peaches, canned	0.4	Shredded wheat	3.8		
Pears, canned	0.2	Whole-grain wheat, uncooked	3.8		
Pineapple, canned	0.6	Barley, pearled	2.0		
Cornstarch	0	Hominy	1.0		
Rye bread	0.8	Macaroni, spaghetti	1.2		
Rice, puffed or flakes	0.9	Noodles	1.9		
Farina	0.8	Tapioca	1.0		
Rice, white	0.7	Sugar, brown, dark	2.6		
Honey	0.9	Syrup, table blends	4.1		
Jams & jellies	0.3	Cocoa	2.7		
Sugar, granulated or powdered (white)	0.1	Coconut, dry, shredded	3.6		
Gelatin dessert powder	0				
Wine	0.3				

* It should be noted that the iron content in these foods is based on dry weight, and that this value will be variably reduced upon preparing the food.

the results obtained with some of these foods. All are better absorbed by iron-deficient subjects than by controls. It should be noted that, contrary to standard teaching, iron in hemoglobin is as well absorbed as that in most foods, and that the difference between normal and deficient subjects is least with hemoglobin iron (Callender *et al.*, 1957).

In general (Finch, 1965) a normal subject on a diet containing 15–20 mg of iron absorbs 5–10% of the ingested dose. In states of deficiency absorption may be doubled or trebled. Absorption thus increases with increased need, and this is equally true of physiological states (pregnancy, lactation) and pathological states (deficiency, loss of blood). It should be added that absorption appears to be increased in all anemias, even when the stores are plentiful (hemolytic anemia), except anemia accompanying infection.

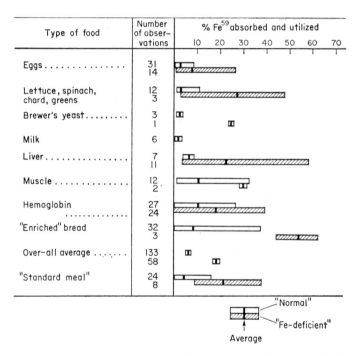

FIG. 11.   Radio-iron measurement of the absorption of iron from foods by adult subjects. The length of the bars indicates the variation among different subjects for each food: the heavy vertical line across each bar indicates the average value. The amount of iron in each feeding varied from 1 to 17 mg. Cross-hatched bars: iron-deficient; white bars normal. (From Moore 1964).

IV. HYPOSIDEROSIS (SIDEROPENIA)

Iron deficiency is probably the commonest nutritional deficiency in the world. It may be isolated or associated with other deficiencies. Experimental hyposiderosis and spontaneous hyposiderosis in man present very similar pictures.

Experimental hyposiderosis can be produced by restricting intake or by causing excessive loss of iron (Morgan, 1964).

In the growing animal, which needs much iron, dietary measures may suffice. The best method is to feed the young animals on a milk diet, with supplementary vitamins and mineral salts. Such a diet should ensure growth and reproduction if iron is added. The amount of iron needed for growth is about 50 mg per kg, but this must be raised to 200 mg per kg for normal reproduction.

In the adult animal the low iron diet has to be combined with venesection, which has the disadvantage of depriving the animal of other factors.

In conditions where the requirements are increased, such as gestation or lactation, there may be some degree of hyposiderosis with a normal diet, iron being mobilized from the stores to meet the demands of the fetus or suckling.

A. HUMAN HYPOSIDEROSIS

1. *Predisposing factors*

Iron deficiency appears when the demand exceeds the supply. The prevalence varies greatly with the region. In countries where the diet is adequate the conditions which promote deficiency are growth, pregnancy, and hemorrhage.

(a) *Growth.* In the first year of life about 150 mg of iron is needed in order to grow from 3 kg to 10 kg. This figure reaches 200–250 mg in case of prematurity (Schulman, 1961). But the iron stores at birth are scanty. Milk is poor in iron, and soon has to be supplemented with a varied diet.

After the first year the risk of iron-deficiency diminishes until puberty.

(b) *Hyposiderosis.* This is much commoner in women than in men; 90% of cases occur in females. Menstrual loss is supposed to amount to 30 mg per month, but in fact the amount is usually unknown, and may be much greater (Moore and Dubach, 1956). During pregnancy the demand is increased: 300 mg of iron is passed on to the fetus. Amenorrhoea almost compensates for this; but a further 100 mg is needed for the placenta, and the loss of blood during parturition is not to be ignored. Hence the prevalence of anemia after repeated pregnancies (Hunter, 1960; Holly, 1955).

(c) *Hyposiderosis.* This, as a result of bleeding, is of considerable importance. The hemorrhage may be single, and the loss made up from stores. It is often repeated, evident or occult, causing hyposiderosis of which hypochromic anemia is the main effect. It has been recognized, and the cause must be found, in order not to give purely symptomatic treatment.

In many countries iron deficiency results from defective and unbalanced diet. Shortage of protein is added to that of iron. Bleeding often makes matters worse. In particular, hookworm infection is very common in India (Chatterjee, 1964).

Certain symptoms apart from anemia are a direct consequence of hyposiderosis; these will be simply enumerated (Kasper *et al.*, 1965; Jasinski and Roth, 1954).

(i) severe asthenia;
(ii) trophic disorders affecting nails, hair, and mucous membranes;
(iii) digestive disturbances, usually subjective but in rare cases leading to sideropenic dysphagia—the so-called Plummer-Vinson syndrome (Kelly, 1919; Paterson, 1919).

B. BIOLOGICAL EFFECTS

1. *Changes in iron stores*

Stored iron is concentrated mainly in liver, spleen, and bone marrow. Other organs, notably the muscles, contain significant amounts. But for practical reasons most studies have been done on the liver and spleen. Hallgren (1953) has shown that there is a close relationship between the levels of iron in the liver and in the spleen, and a satisfactory if less exact relationship between the liver and the "carcass" (muscles and skeleton).

The iron stores are composed essentially of ferritin and hemosiderin. Figure 12 (Morgan, 1961) shows the changes in these reserves in the rat after bleeding. The ratio of hemosiderin to ferritin is seen to be more or less fixed. But even by continued depletion it is not possible to reduce the amount of iron in the organs below a certain level. The iron that resists further depletion is known as "parenchyma iron". It accounts for only 10–20% of the normal content of liver and spleen, but for nearly half that of the "carcass" (Hallgren, 1953).

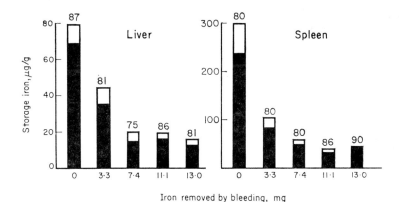

Fig. 12. Mean liver and spleen storage iron concentrations and their relative distribution between ferritin (■) and hemosiderin (□) in rats with hyposiderosis produced by repeated bleeding from the tail over a period of 8 weeks. The severity of hyposiderosis was varied by removing different amounts of iron from different groups of rats as indicated under each column. The figure above each column gives the percentage of the total storage iron which was present as ferritin iron. (From Morgan, 1961).

2. *Effects on iron in blood*

(a) *Hemoglobin.* Shortage of iron naturally causes the level of hemoglobin to fall. This happens when the stores are severely depleted, but begins before they are fully mobilized. Iron-deficiency anemia is hypochromic.

(b) *Plasma iron.* This is lowered with iron deficiency. The fall is a function of the extent of the deficiency, and may reach very low values (10–20 mcg per 100 ml). It is difficult to say how far the stores must be reduced before the serum iron begins to fall. McCall *et al.* (1962) have found a direct relationship between serum iron and stored iron.

(c) *Siderophilin.* In most animals, and especially in man, the level of siderophilin (transferrin), measured as total iron-binding capacity (T.I.B.C.), is raised. The fall in serum iron added to the rise in siderophilin produces a considerable fall in the coefficient of saturation (serum iron ÷ T.I.B.C.).

3. *Absorption*

Absorption is increased in man, as it is in animals. The iron-tolerance test shows a greater rise and much slower return to the initial level than in controls. A comparison between this test and that of serum-iron saturation shows good correlation (Verloop *et al.*, 1958).

4. *Utilization of radioactive iron*

In the absence of stores, injected radioactive iron is almost totally utilized. Iron-deficiency anemia is the only case in which the utilization of iron is greater than normal.

5. *Tissue iron*

The protein most emphatically diminished is hemoglobin, of which the amount in the blood falls from 15 g per 100 ml to 10 g or much less—in extreme cases to 3–5 g. As a result, the mean corpuscular hemoglobin (M.C.H.) falls from the normal 31×10^{-12} g to values of $20–30 \times 10^{-12}$ g; the mean corpuscular hemoglobin concentration (M.C.H.C.) similarly falls to below the normal 32% (Beutler *et al.*, 1963).

However, recent studies show that the levels of other iron-containing proteins in the tissues, particularly enzymes, are also lowered. Beutler (1957) showed that cytochrome *c*, cytochrome oxidase, succinate dehydrogenase, and aconitase could be reduced in the tissues of rats deprived of iron. But the reduction does not affect all tissues: the enzymes mentioned are all reduced in the kidney, but not in the liver. Another enzyme containing iron—catalase—is not affected. In the rat Dallman and Schwartz (1965) have confirmed a reduction in cytochrome *c* in intestinal mucosa and muscle. The same authors also found a fall in the amount of myoglobin. The rate of return to normal depends on the rate of cell production: iron therapy restores the level of hemoglobin to normal in weeks, and that of intestinal cytochrome *c* in two days. On the other hand, the repletion of cytochrome *c* and myoglobin in muscle takes six weeks.

The results in man are less complete. Cytochrome oxidase in leucocytes is moderately depressed, but not aconitase (Beutler, 1959; Tanaka and Valentine, 1961). Jacob (1961) has examined biopsy specimens of buccal mucosa by histochemical means. He has shown the disappearance of cytochrome oxidase and its reappearance after iron therapy.

This research, still in the early stages, shows that numerous enzymes may be affected by iron deficiency. Depression of them may be the cause of some of the symptoms, which are not all due to anemia.

C. OTHER HYPOSIDEROSES AND DYSSIDEROSES

1. *Iron deficiency from defective absorption*

The prevalence of hyposiderosis due to defective intestinal absorption is open to discussion. It may cause chlorosis in adolescents. The anemia is said to be due to inadequate absorption; this would be overcome by large doses of iron, to which chlorosis in fact responds. Absorption is disturbed with intestinal hurry (sprue, idiopathic steatorrhoea) (Badenoch and Callender 1954; Hawkins *et al.*, 1950; Havrani *et al.*, 1965).

2. *Post-gastrectomy anemia*

Summaries are given by several groups (Wells and Welbourn 1951, Baird *et al.*, 1959; Lederer, 1951).

3. *Diaphragmatic hernia*

This is discussed by Mallarmé and Tilquin (1948).

4. *Anemia of infection*

Infection is often accompanied by anemia, of which the following pattern is characteristic:

(i) normochromic anemia;

(ii) low serum iron (Thoenes and Aschaffenburg, 1934);

(iii) low siderophilin; hence no depression of the coefficient of saturation (Laurell, 1947);

(iv) reduced digestive absorption (Gubler *et al.*, 1950);

(v) poor utilization of injected iron; instead of being utilized for hemopoiesis, iron drains to the reticuloendothelial system (Finch *et al.*, 1949); iron therapy is therefore ineffective, and should not be given until the infection has been treated.

5. *Anemia of malignant disease*

Anemia with cancer may be associated with a low serum iron. Utilization of iron is generally increased (Miller *et al.*, 1956).

V. HYPERSIDEROSES

An excess of iron may be experimental or pathological. Findings vary, because of differences in the duration of experiments, and perhaps for other, still unknown, reasons. An experimental overload causes siderosis without cirrhosis. A clinical surfeit causes siderosis with cirrhosis. The role of iron in the development of hepatic lesions is not yet known.

In man, an excess of iron may arise spontaneously, or it may be due to excessive intake of exogenous iron. An exogenous excess may be acute or chronic. It may be dietary or therapeutic.

A. PRIMARY HYPERSIDEROSIS

This is hemochromatosis. The first description of hemochromatosis was by Trousseau in 1856. Sheldon (1935) mentioned 300 cases in his monograph. Although this disease has been much studied, its mechanism and etiology remain obscure. Some authors (MacDonald, 1965) maintain that idiopathic hemochromatosis is very rare, and that nearly all cases are secondary. However, the following account is based on standard descriptions.

Hemochromatosis is a disease of maturity (after the age of 40), and ten times commoner in men than in women. There are four main symptoms, which by no means always occur together:

(i) skin pigmentation;
(ii) enlargement of the liver, with only slight functional disturbance;
(iii) diabetes;
(iv) other endocrine disorders, especially of the gonads.

1. *Metabolic disorders*

Hemochromatosis does not usually cause any hematological disturbance. Only a brief account of the disorders will be given, limited to those which involve iron metabolism. A few tests of diagnostic value have been described.

(a) *Estimation of serum iron.* The serum iron is increased in 80% of patients. (Dreyfus and Schapira, 1964). Absence of hypersideremia does not necessarily exclude the diagnosis.

(b) *Iron-binding capacity of serum* (Finch and Finch, 1955). When the serum iron is raised in hemochromatosis the T.I.B.C. is nearly always lowered. It may fall until the U.I.B.C. disappears. The coefficient of saturation (serum iron ÷ T.I.B.C.) is over 0.8, and may reach 1. The rise in the coefficient of saturation is the surest sign; it is found even when the serum iron is normal. Figure 9 shows serum-iron and iron-binding capacity values in various diseases, indicating the problems which the diagnosis of hemochromatosis raises.

(c) *Absorption studies.* (i) The oral iron tolerance test, with a 3–4 mg per kg dose of a ferrous salt, shows a flattened curve (Fig. 13), in contrast with the rise seen in a normal subject (Dreyfus *et al.*, 1950; Hemmeler, 1951). This curve does not indicate that the iron is not absorbed, but that it does not remain in the plasma, where there is not enough free siderophilin to retain it, so that it promptly passes into the tissues. (ii) The radioactive-iron absorption test shows increased absorption in most cases; this can be accurately shown only by balance studies (Bothwell *et al.*, 1953; Heilmeyer, 1954; Petersen and Ettinger, 1953).

(d) *Utilization studies.* These are made by means of radioactive iron, a tracer dose of which is injected intravenously. The rate at which the plasma iron is replaced is shown to remain normal. The most interesting test is the estimation of corpuscular utilization of radioactive iron, which depends on the level of the stores. The proportion of radioactive iron recovered in hemoglobin is 20–40%, instead of the 80% found in normal subjects. The replacement time of radioactive iron is little changed, which with the raised plasma iron leads to an increase in the total turnover of plasma iron averaging 50% (Finch and Finch, 1955; Bothwell *et al.*, 1953).

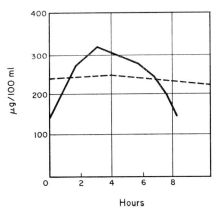

FIG. 13. Normal iron-tolerance curve as compared with the iron-tolerance curve in hemochromatosis: ——— control; – – – – – hemochromatosis.

(e) *Excretion of iron.* Urinary excretion is normally minimal. It is raised in some cases of hemochromatosis but does not exceed 1 mg per day.

With the newer chelating agents, an induced sideruria test has become possible. Intramuscular injection of desferrioxamine is followed by the excretion of 10–50 mg of iron in 24 hr in these patients (not more than 1 mg in controls). This test gives a rough estimate of the iron stores, and allows the effect of treatment with chelating agents to be predicted (Fielding, 1965; Rosen and Tullis, 1966).

(f) *Storage of iron.* The essential metabolic defect in hemochromatosis is an increase of stored iron from 1 g to 10, 20, or occasionally still more (Butt *et al.*, 1956; MacDonald and Pechet, 1965). Various organs are involved (spleen, pancreas, endocrine glands), but puncture-biopsy of the liver is the best diagnostic criterion. The Perls prussian blue reaction shows accumulation of hemosiderin, at first as fine granules in the liver cells, and later as clumps of various sizes. This siderosis is accompanied by progressive fibrosis. The Kupffer cells are only secondarily affected (Fig. 14). Other biopsies (e.g. skin, stomach), and examination of bone marrow, provide interesting but more controversial data.

The mechanism by which iron accumulates is not yet satisfactorily explained.

(a) There is certainly a defect of iron absorption. If absorption is increased by 3 mg daily, there will be a surfeit of 10 g of iron in 10 years. As we shall see, diets over-rich in iron or unbalanced diets can lead to such excessive absorption; but most cases are unexplained.

(b) The degree of saturation of siderophilin has been invoked, but its relevance has not been proved. No qualitative anomaly of this protein has been demonstrated (Saddi, 1962; Bothwell *et al.*, 1962).

(c) An anomaly of storage might be responsible for the disease by attracting an excessive amount of the circulating iron to the tissues. Studies of ferritin (Saddi, 1962) have shown no change in the physico-chemical properties or chemical composition of the protein. We have advanced the suggestion that an excess of apoferritin is produced, which binds a corresponding excess of iron (Dreyfus and Schapira, 1964).

2. *Genetics of hemochromatosis*

Hemochromatosis has been regarded as a hereditary disease since Sheldon put forward the idea in 1935. A few familial cases are known. Hereditary transmission of disturbances of iron metabolism (though not of the complete disease) has been shown in half the male descendants of

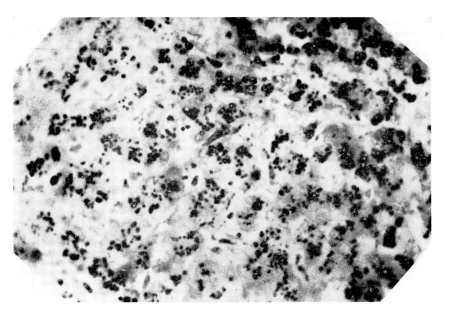

Fig. 14.   Liver biopsy section stained for iron.

patients (Debré *et al.*, 1952; Dreyfus and Schapira, 1964); the proportion may be higher if liver biopsy with electron microscopy is systematically done (Williams *et al.*, 1963). The disorder of iron metabolism is transmitted as a dominant character, but it is possible that the complete picture of the disease is seen only in homozygotes. MacDonald (1965) has criticised the hereditary concept of hemochromatosis, but the strongest arguments are still on its side (editorial, *Lancet* 1966; Charlton and Bothwell, 1966).

Recent studies conducted in our Institute (Saddi and Feingold, 1969) have demonstrated that hemochromatosis is indeed a genetic disease: only homozygotes display the full picture of the disease, while heterozygotes show mild disturbances of iron metabolism.

B. SECONDARY HEMOSIDEROSIS

These have various origins. Hemosideroses may be classified as nutritional, following transfusion, etc.

1. *Nutritional hemosiderosis*

In animals, these can be provoked by an unbalanced diet such as corn grits (Kinney *et al.*, 1948). In man, their prevalence is uncertain. Some authors (MacDonald, 1965) regard them as usual.

The commonest type in our climate is hemosiderosis secondary to alcoholic cirrhosis. This can sometimes be directly proved, when serial liver biopsies in a cirrhotic show the appearance and progressive accumulation of iron (Castelman, 1946). It is usually difficult to distinguish this from idiopathic hemochromatosis. However, Caroli and André (1964) have set out its characteristics, assembled in the following tables, of which the first shows the clinical signs and the second the biological signs.

Lastly, cirrhosis causes anatomical changes in the hepatic lobules, which hemochromatosis on its own, even in the advanced stages, does not produce.

In hemochromatosis secondary to cirrhosis the serum iron is raised and the siderophilin is saturated. But the iron seems to be less easily mobilized, and chelating agents have little effect (Verloop, 1964). Since venesection cannot be considered with cirrhosis, treatment of these cases is almost useless. A kind of hemochromatosis developing rapidly after portacaval shunt has recently been described (Tuttle *et al.*, 1959). Twelve cases were

TABLE 9. COMPARISON BETWEEN IDIOPATHIC AND
POST CIRRHOTIC HEMOCHROMATOSIS

(a) CLINICAL SIGNS

	Hemochromatosis	
	Idiopathic	Alcoholic
Sex		
male	92.3%	80%
female	7.7%	20%
Melanodermia	100.0%	100%
Liver size		
hypertrophic	100.0%	70%
atrophic		5%
normal		25%
Portal hyptertension	0 %	40%
Endocrine symptoms	69.2%	50%
Heart symptoms		
clinical	30.7%	0%
electrical	46.1%	10%
Diabetes	54.0%	30%

(b) BIOLOGICAL SIGNS

	Hemochromatosis	
	Idiopathic	Alcoholic
Hepatic biology		
total cholesterol < 1.5 g	58.3%	66.6%
Flocculations +	7.7%	40.0%
BSP retention	0 %	88.2%
Increase in γ globulins	83.3%	100.0%
Iron metabolism		
mean serum iron	244 gammas	192 gammas
siderophilin saturation	87.5%	68.7%

known in 1964 (Sherlock). Little is known of the mechanism of this excessive absorption.

Callender has shown that iron absorption is increased in cirrhotics, and also in patients with pancreatitis. This absorption can be diminished by giving pancreatic extract, and the active principle of the extract is under study (Malpas and Callender, in Callender (1964). Absorption is also increased in cystic fibrosis of the pancreas (Tonz *et al.*, 1965; Romano, 1966).

2. *Nutritional cytosiderosis*

This was first described by Strachan (1929) in the South African Bantu, and has since been studied by Gillman (1957), and by Bothwell (1960, 1962). It is very common among the Bantu: in a survey involving some hundreds of examinations, 40% of men and 12% of women showed a hepatic siderosis comparable with that of idiopathic hemochromatosis. The iron deposits are confined to the liver; and, within the liver, to the reticuloendothelial system. Only when cirrhosis is added to the siderosis does this affect the parenchymatous cells of the liver, and spread to other organs.

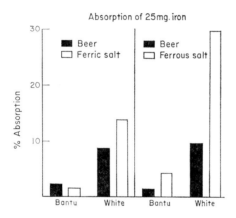

FIG. 15. A comparison in Bantu and white subjects of the absorption of iron in Bantu beer with a similar dose of iron given as ferric chloride or ferrous ascorbate. (From Bothwell, 1964).

The cytosiderosis of the Bantu seems entirely due to dietary imbalance, above all to an excessive amount of iron in the food. These people prepare their food, and in particular their fermented liquor (beer), in iron utensils. Their intake of iron often exceeds 100 mg per day. On the other hand, it has been shown that absorption is less than in Europeans, and that this is accordingly not primarily a disorder of absorption.

3. *Hemosiderosis due to metabolic disorders*

Certain biochemical lesions which interfere with the normal utilization of iron and lead to its accumulation in the tissues have been described in the past few years. These disorders can make repeated transfusion necessary and so give rise to transfusion hemosiderosis.

The most interesting condition is hypersideremic hypochromic anemia, which is often hereditary; Heilmeyer has called it sidero-achrestic anemia (Cooley, 1945; Verloop *et al.*, 1964). The patients have a refractory anemia of varying severity. Cytological examination of the bone marrow shows that the number of sideroblasts among the erythroblasts is much higher than normal. Even if transfusion is unnecessary hemosiderosis is not uncommon, since absorption is very high. Utilization of iron is prevented by a biochemical lesion of the biosynthesis of hem, of which the site has not been determined. Some cases are improved by treatment with large doses of vitamin B_6.

This primary hypersideremic hypochromic anemia has to be distinguished from very similar conditions giving rise to secondary anemias, of which the commonest is thalassemia minor. The presence of increased amounts of fetal hemoglobin or hemoglobin A_2 serves to distinguish them.

Apart from these hypersideremic hypochromic anemias there have been cases, much less common, of hyposideremic anemia producing hypersiderosis. The most interesting example is the case of atransferrinemia described by Heilmeyer (1962, 1964). In this 7-year-old girl the serum iron and the T.I.B.C. did not rise above 30 mcg per 100 ml. The very severe anemia, with very poor utilization of iron, showed the importance of transferrin (siderophilin) as a vehicle for transporting iron from the plasma to the bone marrow. Necropsy showed gross siderosis of all the organs, with the exception of the bone marrow.

4. *Post-transfusion hemosiderosis*

Post-transfusion hemosiderosis has been known since 1920. It has become commoner since a growing number of patients with refractory anemia have had a chance of prolonged survival. Since iron introduced into the body cannot be discharged, and since a liter of blood contains 500 mg of iron, repeated transfusions must inevitably lead to a surfeit of iron in the body. Nevertheless, the amount of iron given does not account for all the observed effects, and susceptibility differs in different individuals.

Two types of refractory anemia are liable to post-transfusion hemosiderosis:

(a) The commoner type is that of the erythroid marrow with defective erythropoiesis (Ellis *et al.*, 1954; Caroli *et al.*, 1957). Intestinal absorption is high, which explains why in some subjects the amount of iron accumulated exceeds the amount transfused (see Cleton and Blok, 1964). In these patients the surplus is mainly parenchymatous, and the histological picture resembles that of idiopathic hemochromatosis.

(b) Patients with hypoplastic marrow receive much larger doses of iron transfusion—sometimes by hundreds of transfusions. This enormous overload is mostly well tolerated. It always starts in the Kupffer cells, and only secondarily reaches the parenchyma.

5. *Focal hemosiderosis*

Two types of focal hemosiderosis are important.

(a) *Renal hemosiderosis.* When intravascular hemolysis exceeds the binding capacity of the plasma haptoglobin, hemoglobin filters across the glomeruli (Laurell, 1958). The iron released from the hemoglobin is stored as ferritin. If the hemolysis is prolonged siderosis of the renal tubular cells develops and hemosiderin appears in the urine. Hemosiderinuria is typically found with paroxysmal nocturnal hemoglobinuria. This renal siderosis does not apparently cause loss of function, probably because the renal tubules, loaded with iron, are constantly desquamated and replaced (Crosby, 1953).

(b) *Pulmonary hemosiderosis.* This was first described by Ceelen in 1931; more than a hundred cases are now known (Soergel and Sommers, 1962). The etiology is obscure. The characteristic feature is intra-alveolar hemorrhage, probably from the alveolar capillaries. There is a considerable increase of iron in the lung, in the form of hemosiderin. A special type of pulmonary siderosis is industrial siderosis. This is not so much an illness as a tattooing, which has usually no pathological effects.

C. EXPERIMENTAL CHRONIC EXCESS

Various workers have produced a surfeit of iron by experimental means but without reproducing the picture of idiopathic hemochromatosis.

(1) The overload is most easily created parenterally. Since the pioneer work of Chevallier (1915) and of Rous and Oliver (1918) numerous preparations have been used: red blood-cells, colloidal iron, saccharated iron oxide, iron ascorbate, iron-dextran. The levels of iron in the body attained in these experiments ranged from 0.1 to 3.3 g per kg, and the follow-up periods from 4 weeks to 7 years (Brown *et al.*, 1957). Iron given in this way was always concentrated in the reticuloendothelial system (Brown *et al.*, 1957; Finch *et al.*, 1950). If the doses given did not exceed those seen in human hemochromatosis no damage to the liver cells was found. Only massive overdoses are likely to be lethal (Brown *et al.*, 1959).

(2) Siderosis can be produced in the monkey and the rat by dietary excess (Lorenz and Menkin, 1936). This arises more readily if rats are given an unbalanced diet. The most effective procedure was devised by Kinney *et al.* (1948), who used a diet based on corn grits. This will produce siderosis of the liver parenchyma with fibrosis but no true cirrhosis. The addition to the diet of an abnormal amino acid, ethionine (an analog of methionine) also greatly increases the absorption of iron (Kinney *et al.*, 1955). A diet rich in iron and deficient in folic acid will produce a picture similar to that of hemochromatosis (MacDonald and Pechet, 1965).

VI. THERAPY

A. HYPOSIDEROSIS

The treatment of iron deficiency has been known for centuries. It is 3200 years since Melampus of Argos restored to Iphiclus, Prince of Phylace, his lost virility by making him drink a cup of wine in which he had soaked the sacrificial knife, from which the rust was thus mixed with the wine. Rust, then, was the first preparation of iron to be used. This was the saffron or crocus of Mars of which Dioscorides wrote. But he also gave iron in another form: he recommended water and wine in which red-hot iron had been quenched for stopping seepages and hemorrhages, fluxes and discharges: he thought it worked by sealing the fibres of the tissues and eliminating surplus fluids.

Treatment with iron did not become established practice until the time of Paracelsus (1493–1554). In 1520 Johannes Lange became the first to treat chlorosis with iron. Sydenham (1624–89) laid down conditions for giving it, usually after blood-letting. During the 17th and 18th centuries the simplest forms were used—iron filings or iron oxide (Lémery). Iron salts were introduced in the 19th century: sulfate, carbonate (Blaud), iron, and ammonium citrate (Trousseau). At the end of the last century Hayem set out the principles of iron therapy. Iron was out of favour during the first quarter of the present century, but, thanks to the work of Fontès and Thivolle (1925), McCance and Widdowson (1937), and numerous studies with radioactive iron, it has become possible to examine the absorption of iron experimentally, and to establish treatment on a bio-chemical basis.

1. *Indications*

Any cause of hyposiderosis provides an indication for iron therapy. The main indication is hypochromic anemia, which is typical of iron deficiency. This treatment has to be given whenever there is anemia with a low red-cell count and microcytosis—which in no way exonerates one from seeking possible causes. But in these cases cell count and hemoglobin level are enough to establish the indication.

These hypochromic anemias are most often due to profuse or repeated hemorrhage; sometimes they are due to disorders of ionization or absorption of iron (achylic and agastric anemias, essential hypochromic anemia, chlorosis). In the period of recovery from pernicious anemia, hemolytic anemias or sprue, the stores may become depleted and require the addition of iron to the specific treatment, but this is a rare indication. Failure to respond to iron occurs only with anemia of infection; these cases are rare, but beyond question.

Besides hypochromic anemia, hyposiderosis without anemia is seen in some women and infants. Particular attention should be paid to women during pregnancy and lactation, babies of women with iron deficiency, and premature babies. Iron may be given either by mouth or parenterally.

2. *Treatment by mouth*

This should always be tried first; it is effective in the great majority of cases.

Preparations in use

The choice of a preparation is based on three criteria:
  (i) time taken to correct anemia;
  (ii) amount of intestinal absorption;
  (iii) gastrointestinal tolerability.

The anemia should be corrected rapidly—the hemoglobin should be raised by 0.5–1 g per 100 ml weekly, after a latent period of two weeks. Intestinal absorption can be estimated only by means of isotopes (Brise and Hallberg, 1962; Pitcher *et al.*, 1965). For a long time the preparation used was reduced iron, which is insoluble and unionized: it had the advantage of being cheap (Reimann and Fritsch, 1931). Its action is weak, so that large doses, liable to cause gastrointestinal upsets, are required. Reduced iron has therefore been given up and replaced by iron salts. The less well absorbed ferric salts have given way to ferrous salts. In France, protoxalate of iron is still in use. But this poorly soluble salt is inferior to the preparations based on soluble ferrous salts. Several of these have come forward.

(a) Ferrous chloride (Lederer, 1951) is highly effective, but too readily oxidized for general use.

(b) Ferrous sulfate is by far the most widely used iron salt; it is effective, generally well tolerated, and cheap. It may be given as the hydrated salt $FeSO_4.7H_2O$, containing 20% of iron, or in the dehydrated form with 29%. Its blue-green colour is changed by oxidation to brownish yellow; it must then be discarded.

The normal adult dose is 200 mg of elemental iron per day, divided into three doses. It is usually taken in tablets, but is also available as syrup, and as drops.

It is well tolerated by 90% of patients. In cases of intolerance treatment can often be continued with smaller doses.

(c) *Ferrous gluconate* (Jasinski and Roth, 1954) has been suggested with the hope of reducing digestive disturbances. It contains 12% of iron. It is available in tablet or in capsule form. To give the same results as the sulfate an equivalent dose in elemental iron must be given. The better tolerability reported is perhaps due simply to the smaller content of iron in a given amount of the substance.

(d) *Ferrous fumarate* is a red-brown salt containing 33% of iron. This salt is perhaps more stable than the sulfate. The daily dose of iron is the same: 200 mg, corresponding to 0.64 g of fumarate.

(e) *Iron succinate* has been suggested on the grounds that succinic acid activates the absorption of the metal (Brise and Hallberg, 1953). Its advantages over the usual salts do not seem great enough for it to be widely adopted.

(f) *Other preparations* which have been recommended are ferrous calcium citrate, ferric ammonium citrate, ferrous glycine sulfate, and ferrous cholinate.

Comparison of different iron salts

Figure 16, taken from Brise and Hallberg, shows the absorption of different iron salts in relation to ferrous sulfate as a standard. Only the succinate is perhaps a little better. Lactate, fumarate, glutamate, gluconate, and glycine-sulfate are equilalent to the sulfate. The nonionized complexes (citrate, pyrophosphate, versenate) and the ferric salts are definitely inferior. Of the usual preparations, then, it appears that sulfate, fumarate, and gluconate can be equally recommended, the first two having the advantage of a higher proportion of iron in the molecule.

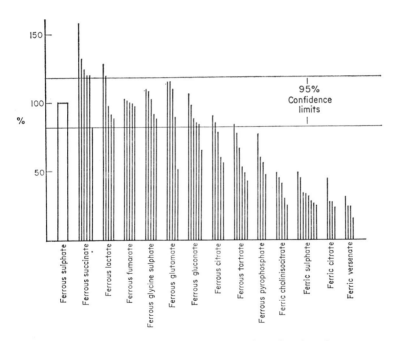

FIG. 16. The relative gastrointestinal absorption of various iron compounds. Note that ferrous salts are better absorbed than ferric salts. (From Brise and Hallberg, 1962).

Duration of treatment

Formerly, treatment lasted no more than a few weeks. In fact only the anemia was recognized, and treatment was limited to correcting it, often incompletely, without considering replenishment of the iron stores. In order to achieve this, which is necessary to a complete cure of hyposiderosis, treatment has to be maintained for a considerable period. There are three criteria to be met:

(a) the anemia must be fully resolved (a reticulocyte response is not enough; even in women one should aim at a red-cell count of 5,000,000 and a hemoglobin level of 15 g per 100 ml);

(b) the serum iron must return to the normal level, above 90 μg per 100 ml.;

(c) the coefficient of saturation must resume a normal value around 40%, and the intestinal absorption of iron must decrease.

These tests are not always done in practice. In this case it is wise to think in terms of four months' treatment if the patient is anemic, or two months if he is not.

Jasinski and Roth, who have contributed largely to the understanding of incomplete hypersideroses, have laid down two rules which serve as a guide to treatment: the worse the anemia the longer the treatment; and when the anemia has been corrected a further six weeks are needed to replenish the stores.

Given these conditions the danger of relapse, even in predisposed subjects, is greatly reduced, though not completely removed. There are patients who need a fresh course of treatment every six months; they are doubtless unable to ionize and absorb dietary iron. This is especially the case after gastrectomy, but a search for occult bleeding must always be made.

Adjuvants

These do not appear to be justified, with the possible exception of ascorbic acid, which increases absorption, and an adequate intake of protein in the diet. Indeed:

(a) If the diagnosis of iron deficiency is certain, and the cause is nutritional (the causes of repeated loss of blood having been excluded), then iron alone will effect a cure. The addition of cobalt, molybdenum, vitamin B_{12}, and folic acid, as in numerous compound preparations, is useless.

(b) If the case is not of iron deficiency, these compound preparations are also apt to be useless if not harmful. With anemia of infection, the iron is not absorbed. With hemolytic or aplastic anemias it is absorbed, but not utilized because there is already a surplus in store, and it merely increases the risk of secondary hemochromatosis. This shows the importance of exact diagnosis, which the doctor is tempted to overlook if he uses these complex, "all-purpose" preparations.

3. *Parenteral treatment*

Until 1947, parenteral iron therapy remained in the experimental stage because of the impossibility of giving doses above 10 mg without provoking toxic reactions. The colloidal ferric hydroxide preparations used by Goettsc h*et al.* (1946) were still very toxic. In 1947 Nissim introduced saccharated iron oxide, allowing intravenous injection of 500 mg of iron. In 1954, Fletcher and London used iron-dextran, which can be given by intramuscular injection.

Indications

The indications for parenteral treatment are few:

(a) poor absorption of iron (with digestive disorders, especially idiopathic steatorrhoea, or after surgical removal of part of the intestine);

(b) compensation for frequent loss of blood;

(c) intolerance of iron by mouth, or more often a suspicion that the patient is not taking his medication correctly.

An inadequate response to treatment by mouth, apart from these causes, should raise a suspicion either of an unrecognized source of bleeding or of a wrong diagnosis.

Preparations in use

Four main types of preparation have been described, two intended for intravenous and two for intramuscular use.

(a) *Saccharated iron oxide.* This was the first to be used. After intravenous injection 100–200 mg is cleared from the plasma in 3–6 hr, being taken up by the reticuloendothelial system and then the liver cells.

Urinary excretion is negligble. Because it is impossible to give more than 200 mg without danger, this preparation is tending to give way to other, less toxic preparations.

(b) *Iron-dextrin* (*dextriferron*). This preparation, introduced by Agner *et al.* in 1948, is a complex of ferric hydroxide with a dextrin of which the molecular weight is 230,000 (Fielding, 1961). It forms a colloidal solution, with an iron content of 2% and a pH of 7.5. The commercial preparation contains 20 mg of iron in 1 ml. In the rabbit doses of 50 mg per kg are tolerated; the fate of the drug is analogos with that of saccharated iron oxide. The plasma iron can be raised to 15,000 mcg per 100 ml. There is no urinary excretion. The customary dose is 100 mg by intravenous injection. Toxic reactions appear to be less common than with saccharated iron oxide. The efficacy of the two substances is comparable.

(c) *Iron-dextran* ("Imferon"®). This is a complex of ferric hydroxide and a dextran with a molecular weight of 180,000. The commercial preparation has a pH of 6, and contains 50 mg of iron in 1 ml. Following intramuscular injection in the rabbit (Goldberg, 1958) the iron enters the lymph and then the plasma. The plasma iron may reach 1 mg per 100 ml without causing trouble, because within the complex the iron is not ionized. The iron is slowly and progressively released from the site of injection. Some remains there: over 20% of the injected dose is found after 50 days. Variations in this respect may depend on the site of injection, and doubtless also on the intensity of hematopoiesis. The serum iron remains raised for a week; accordingly serum-iron estimation should not be requested for some days after the injection. The hematological response to iron-dextran is excellent, and if its use is confined to the intramuscular route adverse reactions are very rare. Because of a carcinogenic effect in certain strains of mice and rats (Richmond, 1957; see editorial *Brit. med. J.*, 1958, and Zuelzer, 1960) this preparation was withdrawn from the market in 1960, but it was reintroduced in 1962. Iron-dextran is certainly the most widely used of all parenteral preparations.

A similar type of preparation, iron-polyisomaltose, with a lower molecular weight, has recently been put forward.

(d) *Iron-sorbitol* and citric acid complex with dextrin as a stabilizer ("Jectofer" ®) contains 50 mg of iron per ml; its pH is 7.5. It diffuses much more rapidly than iron-dextran, and saturates the siderophilin in a few hours. It has the peculiarity that some of it (up to 30%) can be excreted in the urine. Utilization is excellent (Andersson, 1961).

Choice of preparation

Intramuscular preparations cause trouble less often than intravenous. The large amount of iron-dextran remaining at the site of injection is a nuisance. A rapidly absorbed preparation such as iron-sorbitol probably represents an advance, but it is still too soon to judge.

Calculation of total dose to be injected. It is essential to give an adequate dose, but also not to overload the body unduly with iron. These are several ways of calculating the required dose. That of Brown and Moore (1956) is simple: normal hemoglobin minus patient's initial hemoglobin $\% \times 0.255$ = grams of iron needed. This method allows for 50% replacement of tissue stores.

Effect of anemia. With iron-deficiency anemia the level of hemoglobin can be expected to rise by 0.1–0.3 g per 100 ml per day as a result of parenteral therapy. No difference in efficacy between intravenous and intramuscular preparations can be inferred from the studies of Cope *et al.* (1956), and of Scott and Govan (1954). Nor does the response to injected iron appear to be any more rapid than that to iron given by mouth (Pritchard, 1961). But the stores are probably more easily replenished.

The effect of treatment on other symptoms of hyposiderosis is extremely rapid and often dramatic. Lack of energy and digestive disorders vanish in a few days.

The response to iron therapy is remarkable. In view of its efficacy and of the prevalence of latent iron deficiency it is justifiable to insist on the need of investigations for hyposiderosis in all suspect cases, especially in infants and pregnant women.

B. HYPERSIDEROSIS

Until lately no treatment was available for hypersiderosis, but there are now two possibilities: venesection, and chelating agents.

1. *Venesection*

This was the first effective means of treatment (Finch, 1949; Davis and Arrowsmith, 1950). Large quantities of blood must be let for a good response. Typically 500 ml of blood is removed once or twice a week— 25–50 l of blood per year, representing 12–25 g of iron. On the whole patients tolerate these massive depredations well, and regeneration is

J

excellent, showing that hematopoiesis is not affected. The objective must be partial desaturation of siderophilin. Absorption of iron is greatly increased in these patients. If treatment is stopped, the siderophilin is replenished in a few months. Clinical improvement is certain (Davis and Arrowsmith, 1950; Kleckner *et al.*, 1955; Darnis, 1958). Treatment by venesection is restricted to idiopathic hemochromatosis. It cannot be used for hyper-siderosis secondary to cirrhosis, where there is no regeneration; still less with post-transfusion hemosiderosis. It is in these latter cases that the introduction of effective chelating agents may, one hopes, transform the prognosis.

2. *Chelating agents*

The earliest trials involved the experimental use of EDTA in the rat (Foreman *et al.*, 1952), and in man (Klotz *et al.*, 1957; Figueroa *et al.*, 1955). They showed only a slight increase in sideruria. Since 1960, new chelating agents with a much greater affinity for iron have appeared. The most important are two salts related to EDTA—trisodium calcium diethylene-triamine pentaacetate (DTPA) and ethylene diamine di-(*o*-hydroxyphenylacetic acid) (EDDHA)—and desferrioxamine.

(a) *DTPA*. The structures of EDTA and DTPA are compared in Fig. 17. The affinity of DTPA for iron is very close to that of siderophilin. Injection (preferably intravenous) of 1 g of DTPA in patients suffering from hemochromatosis promotes urinary excretion which may attain 40 mg per day (Brick and Rath, 1964). It does not seem possible to continue the treatment for long periods, because the effect wears off. Toxic reactions have been reported.

(b) *EDDHA* (Korman, 1960). This chelate has received less study than DTPA, though the complex may be even more stable.

(c) *Desferrioxamine*. Desferrioxamine was discovered in 1960 in Switzerland (see Prelog, 1964). The formula is discussed on p. 204 above. Desferrioxamine B, with a molecular weight of 597, is used as the methane-sulfonate, which is much more soluble than the chloride originally used (Moeschlin and Schnider, 1964). Its affinity for iron is considerable; the stability constant of 10^{31} is higher than that of transferrin, 10^{29}. Table 10 compares desferrioxamine, EDTA, and DTPA in this respect, and shows that desferrioxamine has both the highest stability constant for iron and the greatest differentiation between iron and other metals.

Experimentally, desferrioxamine is able to increase the urinary excretion of iron in a rat or guinea pig which has been given an injection of iron.

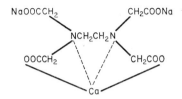

Disodium calcium ethylene-diamine tetra-acetate

(E.D.T.A.)

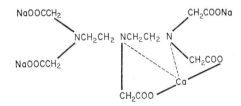

Trisodium calcium diethylene-triamine penta-acetate

(D.T.P.A.)

FIG. 17. Comparison of chemical structure of E.D.T.A. and D.T.P.A.

In man, desferrioxamine is given by intramuscular injection at a daily rate of 1000 mg (in one or two doses) for an adult. In cases of hemochromatosis the daily excretion is usually 10–30 mg. Before starting treatment it is possible to estimate the chances of success by means of an induced hypersideruria test. The patient is given an injection of 500 or 1000 mg of desferrioxamine, and the urine is collected for 24 hr; the

TABLE 10. STABILITY CONSTANTS OF DIFFERENT DESFERRIOXAMINE B-METAL COMPLEXES, COMPARED WITH THE CORRESPONDING FIGURES FOR E.D.T.A. AND D.T.P.A.

Metallic ion	Desferrioxamine	E.D.T.A.	D.T.P.A.
Mg^{2+}	10^4	10^9	10^9
Ca^{2+}	10^2	10^{11}	10^{10}
Sr^{2+}	10	10^9	10^{10}
Fe^{3+}	10^{31}	10^{25}	10^{29}
Co^{2+}	10^{11}	10^{16}	10^{19}
Ni^{2+}	10^{10}	10^{19}	10^{20}
Cd^{2+}	10^8		
Zn^{2+}	10^{11}		

amount of iron excreted indicates the likely effect of treatment (in normal subjects it does not exceed 1 mg in 24 hr). Treatment can be continued for several months, or even years, without its effect wearing off, and without toxic reactions. A daily excretion of 15 mg removes 450 mg in a month, equivalent to a venesection of 1 liter. This means that the effect of this treatment is in general less than that of repeated venesection, but there is no objection to applying both methods simultaneously. With hemo-siderosis secondary to cirrhosis, the results are less satisfactory: excretion does not usually exceed 5 mg per day (Wöhler, 1964; Albahary, 1964). The most interesting cases are the refractory anemias (sidero-achrestic anemia, severe hemolytic anemias, Blackfan-Diamond anemia). In these cases excretion up to 10–20 mg can be obtained even in children, and maintained for months, as we have ourselves observed in two brothers suffering from chronic hemolytic anemia. It is thus possible to counter-balance the effect of transfusions up to 1 liter per month, allowing the patient to survive indefinitely. On the other hand we see no point in starting treatment with chelating agents as soon as it is realized that a child needs repeated transfusions; the urinary excretion does not increase until there is a considerable excess of iron.

VII. PHARMACOLOGY AND TOXICITY

Ingested iron is very well tolerated. Nevertheless, very large doses can cause trouble, and over 100 cases of poisoning in children have been reported. This is very rare in France, but not uncommon in the English-speaking countries. It is nearly always due to ferrous sulfate, and to preparations of which the appearance and taste attract children.

The lethal dose by mouth is of the order of 500 mg (per kg) of elemental iron in the mouse. This dose would correspond with 5 g for a 10-kg child. Serious accidents have been reported with 2 g (Ross, 1953), but also survival after taking 5 g.

The clinical picture includes nausea, vomiting, abdominal pain, diarr-hoea, and hematemesis. The initial asthenia gives way to a state of shock in 4–6 hr. Some cases are fatal in the first few hours; the rest improve and recover. But if infectious or intestinal complications set in, the prognosis deteriorates.

As regards the mechanism of poisoning, there is no longer any doubt about the part which iron itself plays. It acts at two levels: in the alimen-tary canal, it is responsible for necrosis and other intestinal lesions; in the circulation the very high levels, 3000–5000 mcg in most cases (Smith *et al.*, 1950; Amerman *et al.*, 1958), greatly exceed the binding capacity of the siderophilin. Iron has vasodilator and hypotensive properties. It has been suggested that ferritin enters the circulation, but this has not been demonstrated (Smith, 1952; Hoppe *et al.*, 1955; Bronson and Sisson, 1960). Reissmann has shown the occurrence in dogs and rabbits, poisoned with iron salts, of metabolic acidosis (Reissmann and Coleman, 1955).

Treatment

Until the past few years the prognosis of acute iron poisoning has been extremely grave, and some 40% of cases have been fatal. It has much improved since the introduction of specific chelating agents. The treatment now consists of two complementary series of measures.

1. *General measures.* The objects are:

(a) to eliminate the ingested iron: emesis, gastric lavage, administration of sodium bicarbonate to promote the formation of an insoluble bicarbonate;

(b) to maintain the general condition: treatment of shock and acidosis.

2. *Use of chelating agents.* As in the case of hemochromatosis the first trials were made with EDTA. In experiments on the dog Bronson and Sisson (1960) were able to lower the serum iron after poisoning. In 1959 the American Medical Association recommended injection of EDTA in man (Conley, 1959). With the introduction of new chelating agents, however, EDTA has been entirely superseded. DTPA has been used, but the most thorough trials have been made with desferrioxamine. In the guinea pig, treatment with 2000 mg per kg started 30 min after poisoning gives 100% survival of animals after an LD_{50} and 80% after an LD_{100}. Even if treatment is delayed for 6–12 hr 80% of the animals survive an LD_{50}. After 24 hr there is no longer any protective action. In man, Moeschlin and Schnider (1964) suggest the following schedule:

(i) desferrioxamine, 8000–12000 mg (2000 mg in 10 ml of distilled water), by gastric tube;

(ii) intravenous infusion of desferrioxamine, 2000 mg, dissolved in 5% laevulose; the dose to be continued for two days.

Reports of the successful use of this treatment have recently been published.

REFERENCES

a. BOOKS, REVIEWS, AND MONOGRAPHS

BEUTLER, E., FAIRBANKS, V. F. and FAHEY, J. L. (1963). *Clinical disorders of iron metabolism.* Grune and Stratton, New York.

BOTHWELL, T. H. and FINCH, C. A. (1962). *Iron metabolism.* Little, Brown and Co., Boston.

DREYFUS, J. C. and SCHAPIRA, G. (1958). *Le fer: biochimie, physiologie, pathologie.* Expansion Scientifique Française, Paris, p. 368.

Eisenstoffwechsel, ed. by KEIDERLING, W. (1959). Georg Thieme, Stuttgart (referred to as *Eisenstoffwechsel*).

HEILMEYER, L. and PLOTNER, K. (1937). *Das Serumeisen und die Eisen-mangelKrankheit.* Fischer, Iena.

HEMMELER, G. (1951). *Métabolisme du fer.* Masson et Cie, Paris.

Iron Metabolism, an international symposium. DREYFUS, J. C. and SCHAPIRA, G., chairmen; ed. by GROSS, F. (1964). Springer-Verlag, Berlin. (Referred to as *Iron metabolism*).

JASINSKI, B. and ROTH, O. (1954). *Larvierte Eisenmangel Krankheit.* Benno Schwabe, Basle.

MACDONALD, R. A. (1964). *Hemochromatosis and hemosiderosis.* Charles Thomas, Springfield.

SHELDON, J. H. (1935). *Haemochromatosis.* Oxford Univ. Press, London.

b. ORIGINAL PAPERS

AEBI, H., HEINIGER, J. P. and SUTER, H. (1963). Some properties of red cells and other tissues from normal and acatalatic humans. *Biochem. J.*, **89**: 63.

AGNER, K. (1958). Crystalline myeloperoxidase. *Acta chem. Scand.*, **12**: 89–94.

AGNER, K., ANDERSSON, N. S. E. and NORDENSON, N. G. (1948). Intravenöse Eisentherapie. *Acta haematol.*, **1**, 193–211.

ALBAHARY, C. (1964). Introduction to the general discussion on iron chelation. In: *Iron metabolism*, pp. 580–87 (q.v. in list of books).

AMERMAN, E. E., BRESCIA, M. A. and AFTAHI, F. (1958). Ferrous sulfate poisoning. *J. Pediatrics*, **53**: 476–80.

ANDERSSON, N. S. E. (1961). Clinical investigation on a new intramuscular haematinic. *Brit. Med. J.*, **1**: 275–9.

ARNON, D. I., TSUJIMOTO, H. Y. and ME SWAIN, B. S. (1967). Ferredoxin and photosynthetic phosphorylation. *Nature*, **214**, 562–6.

ARNON, D. I. (1965). Ferredoxin and photosynthesis. *Science*, **149**: 1460–70.

ARROWSMITH, W. and MINNICH, V. (1941). Site of absorption of iron from the gastrointestinal tract. *J. Amer. med. Ass.*, **116**: 2427–8.

BADENOCH, J. and CALLENDER, S. T. (1954). Iron metabolism in steatorrhea. The use of radioactive iron in studies of absorption and utilisation. *Blood*, **9**: 123–33.

BAIRD, I. M., BLACKBURN, E. K. and WILSON, G. M. (1959). The pathogenesis of anaemia after partial gastrectomy. *Quart. J. Med.*, **28**: 21–34.

BANNERMAN, R. M. (1965). Quantitative aspects of hemoglobin iron absorption. *J. lab. clin. Med.*, **65**: 944–50.

BEARN, A. G. and PARKER, W. C. (1963). Some observations on transferrin. In: *Iron metabolism*, pp. 60–71 (q.v. in list of books).

BERGEIM, O. and KIRCH, E. R. (1949). Reduction of iron in the human stomach. *J. biol. Chem.*, **177**: 591–6.

BESSIS, M. and BRETON-GORIUS, J. (1959). Ferritin and ferruginous micelles in normal erythroblasts and hypochromic hypersideremic anaemias. *Blood*, **14**: 423–32.

BESSIS, M. and BRETON-GORIUS, J. (1961). L'ilot érythroblastique et la rhophéocytose de la protéine dans l'inflammation. *Nouv. Rev. Fr. Hématol.*, **1**: 569–82.

BEUTLER, E. (1957). Iron enzymes in iron deficiency. Cytochrome C. *Amer. J. med. Sci.*, **234**: 517–27.

BEUTLER, E. (1959). Iron enzymes in iron deficiency. IV. Cytochrome oxidase in rat kidney and heart. *Acta haematd.*, **21**: 371–7.

BEUTLER, E. (1964). Tissue effects of iron deficiency. In: *Iron metabolism*, pp. 256–72 (q.v. in list of books).

BLAUD, P. (1832). Sur les maladies chroniques, et sur un mode de traitement spécifique dans ces affections. *Rev. méd. franç. Etrang.*, **45**: 341–67.

BOTHWELL, T. H. and BRADLOW, B. A. (1960). Siderosis in the Bantu. *Arch. Path.*, **70**: 279–92.

BOTHWELL, T. H., JACOBS, P. and TORRANCE, J. D. (1962). Studies on the behaviour of transferrin in idiopathic haemochromatosis. *South afr. med. J.*, **27**: 35–9.

BOTHWELL, T. H., VAN DOORN-WITTKAMPF, H., DU PREEZ, M. L. and ALPER, T. (1953). The absorption of iron-radioiron studies in idiopathic hemochromatosis malnutritional cytosiderosis and transfusional hemosiderosis. *J. lab. clin. Med.*, **41**: 836–48.

BRAUNITZER, G., GEHRING-MULLER, R., MILSCHMANN, N., HILSE, K., HOBOM, B., RUDLOFF, V. and WITTMAN-LIEBOLD, B. (1961). Die Struktur des normalen menschlichen Häemoglobins. *Z. physiol. Chem.*, **325**: 283–6.

BRICK, I. B. and RATH, C. E. (1964). Evaluation of trisodium calcium diethylenetriamine penta-acetate in hemochromatosis and transfusion hemosiderosis. In: *Iron Metabolism*, pp. 568–79 (q.v. in list of books).

BRISE, H. and HALLBERG, L. (1962). Absorbability of different iron compounds. *Acta Med. Scand.*, **171**: (suppl. 376), 23–8.

BROCK J. F. and HUNTER, D. (1937). *Quart. J. Med.*, **6**: 5 quoted by Dreyfus and Schapira (1958).

BRONSON, W. R. and SISSON, T. R. C. (1960). Studies on acute iron poisoning. *A.M.A.J. Dis. Child.*, **99**: 18–26.

BROWN, E. B., JR., DUBACH, R. and MOORE, C. V. (1958). Studies in iron transportation and metabolism. XI. Critical analysis of mucosal block by large doses of inorganic iron in human subjects. *J. lab. clin. Med.*, **52**: 335–55.

BROWN, E. B., JR., DUBACH, R., SMITH, D. E., REYNAFARJE, C. and MOORE, C. V. (1957). Studies in iron transportation and metabolism. X. Longterm iron overload in dogs. *J. lab. clin. Med.*, **50**: 862–93.

BROWN, E. B. and MOORE, C. V. (1956). Parenterally administered iron in the treatment of hypochromic anemia. In: *Progress in Hematology*. Grune and Stratton, p. 22–46.

BROWN, E. B., JR., SMITH, D. E., DUBACH, R. and MOORE, C. V. (1959). Lethal iron overload in dogs. *J. lab. clin. Med.*, **53**: 591–606.

BUTT, E. M., NUSBAUM, R. E., GILMOUR, T. C. and DIDIO, S. (1956). Trace metal patterns in disease states; hemochromatosis and refractory anemia. *Amer. J. clin. Path.*, **26**: 225–42.

CALLENDER, S. T. (1964). Digestive absorption of iron. In: *Iron metabolism*, pp. 89–96 (q.v. in list of books).

CALLENDER, S. T., MALLETT, B. J. and SMITH, M. D. (1957). Absorption of haemoglobin iron. *Brit. J. Haematol.*, **3**: 186–92.

CAROLI, J. and ANDRÉ, J. (1964). Surcharge ferrique dans les cirrhoses (à l'exclusion de l'hémochromatose idiopathique). In: *Iron metabolism*, pp. 326–39 (q.v. in list of books).

252   *Hematopoietic Agents*

CAROLI, J., BERNARD, J., BESSIS, M., COMBRISSON, A., MALASSENET, R. and BRETON, J. (1957). Hémochromatose avec anémie hypochrome et absence d'hémoglobine anormale. Etude au microscope électronique. *Presse méd.*, **2**: 1991.

CASTELMAN, P. (1946). In: Case Records of the Massachusetts General Hospital. Case 32481. *New Engl. J. Med.*, **235**: 798.

CEELEN, W. (1931). Die Kreislaufstörungen der Lungen. In: *Henke-Lubarsch: Handbuch der speziellen pathologischen Anatomie und Histologie*. Vol. III, p. 20.

CHATTERJEE, J. B. (1964). Some aspects of iron deficiency anaemia in India. In: *Iron metabolism*, pp. 219–40 (q.v. in list of books).

CHARLTON, R. W. and BOTHWELL, T. H. (1966). Hemochromatosis: dietary and genetic agents. In: *Progress in Hematology*, GRUNE and STRATTON (Ed.), p. 298–323.

CLAYTON, R. K. (1960). The induced synthesis of catalase in *Rhodopseudomonas spheroides*. *Biochim. biophys. Acta.*, **37**: 503–12.

CHEVALLIER, P. (1915). *Ann. Med.*, **2**: 229 quoted by DREYFUS and SCHAPIRA (1958).

CLETON, F. J. and BLOK, A. P. R. (1964). Post transfusional haemosiderosis. In: *Iron metabolism*, pp. 347–58 (q.v. in list of books).

CONLEY, B. E. (1959). Accidental iron poisoning in children. *J. Amer. med. Ass.*, **170**: 676–77.

COOK, S. F. (1929). The structure and composition of hemosiderin. *J. biol. Chem.*, **82**: 595–609

COOLEY, T. B. (1945). A severe type of hereditary anemia with elliptocytosis. *Amer. J. med. Sci.*, **209**: 561–68.

COPE, E., GILLHESPY, R. O. and RICHARDSON, R. W. (1956). Treatment of iron deficiency anemia: comparison of methods. *Brit. Med. J.*, **2**: 638–40.

CROSBY, W. H. (1953). Paroxysmal nocturnal hemoglobinuria. Relation of the clinical manifestations to underlying pathogenic mechanisms. *Blood*, **8**: 769–812.

CURZON, G. (1960). The effects of some ions and chelating agents on the oxidase activity of caeruloplasmin. *Bioch. J.*, **77**: 66–73.

DALLMAN, P. R. and SCHWARTZ, H. G. (1965). Myoglobin and cytochrome response during repair of iron deficiency in the rat. *J. clin. Invest.*, **44**: 1631–8.

DARNIS, F. (1958). Pathogénie et traitement des hémochromatoses. *Pathol. Biol.*, **34**: 873–90.

DAVIS, N. D. and ARROWSMITH, W. R. (1950). The effect of repeated bleedings in hemochromatosis. *J. lab. clin. Med.*, **36**: 814–5.

DAVIS, P. S., LUKE, C. G. and DELLER, D. J. (1966). Reduction of gastric iron binding protein in hemochromatosis. A previously unrecognized metabolic defect. *Lancet*, **2**: 1431–83.

DAVIS, P. S, LUKE, C. G. and DELLER, D. J. (1967). Gastric iron binding protein in iron chelation by gastric juice. *Nature*, **214**: 1126.

DEBRÉ, R., DREYFUS, J. C., FREZAL, J., LABIE, D., LAMY, M., MAROTEAUX, P., SCHAPIRA, F. and SCHAPIRA, G. (1958). Genetics of haemochromatosis. *Ann. hum. Genet.*, **23**: 16–30.

DEBRÉ, R., SCHAPIRA, G., DREYFUS, J. C. and SCHAPIRA, F. (1952). Métabolism du fer chez les descendants de malades atteints de cirrhose bronzée. *Bull. Mém. Soc. Méd. Hôp. Paris*, **18**: 665–9.

DICKMANN, S. R. and CLOUTIER, A. A. (1951), *J. biol. Chem.*, **188**: 379 quoted by DREYFUS and SCHAPIRA (1958).

DREYFUS, J. C. and SCHAPIRA, G. (1955). Sidérophiline. *Bull. Soc. Chim. Biol.*, **37**: 541–62.

DREYFUS, J. C. and SCHAPIRA, G. (1964). The metabolism of iron in haemochromatosis. In: *Iron metabolism*, pp. 296–326 (q.v. in list of books).

DREYFUS, J. C., SCHAPIRA, G. and SCHAPIRA, F. (1950). Le métabolisme due fer au cours de la cirrhose bronzée. Fer sérique et épreuve d'hypersidérémie provoquée. *Bull. Acad. nat. Méd.*, pp. 302–303.

DREYFUS, J. C. (1950). Ph.D. thesis quoted by DREYFUS and SCHAPIRA (1958).

EDITORIAL (1960). Carcinogenic risks of iron-dextran. *Brit. med. J.*, **1**: 788–9.

EDITORIAL (1966). Haemochromatosis: hereditary or acquired. *Lancet*, **i**, 750–51.

EICHHORN, G. L. (1960). The function of iron in biochemistry. In: *Iron metabolism*, pp. 9–21 (q.v. in list of books).

ELLIS, J. T., SCHULMAN, I. and SMITH, CH. (1954). Generalized siderosis with fibrosis of liver and pancreas in Cooley's anemia. *Amer. J. Path.*, **30**: 287–309.

ELVEHJEM, C. A. (1935). The biological significance of copper and its relation to iron metabolism. *Physiol. Rev.*, **15**: 471–507.

FARRANT, J. L. (1954). An electron microscopic study of ferritin. *Biochim. biophys. Acta*, **13**: 569–76.

FEIGELSON, P. and GREENGARD, O. (1961). A microsomal iron-porphyrin activator of rat liver tryptophan pyrrolase. *J. biol. Chem.*, **236**: 153–7.

FIELDING, J. (1961). Intravenous iron dextrin in iron deficiency anemia. *Brit. med. J.*, **2**: 279–83.

FIELDING, J. (1965). Differential ferrioxamine test for measuring chelatable body iron. *J. clin. Path.*, **18**: 88–97.

FIGUEROA, W. G., ADAMS, W. S., DAVIS, F. W. and BASSETT, S. H. (1955). A study of the effect of disodium calcium versenate (Ca EDTA) on iron excretion in man. *J. lab. clin. Med.*, **46**: 534.

FINCH, C. A. (1949). Iron metabolism in hemochromatis. *J. clin. Invest.*, **28**: 780.

FINCH, C. A. (1959). Some quantitative aspects of erythropoiesis. *Ann. N.Y. Acad. Sci.*, **77**: 410–16.

FINCH, C. A. (1960). Physiopathologic mechanisms of iron excretion. In: *Iron metabolism*, pp. 452–60 (q.v. in list of books).

FINCH, C. A. (1965). Iron balance in man. *Nutr. Rev.*, **23**: 129–31.

FINCH, C. A., GIBSON, J. G., PEACOCK, W. C. and FLUHARTY, R. G. (1949). Iron metabolism. Utilization of intravenous radioactive iron. *Blood*, **4**: 905–27.

FINCH, S. C. and FINCH, C. A. (1955). Idiopathic hemochromatosis, an iron storage disease. *Medicine*, **34**: 381–430.

FLETCHER, F. and LONDON, E. (1951). Intravenous iron. *Brit. med. J.*, **1**: 984.

FOLDBERG, L. (1958). Pharmacology of parenteral iron preparation. In: *Iron in clinical medicine*. Univ. Calif. Press, p. 74.

FONTÈS, G. and THIVOLLE, L. (1925). Sur la teneur du sérum en fer non hémoglobinique et sur sa diminution au cours de l'anémie expérimentale. *C.R. Soc. Biol.*, **93**: 687–9.

FOREMAN, H., HUFF, R., ODA, J. and GARCIA, J. (1952). Use of a chelating agent for accelerating excretion of radio-iron. *Proc. Soc. exp. biol. Med.*, **79**: 520–24.

FRAENKEL-CONRAT, H. and FEENEY, R. E. (1950). *Arch. Biochem.*, **28**: 452 quoted by DREYFUS aud SCHAPIRA (1958).

GERALD, P. S., COOK, C. D. and DIAMOND, L. K. (1957). Hemoglobin M. *Science*, **126**: 300–301.

GILLMAN, T., LAMONT, N., HATHORN, M. and CANHAM, P. A. S. (1957). Haemochromatosis: African nutritional siderosis and experimental siderosis in animals. *Lancet*, **273**: 173–75.

GOETTSCH, A. T., MOORE, C. V. and MINNICH. V. (1946). Observations on the effect of massive doses of iron given intravenously to patients with hypochromic anemia. *Blood*, **1**: 129–42.

GOLDBERG, L. (1958). Pharmacology of parenteral iron preparation, quoted by BEUTLER, FAIRBANKS and FAHEY (1963)

J*

GRANICK, S. (1946). Ferritin: its properties and significance for iron metabolism. *Chem. Rev.*, **31**: 489–511.

GRAYZEL, A. I., HORCHNER, P. and LONDON, I. M. (1966). The stimulation of globin synthesis by heme. *Proc. nat. Acad. Sci., Wash.*, **55**: 650–55.

GRIBBLE, T. J. and SCHWARTZ, H. C. (1965). Effect of protoporphyrin on hemoglobin synthesis. *Biochim. biophys. Acta*, **103**: 333–8.

GRUNBERG, H. (1941). Siderocytes: a new kind of erythrocyte. *Nature*, **148**: 114–15.

GUBLER, C. J., CARTWRIGHT, G. E. and WINTROBE, M. M. (1950). Anemia of infection. X. Effect of infection of the absorption and storage of iron by the rat. *J. biol. Chem.*, **184**: 563–74.

HAGGIS, G. H. (1965). The iron oxide core of the ferritin molecule. *J. mol. Biol.*, **14**: 598–602.

HAHN, P. F., BALE, V. F., LAURENCE, E. O. and WHIPPLE, G. H. (1939). Radioactive iron absorption by the gastrointestinal tract; influence of anemia, anoxia and antecedent feeding; distribution in growing dogs. *J. exp. Med.*, **78**: 169–88.

HAHN, P. F., GRANICK, S., BALE, W. F. and MICHAELIS, L. (1943). Ferritin conversion of inorganic and hemoglobin iron into ferritin iron in animal body. *J. biol. Chem.*, **156**: 407–12.

HALLBERG, L., BRISE, H. and SOLVELL, L. (1960). A new method for studies on iron absorption in man. In: *Proc. VIIth Intern. Cong. Rome, 1958. Intern. Soc. Hematol.* Vol. 2. New York, Grune and Stratton, pp. 524–8.

HALLBERG, L. and SOLVELL, L. (1960). Iron absorption studies. *Acta med. Scand.*, **168**: (suppl. 358); 3–108.

HALLGREN, B. (1953). (Quoted by MORGAN (1964)). *Acta Soc. med. Uppsal.*, **59**: 79.

HARRISON, P. M. (1964). Ferritin and haemosiderin. In: *Iron metabolism*, pp. 40–56 (q.v. in list of books).

HAVRANI, F. S., BURKE, W. and MARTINEZ, E. J. (1965). Defective reutilization of iron in the anemia of inflammation. *J. lab. clin. Med.*, **65**: 560–70.

HAWKINS, C. F., FEENEY, A. L. P. and COOKE, W. T. (1950). Refractory hypochromic anaemia and steatorrhea; treatment with intravenous iron. *Lancet*, **2**: 387–91.

HAYAISHI, O. (1963). Direct oxygenation by O_2: oxygenases. In: *The Enzymes*. Acad. Press, vol. 8, pp. 353–71.

HEATH, C. W., STRAUSS, M. G. and CASTLE, W. B. (1932). Quantitative aspects of iron deficiency in hypochromic anemia. *J. clin. Invest.*, **11**: 1293–312.

HEILMEYER, L. (1954). Die Hämochromatose: Klinik, Eisenstoffwechsel und Pathogenese. *Acta haematol.*, **11**: 137–51.

HEILMEYER, L. (1960). Human hyposideraemia. In: *Iron metabolism*, pp. 201, 213 (q.v. in list of books).

HEILMEYER, L., EMMRICH, J., HENNEMANN, H. H., SCHUBOTHE, H., KEIDERLING, W., LEE, M. M., BILGER, R. and BERNAUER, W. (1957). Uber eine neuartige hypochrome Anämie bei zwei Geschwistern auf der Grundlage einer Eisenverwertungsstörung: anaemia sideroachrestica hereditaria. *Schweiz. med. Wschr.*, **87**: 1237–8.

HEILMEYER, V. L., KELLER, W., VIVELL, O., BETKE, K., WOHLER, F. and KEIDERLING, W. (1961). Die kongenitale Atransferrinämie. *Schweiz. med. Wschr.*, **91**: 1203.

HEILMEYER, L. (1964). Human hyposideraemia, in *Iron Metabolism*. 1964, 201–213,

HEMMELER, G. (1944). Nouvelles recherches sur le métabolisme du fer: les oscillations du fersérique dans la journée. *Helv. med. Acta*, **11**: 201–7.

HOLLY, R. G. (1955). Anemia in pregnancy. *Obstet. Gynec.*, **5**: 562–8.

HOLMBERG, C. G. and LAURELL, C. B. (1945). Studies on the capacity of serum to bind iron. *Acta physiol. Scand.*, **10**: 307–19.

HOPPE, J. O., MARCELLI, G. M. A. and TAINTER, M. L. (1955). A review of the toxicity of iron compounds. *Amer. J. med. Sci.*, **230**: 558–71.

HUFF, R. L., LAWRENCE, J. H., SIRI, W. E., WASSERMAN, L. R. and HENNESSY, T. G. (1951). Effects of changes in altitude on hemopoietic activity. *Medicine*, 30: 197–217.

HUNTER, C. A. (1960). Iron deficiency anemia in pregnancy. *Surg. Gynec. Obstet.*, 110: 210–14.

JACOB, A. (1961). Iron containing enzymes in the buccal epithelium. *Lancet*, 2: 1331–3.

KARIBIAN, D. and LONDON, I. M. (1965). Control of heme synthesis by feedback inhibition. *Biochem. Biophys. Res. Comm.*, 18: 243–9.

KASPER, C. K., WHISSEL, D. Y. E. and WALLERSTEIN, R. O. (1965). Clinical aspects of iron deficiency. *J. Amer. med. Ass.*, 191: 359–63.

KATZ, J. H. and JANDL, J. H. (1964). The role of transferrin in the transport of iron into the developing red cell. In: *Iron metabolism*, pp. 103–117 (q.v. in list of books).

KELLY, A. B. (1919). Spasm at the entrance to the esophagus. *J. Laryngol. Rhinol. Otol.*, 34: 285–89.

KENDREW, J. C. (1962). *Brookhaven. Symp. Biol.*, No. 15.

KINNEY, T. D., HAUFMANN, N. and KLAVINS, J. (1955). *J. exp. Med.*, 102: 157 quoted by DREYFUS and SCHAPIRA (1958).

KINNEY, T. D., HEGSTED, D. M. and FINCH, C. A. (1949). The influence of diet on iron absorption. The pathology of iron excess. *J. exp. Med.*, 90: 137–46.

KINNEY, T. D., HEGSTEDT, D. M. and FINCH, C, A. (1948). *Amer. J. Pathol.*, 24: 699 quoted by DREYFUS and SCHAPIRA (1958).

KINNEY, T. D., KAUFMAN, N. and KLAVINS, J. (1965). Effects of ethionine induced pancreatic damage on iron absorption. *J. exp. Med.*, 102: 151–56.

KLECKNER, M. S., JR., BAGGENSTOSS, A. H. and WEIR, J. F. (1955). Iron-storage diseases. *Amer. J. clin. Path.*, 25: 915–31.

KLOTZ, H. P., AVRIL, J. and PARIENTE, R. (1957). Aggravation rapide de deux cirrhoses bronzées après l'essai thérapeutique d'un chelateur (EDTA calcique). *Bull. Mem. Soc. Med. Hop. Paris*, 73: 1001–3.

KNOX, W. E. and MEHLER, A. H. (1951). The adaptive increase of the tryptophan peroxidase-oxidase system of liver. *Science*, 113: 237–8.

KONIGSBERG, W., GUIDOTTI, G. and HILL, R. J. (1961). The amino acid sequence of the α chain of human hemoglobin. *J. biol. Chem.*, 236: PC, 55–6.

KORMAN, S. (1960). Iron metabolism in man. *Ann. New York Acad. Sci.*, 88: 460–73.

LAUFBERGER, M. V. (1937). Sur la cristallisation de la ferritine. *Bull. Soc. Chim. biol.*, 19: 1575–82.

LAURELL, C. B. (1947). *Acta. Physiol. Scand.*, 14: Suppl. 46 quoted by DREYFUS and SCHAPIRA (1958).

LAURELL, C. B. (1951). What is the function of transferrin in plasma? *Blood*, 6: 183–7.

LAURELL, C. B. (1958). Iron transportation. In: *Iron in clinical medicine*. Univ. Calif. Press, Berkeley, pp. 8–23.

LEDERER, J. (1951). L'anémie agastrique. *Sem. Hop. Paris*, 27: 1975–9.

LINTZEL, W. (1931). Neuere Ergebnisse der Erforschung des Eisenstoffwechsels. *Ergeb. Physiol.*, 31: 844–919.

LOFTFIELD, R. B. and HARRIS, A. (1956). Participation of the amino acids in protein synthesis. *J. biol. Chem.*, 219: 151–9.

LORENZ, E. and MENKIN, V. (1936). Experimental siderosis. *Arch. Pathol.*, 22: 82–5.

LUKE, C. G., DAVIS, P. S. and DELLER, D. J. (1967). Change in gastric iron binding protein (gastroferrin) during iron deficiency anemia. *Lancet*, 1: 926–7.

LWOFF, A., (1943). *L'évolution physiologique*. Hermann et Cie Paris.

MCCALL, M. G., NEWMAN, G. E., O'BRIEN, J. R. P. and WITTS, L. J. (1962). Studies in iron metabolism. The effects of experimental iron deficiency on the growing rat. *Brit. J. Nutrit.*, 16: 305–23.

MCCANCE, R. A. and WIDDOWSON, E. M. (1937). Absorption and excretion of iron. *Lancet*, 233: 680–4.

256 *Hematopoietic Agents*

MacDonald, R. A. (1963). Idiopathie hemochromatosis: genetic or acquired. *Arch. int. Med.*, **112**: 184–90.

MacDonald, R. A. and Pechet, G. S. (1965). Tissue iron and hemochromatosis. Comparative geographic studies. *Arch. int. Med.*, **116**: 381–91.

MacDonald, R. A. (1966). Primary hemochromatosis: inherited or acquired. In: *Progress in Hematology.* Grune and Stratton, pp. 324–53.

Mallarmé, J. and Tilquin, R. (1948). Étude sur dix cas d'anémie hypochrome tardive observés en 1947, dont six relevant de hernie diaphragmétique. *Sang*, **19**: 282–98.

Margoliash, E., Smith, E. L., Kreil, G. and Tuppy, H. (1961). Amino-acid sequence of horse heart cytochrome *c*. *Nature*, **192**: 1121–7.

Massey, V. (1958). The role of iron in beef-heart succinie dehydrogenase. *Biochim. biophys. Acta*, **30**: 500–9.

Matsubara, H., Sasaki, R. M. and Chain, R. K. (1967). The amino acid sequence of spinach ferredoxin. *Proc. natl. Acad. Sci., Wash.*, **57**: 439–45.

Mazur, A., Litt, I. and Shorr, E. (1950). The relation of sulfhydryl groups in ferritin to its vasodepressor activity. *J. biol. Chem.*, **187**: 485–95.

Michaelis, L. (1947). Ferritin and apoferritin. *Advanc. Protein Chem.*, **3**: 53–66.

Miller, A., Chodos, R. B., Emerson, C. P. and Ross, J. F. (1956). Studies of the anemia and iron metabolism in cancer. *J. clin. Invest.*, **35**: 1248–62.

Mitchell, H. H. and Hamilton, T. S. (1949). The dermal excretion under controlled environmental conditions of nitrogen and minerals in human subjects, with particular reference to calcium and iron. *J. biol. Chem.*, **178**: 345–61.

Moeschlin, S. and Schnider, V. (1964). Treatment of primary and secondary hemochromatosis and acute iron poisoning with a new, potent iron chimirating agent (desferrioxamine B). In: *Iron metabolism*, pp. 525–50 (q.v. in list of books).

Moore, C. V. (1960). Iron nutrition. In: *Iron metabolism*, pp. 241–55 (q.v. in list of books).

Moore, C. V. and Dubach, R. (1951). Observations on the absorption of iron from foods tagged with radio-iron. *Trans. Ass. Amer. Physiol.*, **64**: 245–56.

Moore, C. V. and Dubach, R. (1956). Metabolism and requirements of iron in the human. *J. Amer. med. Ass.*, **162**: 197–204.

Morgan, E. H. (1961). Iron storage and transport in iron depleted rats, with notes on combined iron and copper deficiency. *Austr. J. exp. Biol.*, **39**: 371–9.

Morgan, E. H. (1964). Experimental hyposiderosis. In: *Iron metabolism*, pp. 185–200 (q.v. in list of books).

Morgan, E. H., Marsaglia, G., Giblett, E. R. and Finch, C. A. (1967). A method of investigating internal iron exchange utilizing two types of transferrin. *J. lab. clin. Med.*, **69**: 370–81.

Mouriquand, C. (1958). Le sidéroblaste. Étude morphologique et essai d'interprétation. *Rev. Hématol.*, **13**: 79–99.

Najean, N. (1967). Acquisitions récentes sur le métabolisme du fer. In: *Progrès En Hématologie.* Flammarion, pp. 93–112.

Nason, A. (1963). Nitrate reductases. In: *The Enzymes.* Acad. Press, vol. 7, pp. 587–607.

Nicholls, P. (1963). Cytochromes. A survey. In: *The Enzymes.* Acad. Press, vol. 8, pp. 3–39.

Nicholls, P. and Schonbaum, G. R. (1963). Catalases. In: *The Enzymes.* Acad. Press, vol. 8, pp. 147, 225.

Nishimura, E. T., Hamilton, H. B., Kobara, Ty., Takahara, S., Ogura, Y. and Doi, K. (1959). Carrier state in human acatalasemia. *Science*, **130**: 333–4.

Nissim, J. A. (1947). Intravenous administration of iron. *Lancet*, **2**: 49–51.

Osaki, S., (1966). Kinetic studies of ferrous iron oxidation with crystalline human ferroxidase (ceruloplasmin). *J. biol. Chem.*, **241**: 5053–9.

OSAKI, S. and WAALAS, O. (1967). Kinetic studies of ferrous iron oxidation with crystalline human ferroxidase. *J. biol. Chem.*, **242**: 2653–8.

OZOLS, J. and STRITTMATTER, P. (1967). The homology between cytochrome b5, hemoglobin and myoglobin. *Proc. nat. Acad. Sci., Wash.*, **58**: 264–7.

PALEUS, S. and PAUL, K. G. (1963). Mammalian cytochrome *c*. In: *The Enzymes*. Acad. Press, vol. 8, pp. 97–112.

PATERSON, D. R. (1919). A clinical type of dysphagia. *J. Laryng. Rhinol. Otol.*, **34**: 289–91.

PAUL, K. G. (1963). Peroxidases. In: *The Enzymes*. Acad. Press, vol. 8, pp. 227–73.

PAULING, L. and CORYELL, C. B. (1936). The magnetic properties and structure of hemoglobin, oxyhemoglobin and carbonmonoxyhemoglobin. *Proc. nat. Acad. Sci., Wash.*, **22**: 210–6.

PERUTZ, M. F. (1962). *Proteins and nucleic acids. Structure and functions.* Elsevier.

PERUTZ, M. F. (1964). The hemoglobin molecule. *Scient. Amer.*, **211**: 64–76.

PETERSEN, R. E. and ETTINGER, R. H. (1953). Radioactive iron absorption in siderosis (hemochromatosis) of the liver. *Amer. J. Med.*, **15**: 518–24.

PITCHER, C. S., WILLIAMS, H. S., PARSONSON, A. and WILLIAMS, R. (1965). The measurement of iron absorption by the double isotope technique. *Brit. J. Haematol.*, **11**: 633–41.

POLIS, B. D. SHMUCKLER, H. W. (1953). *J. biol. Chem.*, **201**: 475 quoted by PAUL (1963).

POLLYCOVE, M. (1964). Iron kinetics. In: *Iron metabolism*, pp. 148–70 (q.v. in list of books).

POLLYCOVE, M. and MORTIMER, R. (1961). The quantitative determination of iron kinetics and hemoglobin synthesis in human subjects. *J. clin. Invest.*, **40**: 753–82.

POLONOVSKI, M. and JAYLE, M. F. (1939). Peroxydases animales. Leur spécificité et leur rôle biologique. *Bull. Soc. Chim. Biol.*, **21**: 66–91.

PRELOG, I. V. (1964). Iron containing compounds in micro-organisms. In: *Iron metabolism*, pp. 73–83 (q.v. in list of books).

PRITCHARD, J. A. (1961). The response to iron deficiency. *J. Amer. med. Ass.*, **175**: 478–482.

RATH, C. E. and FINCH, C. A. (1948). Sternal marrow hemosiderin. A method for the determination of available iron stores in man. *J. lab. clin. Med.*, **33**: 81–6.

REIMANN, F. and FRITSCA F. (1931). *Z. Klin. Med.*, **117**: 304 quoted by DREYFUS and SCHAPIRA (1958).

REISSMANN, K. R. and COLEMAN, T. J. (1955). Acute intestinal iron intoxication. *Blood*, **10**: 46–51.

REISSMANN, K. R. and DIETRICH, M. R. (1956). On the presence of ferritin in the peripheral blood of patients with hepatocellular disease. *J. clin. Invest.*, **35**: 588–95.

RICHMOND, H. G. (1957). Induction of sarcoma in rats by an iron-dextran complex. *Scottish Med. J.*, **2**: 169.

RICHTER, G. W. (1958). Electron microscopy of hemosiderin; presence of ferritin and occurrence of crystalline lattices in hemosiderin deposits. *J. biophys. biochem. cytol.*, **4**: 55–8.

RINGLER, R. L. (1961). Studies on the mitochondrial α-glycerophosphate dehydrogenase. *J. biol. Chem.*, **236**: 1192–8.

ROMANO, C. (1966). Iron absorption in cystic fibrosis. *Lancet*, **1**: 657.

ROSEN, B. J. and TULLIS, J. L. (1966). Simplified deferrioxamine test. *J. Amer. med. Ass.*, **195**: 261–4.

ROSS, F. G. M. (1953). Pyloric stenosis and fibrous stricture of the stomach due to ferrous sulfate poisoning. *Brit. med. J.*, **2**: 1200–2.

ROTHEN, A. (1944). Ferritin and apoferritin in the ultracentrifuge. *J. biol. Chem.*, **152**: 679–93.

Rous, P. and Oliver, J. (1918). Experimental hemochromatosis. *J. exp. Med.*, **28**: 629–44.

Saddi, R. (1962). Ferritine et hémochromatose idiopathique. *Rev. franç. Et. clin. biol.*, **7**: 408–10.

Saddi, R., Schapira, G. and Dreyfus, J. C. (1961). Sur l'existence de subunités dans la molécule de ferritine. *Bull. Soc. Chim. Biol.*, **43**: 409–13.

Saddi, R. and von der Decken (A.) (1964). Specific stimulation of amino acid incorporation into ferritin by rat-liver slices after injections of iron *in vivo*. *Biochim. biophys. Acta*, **80**: 196–8.

Saddi, R. and von der Decken, A. (1965). The effect of iron administration on the incorporation of ^{14}C leucine into ferritin by rat liver systems. *Biochim. biophys. Acta*, **111**: 124–33.

Schade, A. L. and Caroline, L. (1946). Iron binding component in human blood plasma. *Science*, **104**: 340–1.

Schaeffer, K. H. (1964). Neuroendocrine control of iron metabolism. In: *Iron metabolism*, pp. 280–8 (q.v. in list of books).

Schapira, G. (1964). Iron metabolism, past, present and future. In: *Iron metabolism*, pp. 1–8 (q.v. in list of books).

Schapira, G. and Dreyfus, J. C. (1948). *Bull. Soc. Chim. biol.*, **30**: 82 quoted by Dreyfus and Schapira (1958).

Schapira, G. and Dreyfus, J. C. (1955). Fer et nutrition. *Ann. Nutrit.*, **9**: 39–92.

Schapira, G. and Dreyfus, J. C. (1959). L'hémochromatose et son hérédité. In: *Eisenstoffwechsel*. pp. 238–44.

Schulman, I. (1961). Iron requirement in infancy. *J. Amer. med. Ass.*, **175**: 118–23.

Schwarzenbach, G. and K. (1963). HydroxamatKomplexe. I. Die Stabilität der EisenKomplexe einfacher Hydroxamsaüren und des Ferrioxamins B. *Helv. chim. Acta*, **46**: 1390–400.

Scott, J. M. and Govan, A. D. T. (1954). Anemia of pregnancy treated with intramuscular iron. *Brit. med. J.*, **2**: 1257.

Serif, G. S. and Kirkwood, S. (1958). *J. biol. Chdm.* **233**: 109 by Paul (1763).

Sherlock, S. (1964). Discussion. In: *Iron metabolism*, pp. 392–9. (q.v. in list of books).

Shoden, A. and Sturgeon, P. (1960). Hemosiderin. I. A physico-chemical study. *Acta haemat.*, **23**: 376–92.

Singer, T. P. (1963). Flavoprotein dehydrogenase of the electron transport chain In: *The Enzymes*. Acad. Press, vol. 7, pp. 345–81.

Singer, T. P. and Kearney, E. B. (1963). Succinate dehydrogenase. In: *The Enzymes*. Acad. Press, vol. 7, pp. 384–445.

Smith, J. P. (1952). The pathology of ferrous sulfate poisoning. *J. Path. Bact.*, **64**: 467–72.

Smith, R. P., Jones, C. W. and Cohran, W. E. (1950). Ferrous sulfate toxicity: report of a fatal case. *New Engl. J. Med.*, **243**: 641–5.

Smithies, O. (1957). Variations in human serum β-globulins. *Nature*, **180**: 1482–3.

Soergel, K. H. and Sommers, S. C. (1962). Idiopathic pulmonary hemosiderosis and related syndromes. *Amer. J. Med.*, **32**: 499–511.

Strachan, A. S. (1929). Haemosiderosis and haemochromatosis in South African natives, with a comment on the etiology of haemochromatosis. M.D. Thesis, Glasgow.

Sunderman, F. W. and Boerner, F. (1949). *Normal values in clinical medicine*. W. B. Saunders Company, Philadelphia (quoted by Beutler et al., 1963).

Surgenor, D. M., Kochlin, B. A. and Strong, L. E. (1949). Chemical, clinical and immunological studies on the products of human plasma fractionation. The metal combining globulin of human plasma. *J. clin. Invest.*, **28**: 73–8.

TANAKA, K. R. and VALENTINE (1961). Aconitase activity of human leucocytes. *Acta haematol.* (*Switz.*). **26**: 12–20.

THOENES, F. and ASCHAFFENBURG, R. (1934). Der Eisenstoffwechsel des wachsenden organismus. *Abh. Kinderheilk, Berlin*, 103.

TONZ, O., WEISS, S., STRAHM, H. W. and ROSSI, E. (1965). Iron absorption in cystic fibrosis. *Lancet*, **2**: 1096–9.

TROUSSEAU, A. (1856). Glycosurie; diabète sucré. *Clin. Med. Hôtel Dieu Paris*, **5**: (2) 663–98.

TUTTLE, S. G., FIGUEROA, W. G. and GROSSMAN, M. I. (1959). Development of hemochromatosis in a patient with Laënnec's cirrhosis. *Amer. J. med.*, **26**: 655–58.

VAHLQUIST, B. C. (1950). The cause of sexual differences in erythrocyte hemoglobin and serum iron levels in human adults. *Blood*, **5**: 874–5.

VERLOOP, M. C. (1964). Discussion. In: *Iron metabolism*, p. 342 (q.v. in list of books).

VERLOOP, M. C., MEEUWISSEN, J. E. T. and BLOKHUIS, E. W. M. (1958). Comparison of the iron absorption test with the determination of the iron binding capacity of serum in the diagnosis of iron deficiency. *Brit. J. Haematol.*, **4**: 70–81.

VERLOOP, M. C., PLOEM, W. and LEUNIS, J. (1964). Hereditary hypersideraemia anaemia. In: *Iron metabolism*, pp. 376–87 (q.v. in list of books).

WASSERMAN, L. R., RASHKOFF, I. A., LEAVITT, D., MAYER, J. and PORT, S. (1952). The rate of removal of radioactive iron from the plasma, an index of erythropoiesis. *J. clin. Invest.*, **31**: 32–9.

WAXMAN, H. S. and RABINOWITZ, M. (1965). Iron supplementation *in vitro* and the state of aggregation and function of reticulocyte ribosomes in hemoglobin synthesis. *Biochem. biophys. Res. Comm.*, **19**: 538–45.

WEINTRAUB, L. R., CONRAD, M. E. and CROSBY, W. H. (1965). Regulation of the intestinal absorption of iron by the rate of erythropoiesis. *Brit. J. Haematol.*, **11**: 432–8.

WELLS, C. and WELBOURN, R. (1951). Post-gastrectomy Syndromes; study in applied physiology. *Brit. med. J.*, **2**: 546–54.

WIDDOWSON, E. M. and McCANCE, R. A. (1948). Sexual differences in the storage and metabolism of iron. *Biochem. J.*, **42**: 577–81.

WILLIAMS, R., SCHEUER, P. J. and SHERLOCK, S. (1963). The inheritance of idiopathic hemochromatosis: a clinical and liver biopsy study of 16 families. *Quart. J. Med.*, **31**: 249–65.

WOHLER, F. (1964). The treatment of hemochromatosis with desferrioxamine. In: *Iron metabolism*, pp. 551–67 (q.v. in list of books).

WORLD HEALTH ORGANISATION. *Study Group on Anaemia*, working paper 10 (5 September 1958).

YU FU LI and FINEBERG, R. A. (1965). Biosynthesis of ferritin by rat liver slices. *J. biol. Chem.*, **240**: 2083–7.

ZUELZER, W. W. (1960). The case of Imferon: convenience and conscience. *A.M.A.J. Dis. Child.*, **100**: 3–5.

SUPPLEMENTARY BIBLIOGRAPHY

LU, A. Y. H., JUNK, K. W. and COON, M. J. (1969). Resolution of the cytochrome P 450 containing co-hydroxylation system of liver microsomes into three components. *J. biol. Chem.*, **244**: 3714–3721.

MASSON, P. L., HERREMANS, J. F. and SCHONNE, E. (1969). Lactoferrin, and iron binding protein in neutrophilic leucocytes. *J. Exp. Med.*, **190**: 643–58.

MORGAN, O. S., WEIR, D. G., GATTENAY, P. B. B. and SCOTT, J. M. (1970). Studies on an iron-binding component in human gastric juice. *Lancet*, p. 861–3.

Symposium on Electron Transport system in microsomes (1965). *Feder. Proc.*, **24**: 1153–99.

SADDI, R. and FEINGOLD, J. (1969). Hémochromatose idiopathique: maladie récessive autosomique. *Rev. franç. Et. Clin. biol.*, **14**: 238–51.

WESTERHAUSEN, M., KELLER, E., MAAS, D., GERMAN, H. J., KLEMENC-LIPPKAN, G. and SCHUROTHE, H. (1969). Atypisches Transferrin mit extrem hohem Serumeisenspiegel. *Klin. Wschr.* **47**: 1279–80.

CHAPTER 5

PROTEINS AND HEMATOPOIESIS

A. Aschkenasy

*Centre National de la Recherche Scientifique, Laboratoire
d'Hématologie Nutritionnelle, 45-Orléans-La Source, France*

I. INTRODUCTION

LARGE amounts of proteins and related substances are used in the formation of blood cells. They are needed for the synthesis of nucleic acids and proteins other than hemoglobin—especially enzymes—in erythroblasts and leucocytes, as well as for the formation of hemoglobin itself, which consumes one-seventh of the total nitrogen requirements (Drabkin, 1951).

The greatest demand is for the synthesis of the polypeptide chains of globin, but even the biosynthesis of heme from simple substances such as iron, glycine, and succinic acid (Shemin, 1954/5) requires the action of specific enzymes at each stage, and these are proteins.

Leucocytes are not only provided with numerous proteinic enzymes; some of these cells (plasma cells and probably certain lymphocytes) also elaborate specific proteins—the immunoglobulins which are released into the circulation.

Hematopoiesis thus makes heavy demands on nitrogen supplies, which the comparative rarity and late onset of pure protein-deficiency anemia would hardly suggest. But with protein deficiency, it is in fact only the concentration of red cells per unit of blood volume that remains unaffected for any length of time, as opposed to the total mass of blood, which decreases more or less in proportion to body weight.

Erythropoiesis would be much more seriously impaired if nitrogen released by hemolysis were not partly re-used for hematopoiesis.

The development of protein-deficiency anemia is also delayed by the transfer, under the control of certain hormones, of amino acids from other tissues to the blood-forming organs.

On the other hand, anemia may seem more pronounced than the actual disturbance of erythropoiesis if the protein deficiency causes edema with hydremia. This commonly occurs in man, but only rarely in the rat unless the deficiency involves not only protein but also methyl groups and vitamin B_{12} (Alexander and Sauberlich, 1957).

In the majority of cases of human nutritional anemia there is in fact a deficiency not only of protein but also of iron and certain hematopoietic vitamins, particularly folic acid, vitamin B_{12}, and niacin.

This is undoubtedly why deficiency anemias, apart from sideropenic anemia, are nearly always normocytic or macrocytic, and normochromic or hyperchromic—even, in some cases, with a megaloblastic bone marrow (Altmann and Murray, 1948; Mehta and Gopalan, 1956); whereas (at least in the rat) experimental protein-deficiency anemia is microcytic and hypochromic.

Furthermore, in man anemia of malnutrition is often aggravated by concurrent infection or infestation, as for instance in kwashiorkor (Gounelle, 1953).

Indeed, it is not only in cases of multiple deficiency in man, but even in laboratory animals deprived solely of protein, that the effect of actual protein deficiency in causing anemia and leucopenia is difficult to distinguish from that of hypovitaminosis: the latter is determined both by the metabolic interdependance between certain amino acids and vitamins, and by the cessation of vitamin synthesis by intestinal microbes affected by lack of protein.

The same lack also reduces dietary intake and thus leads to secondary deficiency of calories, as well as of vitamins and minerals.

Finally, as will be seen later, the hematopoietic action of protein itself does not consist simply of providing specific raw materials but also of stimulating the production of certain hormones and humoral hematopoietic factors such as erythropoietin.

The following account deals successively with the characteristics of experimental protein-deficiency anemia and leucopenia, the hematopoietic effects of dietary and tissue proteins and amino acids, and the interaction between these and the vitamins, between proteins and other foods (carbohydrates, fats, iron), and between proteins and hormones. It ends with a discussion of the mechanisms of protein-deficiency anemia and leucopenia.

II. HEMATOLOGICAL CHARACTERISTICS OF
PROTEIN-DEFICIENCY ANEMIA AND LEUCOPENIA

1. *Low-protein diet*

Even partial deprivation of protein always causes a reduction of the total blood volume (Weech *et al.*, 1937; Metcoff *et al.*, 1945; Benditt *et al.*, 1946), but in the absence of edema the reduction is generally proportional to weight loss, and the ratio of blood mass to body weight remains constant (Benditt *et al.*, 1946; Bethard *et al.*, 1958). Yet according to Hallgren (1954) the total hemoglobin in the rat is proportionally more reduced than the "carcass" protein, so that the priority of erythropoiesis in bled dogs observed by Whipple and Robscheit-Robbins (1951) has not been confirmed in protein-deficient rats, at least as regards the maintenance of total hemoglobin mass.

The concentration of hemoglobin in the blood is also reduced with a low-protein diet, but not nearly to the same extent as the total hemoglobin. The red-cell count, on the other hand, remains normal for a long time if the protein content of the diet exceeds 4% (Pearson *et al.*, 1937; Orten and Orten, 1943; Aschkenasy and Aschkenasy-Lelu, 1947; Aschkenasy and Benhamou, 1950); hence hypochromia without erythrocytopenia.

At a late stage there is moderate reticulocytosis (Orten and Orten, 1943), analogous to that seen in very advanced nitrogen deprivation (Aschkenasy, 1946) and certainly reflecting a compensated hemolysis, the erythrocyte count remaining normal as a rule.

Any kind of protein malnutrition, whether quantitative or purely qualitative, increases anemia caused not only by bleeding (Hahn and Whipple, 1939) but also by various non-specific aggressions.

In this way a diet lacking protein favors the development of anemia in the course of infections (Robscheit-Robbins *et al.*, 1945), after extensive burns or surgical operations (Hallgren, 1954) or in various kinds of experimental poisoning, for instance with sulfonamides (Aschkenasy *et al.*, 1948), aminoacetonitrile (a lathyrogenic compound) (Aschkenasy, 1961c), or lead (Gontzea *et al.*, 1964).

Any physiological condition under which the nitrogen requirements are increased (rapid growth in childhood, muscular work, pregnancy, lactation) is liable to produce anemia if the diet is deficient in protein (Bethell *et al.*, 1943; Hallgren, 1954).

2. *Protein-free diet*

(a) *Anemia.* In the absence of any of the predisposing causes mentioned, anemia involving reduction of both hemoglobin and red-cell count is seen only if protein is completely excluded from the diet.

In adult rats this anemia begins late (after 60–80 days in most strains) and remains mild (as a rule about 6 million red cells and 8 g per 100 ml of hemoglobin). It is hypochromic and microcytic (Aschkenasy, 1946;

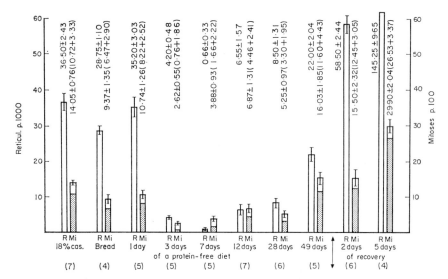

FIG. 1. Mean reticulocyte counts (R) and mitotic indices (Mi) of the bone marrow (after colchicine) ±S.E.M. in rats submitted to a balanced 18% casein diet, a poor natural diet (bread and carrots), a protein-free diet of various duration, or a recovery diet (18% casein) started after 7 weeks of protein deprivation. The upper part of each column of mitotic indices corresponds to myelocytes, the lower part to erythroblasts. Below: numbers of rats in parentheses. Reproduced from *C.R. Acad. Sci.*, **256**: 1155–7 (1963).

Aschkenasy and Pariente, 1951, 1953; Hallgren, 1954), but this is not necessarily the case with species other than the rat: in the monkey, for example, the anemia is normocytic and normochromic (Sood *et al.*, 1965). In man, however, the anemia is hypochromic and microcytic, as in the rat, if it is due solely to protein deficiency (Layani *et al.*, 1949).

At the beginning of a protein-free regimen, the red-cell count, instead of falling, actually rises for a time—the total red-cell mass being too large for the blood volume, which is abruptly reduced because of weight loss. But the reticulocyte count is greatly diminished, reaching a minimum after 7 days: less than 5 per 1000 as against 30–40 per 1000 before the start of the deficiency (Aschkenasy, 1946, 1961b, 1962b,c,d) (Fig. 1).

At the same time the uptake by the red cells of ^{59}Fe given intravenously (Bethard *et al.*, 1958a,b; Aschkenasy, 1962b,c,d) (Fig. 2) or orally (Aschkenasy, 1965f) (Table 1) is almost completely blocked.

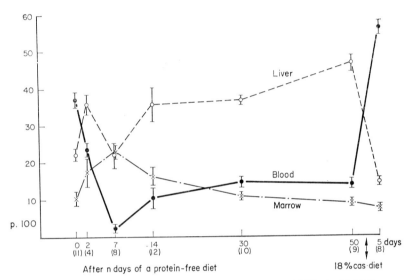

FIG. 2. Evolution of the percentage incorporation of ^{59}Fe ($\pm$S.E.M.) into the erythrocytes (●——), the bone marrow (○ – –) and the liver (× – · –) during 50 days of a protein-free diet and after 5 days of a recovery diet with 18% casein. Numbers of rats in parentheses. Reproduced from *Ann. Nutr. Aliment.*, **17**: B207–24 (1963).

In the bone marrow, mitotic activity of erythroblasts almost ceases from the 4th day of the regimen, reaching its minimum before that of the reticulocyte count, which does not appear until the 8th day (Aschkenasy, 1963a) (Fig. 1). Ito *et al.* (1964) have reported a simultaneous reduction of the number of erythroblasts.

Transitory erythroblastopenia has been reported in children suffering from kwashiorkor, but lack of protein does not appear to be the sole cause of this (Kho *et al.*, 1962).

Paradoxically, as experimental protein deficiency is continued and anemia develops, both the reticulocyte count and the uptake of ^{59}Fe by the red cells tend to increase again (Aschkenasy, 1946, 1962c) (Figs. 1 and 2; Table 1).

The same applies to mitotic activity in bone marrow, estimated by the stathmokinetic (colchicinic) method (Aschkenasy, 1963a) (Fig. 1). When the anemia becomes serious shortly before the death of the animals, the reticulocyte count may even exceed the values in normal rats, while increasing numbers of pyknotic erythroblasts appear in the blood.

TABLE 1. GASTRO-INTESTINAL ABSORPTION AND DISTRIBUTION OF THE ABSORBED ^{59}FE ONE WEEK AFTER THE INTRA-GASTRIC ADMINISTRATION OF THE ^{59}FE IN CONTROLS (18% CASEIN DIET), IN PROTEIN DEPRIVED RATS, AND IN RATS RESTORED WITH 18% CASEIN AFTER 7 WEEKS OF PROTEIN STARVATION

Diet (6 rats per group)	Total ^{59}Fe absorbed (%) ± S.E.M.	Percentages (± S.E.M.) ^{59}Fe incorporation			
		Blood	Liver	Spleen	Bone marrow
18% caseine	33.60 ±4.91	7.32 ±1.68	1.93 ±0.49	0.14 ±0.03	0.73 ±0.11
Without protein; ^{59}Fe given the 8th day of the diet	24.64 ±4.15	0.10 ±0.03	1.10 ±0.18	0.03 ±0.006	0.32 ±0.06
Without protein; ^{59}Fe given the 50th day of the diet	10.23 ±3.52	1.87 ±0.27	0.40 ±0.09	0.03 ±0.003	0.39 ±0.05
18% casein after 7 weeks of protein starvation; ^{59}Fe given the 4th day of the diet	22.96 ±2.42	10.22 ±0.79	1.98 ±0.51	0.13 ±0.01	0.36 ±0.02

During the anemic phase the bone marrow is filled with immature red cells (Fig. 3), hence showing a picture of regeneration—somewhat surprisingly with an anemia due to lack of blood-forming material—not unlike that of iron-deficiency anemia.

As will be shown later, this picture may be attributed both to a partial blockage of the transformation of erythroblasts into reticulocytes and to stimulation of the marrow as a response to excessive hemolysis.

The graphs of the distribution of ^{59}Fe (injected intravenously) between blood, bone marrow, and liver show that the blockage of iron utilization for erythropoiesis after the first week of protein starvation is accompanied by storage of iron, especially in the liver. The liver, however, doubtless

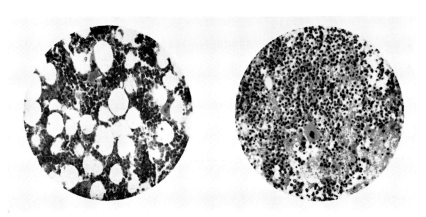

FIG. 3. Histologic sections of femoral marrows of a normal rat (left) and of a rat made anemic by a protein-free diet (right). Note, in the latter, the profusion of normoblasts in the marrow and the disappearance of fat vesicles. (Hematoxylin-eosin × 180). Reproduced from *Amer. J. Clin. Nutr.*, **5**: 14–25 (1957).

because of progressive fatty infiltration, gives way to bone marrow as a site of storage when the deficiency is continued and erythropoiesis is to some extent reactivated (Aschkenasy, 1962c, 1963d) (Fig. 2).

(b) *Leucopenia*. The onset of protein-deficiency leucopenia (Aschkenasy, 1946; Kornberg, 1946; Guggenheim and Buechler, 1949; Aschkenasy and Dray, 1953/4) is earlier than that of anemia. In the terminal phase the lymphocytic series is more reduced than the neutrophil series. The eosinophils almost completely disappear.

Of the lymphocytes the large-and medium-sized ones are at first reduced in number, while the small lymphocytes are preserved for some time (Fig. 4).

To some extent these are really the same cells, of which both cytoplasm and nuclei contract under the influence of lack of dietary protein, as shown by the general shift to the left of the histogram of lymphocyte size (Aschkenasy, 1964d, 1965d,e) (Fig. 5a,b).

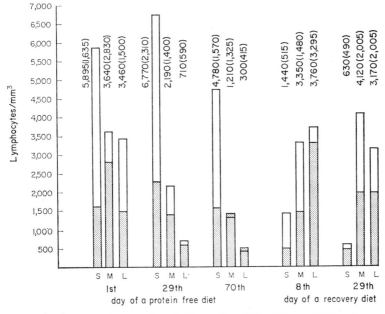

FIG. 4. Average levels of small (S), medium (M) and large (L) lymphocytes in intact (the entire columns) or thymectomized (the stippled segments of the columns and values in parentheses) male rats fed protein-free and recovery diets. In the 8th and 9th columns the cell levels in thymectomized rats exceeded those in intact rats. Reproduced from *Israel J. med. Sci.*, **1**: 552–62 (1965).

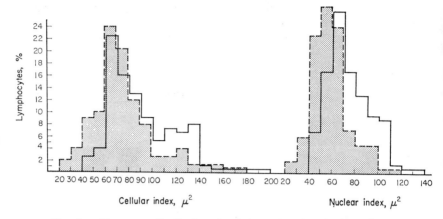

FIG. 5a.   Frequency distribution of cellular and nuclear indices (μ^2) of lymphocytes of male rats on the first (uninterrupted outline) and 29th days (stippled surface; interrupted outline) of a protein-free diet.

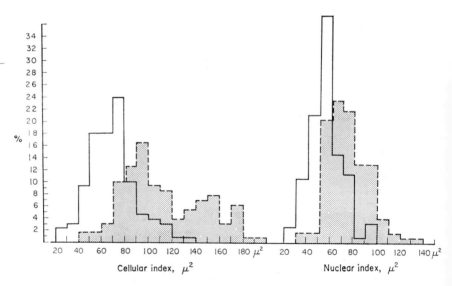

FIG. 5b.   Cellular and nuclear indices of lymphocytes in male rats after 70 days of a protein-free diet and after 7 days of a recovery diet (stippled surface).   Reproduced from *Israel J. med. Sci.*, **1**: 552–62 (1965).

Of all the lymphoid organs, the thymus is the first to undergo atrophy (Aschkenasy, 1954b, 1964a); this atrophy seems to play a role in the disappearance of large- and medium-sized lymphocytes in the course of protein deficiency. These cells are much more numerous in intact rats than in rats after thymectomy, as long as the diet is balanced, while after prolonged nitrogen deprivation the numbers become similar in the two groups of animals (Aschkenasy, 1965b,d,e) (Fig. 4).

However, the number of large and medium lymphocytes is reduced as a result of deficiency even in thymectomized rats, and the same is true of small lymphocytes: the production of thymus-independent lymphocytes is therefore also inhibited by protein starvation.

Inhibition of leucopoiesis weakens phagocytic and immunological defence mechanisms in protein deficiency.

According to most authors, though not to Metcoff *et al.* (1948), animals deprived of protein produce less antibodies than controls (Cannon *et al.*, 1943; Wissler, 1947; Benditt *et al.*, 1949; Delmonte *et al.*, 1962).

However, it is mainly the phagocytic reactions that are weakened, as much in respect of microbial antigens (Mills and Cottingham, 1943; Guggenheim and Buechler, 1948; Delmonte *et al.*, 1962) as of red blood cells (Sós, 1964) or foreign proteins (Gray, 1964).

Furthermore, γ-globulins are reduced after prolonged nitrogen deprivation (Aschkenasy and Blanpin, 1959; Aschkenasy, 1965c,d,e), but this reduction occurs later than that of serum albumin.

3. *Recovery from blood disorders of protein deficiency*

The ill-effects of protein depletion on the blood can be cured until a very advanced stage by a diet containing enough of a complete protein such as casein or lactalbumin.

Between the 4th and 11th days (usually with a maximum at the 6th day) there is a considerable but transitory release of reticulocytes into the circulation (Fig. 6), and also, to a smaller extent, of pyknotic erythroblasts (Aschkenasy and Aschkenasy-Lelu, 1947; Aschkenasy and Pariente, 1951).

At the same time, there is a strong increase in mitotic activity in the erythroblasts of the bone marrow (Fig. 1).

The total mass of circulating red cells and hemoglobin increase as soon as recovery begins, but during the first few days the increase only keeps pace with the weight gain; the red-cell count actually falls for a time, because the restoration of erythropoiesis lags behind that of the plasma volume.

The rate at which erythrocytes and hemoglobin recover depends, of course, on the protein content of the diet. With casein the optimum is 30%, but 15% suffices to produce the maximum release of reticulocytes and erythroblasts. With as little as 7% erythropoiesis recovers only slowly, but still keeps ahead of body-weight gain (Aschkenasy and Aschkenasy-Lelu, 1947).

The mean corpuscular volume rises sharply with the release of reticulocytes, because of the larger volume of these cells, then falls again before its definitive rise (Aschkenasy and Pariente, 1951).

Hemoglobin is formed in large quantities as soon as an adequate diet is given (with 18% of casein), as shown by a large increase in the uptake by the red cells of ^{59}Fe injected intravenously (Aschkenasy, 1962c) (Fig. 2).

Both intestinal absorption of oral ^{59}Fe and utilization for erythropoiesis of the absorbed ^{59}Fe are rapidly increased: in 7 days, 23% of the isotope is absorbed if it is given on the 4th day of recovery, as against only 10%

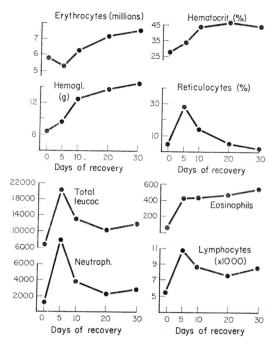

FIG. 6. Changes in the levels of erythrocytes, hemoglobin, hematocrit, reticulocytes and leucocytes during the recovery of protein starved rats with a 18% casein diet. Graph partly reproduced from *Sang*, **30**: 168–75. (1959)

before recovery, and the amount found in the blood at the same times averages 10% of the ^{59}Fe during recovery, as against 2% in rats still deprived of protein (Aschkenasy, 1965f) (Table 1).

Recovery is always accompanied by the release into the circulation not only of reticulocytes, but of neutrophils, lymphocytes, and eosinophils (Aschkenasy and Aschkenasy-Lelu, 1947; Aschkenasy and Dray, 1953/4; Aschkenasy, 1959) (Fig. 6).

The lymphocytes are increased in number, and also in size (Fig. 5b), the volume of the cytoplasm increasing more than that of the nucleus; hence the proportion of medium and large lymphocytes increases at the expense of the small lymphocytes (Aschkenasy, 1964d, 1965d) (Fig. 4).

At the same time there is regeneration of the lymphoid organs, in particular of the thymus.

III. HEMATOPOIETIC ACTION OF PROTEINS

A. DIETARY PROTEINS

1. *Erythropoietic action*

Casein, liver and muscle proteins, hemoglobin, and globin itself (Robscheit-Robbins and Whipple, 1937, 1949) are all strongly hematopoietic in dogs rendered anemic both by repeated bleeding and by a protein-deficient diet.

In dogs, regeneration of hemoglobin generally precedes that of the plasma proteins, even if they are fed with the latter. Only egg proteins and lactalbumin favor the regeneration of plasma proteins rather than hemoglobin (Robscheit-Robbins and Whipple, 1949; Whipple and Robscheit-Robbins, 1951).

These results in dogs do not seem to apply to rats, in which Orten and Orten (1946) produced similar regeneration of hemoglobin, after bleeding, with diets containing 18% of casein or of lactalbumin; indeed, the latter is more effective than casein if the amount of protein in the diet does not exceed 2.8%.

According to Buechler and Guggenheim (1949), egg and meat proteins are more beneficial than casein to rats rendered anemic by protein deficiency.

However, in these experiments proteins were given only at a level of 9 g per 100 g of food, which in turn was limited to a total of 9 g per day.

It is of some interest that mice, and sometimes also rats, develop severe anemia if they are fed entirely on meat for long periods. This anemia has been ascribed to deficient absorption of iron due to lack of calcium

(Moore *et al.*, 1962) and to an excess of zinc (Guggenheim, 1964), since meat has a high content of this element, while lacking copper and calcium, which are physiological antagonists of zinc.

Human and bovine hemoglobin have little erythropoietic activity in the rat, perhaps because they are deficient in isoleucine, which is essential to hemoglobin synthesis in this animal (Orten *et al.*, 1945).

Vegetable proteins are unsuitable for erythropoiesis, in so far as they are deficient in essential amino acids, as, for instance, gliadine, which is short of lysine, or zein, which lacks both lysine and tryptophan (Harris *et al.*, 1943; Gillespie *et al.*, 1945; Bevan *et al.*, 1950).

Ground-nut protein contains too little methionine, lysine, threonine, and tryptophan. All these amino acids have to be added for it to become as effective an erythropoietic agent as casein (Tasker *et al.*, 1963).

The results with soya vary according to experimental conditions and the species of animal. The biological value of this protein is known to be enhanced by cooking, which seems to facilitate the release of certain amino acids (especially methionine, but also valine and threonine) (Borchers, 1961).

Soya does little to restore hemoglobin in dogs rendered anemic by bleeding and protein deficiency (Whipple and Robscheit-Robbins, 1951). Prolonged administration of this protein to monkeys (for 2–7 months) actually produces a hypochromic anemia, which may be due to inhibition of intestinal absorption of iron by phytates contained in soya, and to consequent iron deficiency (Fitch *et al.*, 1964). In the rat, on the other hand, soya protein may be even more effective than casein if each of them is given to protein-deficient rats, in small amounts and with a restricted diet (Buechler and Guggenheim, 1949).

In such a restricted diet, wheat protein is less effective than casein, although if it is given *ad libitum* it is the only vegetable protein which can compete with casein in respect of effects on growth and on the formation of hemoglobin and plasma proteins (Chitre and Vallury, 1956).

2. *Leucopoietic action*

Guggenheim and Buechler (1949) found that in rats previously subjected to nitrogen deficiency, proteins from eggs, meat, ground-nut, and soya had greater leucopoietic activity than casein, which in turn was better than maize or wheat proteins.

These results, obtained with a restricted diet (9 g per day) and a sub-optimal protein content (9 %) would probably not apply to an unlimited diet with 18 %.

The hematopoietic potency of a protein, like its biological value, depends not only on the nature of its constituent amino acids but on their proportions, and also on the method of preparation—industrial or culinary—on its digestibility, and lastly on the conditions under which it is given: in one or more daily amounts, alone or together with other foods.

A diet containing various inadequate proteins may still exert hematopoietic activity by virtue of compensation for the amino-acid deficiencies of each particular protein by the others.

B. TISSUE PROTEINS AND CATABOLIC PRODUCTS OF HEMOLYSIS

1. In the complete absence of protein from the diet, erythropoiesis is at first almost completely suppressed, but is to some extent resumed at an advanced stage of deficiency. This can only be explained by utilization of stored protein.

These tissue proteins also account for the transient erythropoietic response of the protein-deficient organism to bleeding (Hallgren, 1954), calorigenic hormones (Aschkenasy, 1954b, 1961b), cobalt (Orten and Orten, 1945), or hypoxia (Reissmann, 1964b). In the early stages of deficiency all these factors appear to act mainly by causing release of erythropoietin, of which production is arrested at this time (Aschkenasy, 1963d).

2. The nitrogenous products of hemolysis do not seem to be preferentially utilized for erythropoiesis (Madden *et al.*, 1945; Yuile, 1949). However, they may be involved by stimulating the erythropoietic tissues either *directly* (Sanchez-Medal *et al.*, 1963) or *indirectly*, by acting on erythropoietin production, which would explain the apparent return of this activity in advanced nitrogen deprivation (Aschkenasy, 1964c).

IV. HEMATOPOIETIC ACTION OF AMINO ACIDS

A. ERYTHROPOIETIC ACTION

1. *Comparison of casein with "equivalent" mixtures of amino acids*

Hemoglobin appears to be synthesized mainly from free amino acids transported by the immature red cells themselves. Piha (1954) has in fact shown that reticulocytes have a much larger free amino acid content than adult erythrocytes.

Benditt *et al.* (1947) found that a mixture of 10 essential amino-acids was as effective as casein in restoring the levels of serum proteins and erythrocytes, when given for 10 days to protein-deficient rats. But in the absence of any one amino acid (except arginine) the mixture lost its effect.

Studies in our laboratory have confirmed that the erythropoietic effect of a complete mixture of synthetic amino acids is equivalent to that of casein:

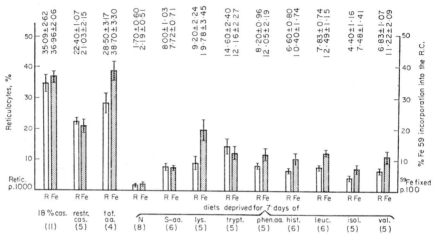

FIG. 7. Mean reticulocyte counts p. 1000 red cells ($\pm$ S.E.M.) and percentage incorporation of ^{59}Fe ($\pm$ S.E.M.) in control rats on a 18% casein diet and in rats which received for one week either the same balanced diet but restricted to $\frac{1}{3}$ of the *ad libitum* ingested one, or a diet entirely deprived of nitrogen, or containing an amino acid mixture: complete (tot. aa.), or lacking certain essential amino acids (sulfur amino acids, lysine, tryptophan, phenolic amino acids, histidine, leucine, isoleucine, valine). Blank columns, reticulocytes; stippled columns, ^{59}Fe. Reproduced from *C.R. Soc. Biol.*, **156**: 1971–6 (1962).

(1) After a week on a diet containing 17% of a mixture of 19 amino acids (made up according to Rose *et al.*, 1948) the rats showed no reduction of reticulocyte count or uptake of ^{59}Fe by red cells, in contrast to the results of a diet without nitrogen or lacking any one of the essential amino acids in rats (Aschkenasy, 1962d) (Fig. 7).

(2) If a diet with the same complete mixture of amino acids is given after 7 weeks of nitrogen deprivation, the release of reticulocytes is rather less than with casein—the same phenomenon has been observed when casein is replaced by an acid hydrolysate supplemented with tryptophan (Bourgeat and Aschkenasy, 1948)—but the utilization for erythropoiesis

of oral ^{59}Fe is at least as great with the amino acids (15.7%) as with casein (10.4%) (Aschkenasy, 1966c).

2. *Effects of single amino-acid deficiencies*

(1) *Previous reports*

(a) *Tryptophan.* A diet including an acid hydrolysate of casein, supplemented with cystine but lacking tryptophan, causes only a moderate and delayed (after 3 months) fall in hemoglobin in the rat, without affecting the erythrocytes (Albanese *et al.*, 1943). But if tryptophan is absent it is impossible to restore either protein-deficiency anemia (Benditt *et al.*, 1947) or hemorrhagic anemia (Sebrell and McDaniel, 1952).

Even if given alone, tryptophan facilitates regeneration of hemoglobin in bled dogs (Whipple and Robscheit-Robbins, 1940; Sós, 1964), and it reinforces the anti-anemic effect of an acid hydrolysate of casein in phenyl-hydrazine-poisoned rats (Yeshoda and Damodaran, 1947). Fontès and Thivolle (1930) have even found an erythropoietic effect of tryptophan in normal dogs and rabbits.

Tryptophan metabolism is disturbed in congenital hypoplastic anemia (erythrogenesis imperfecta). But the anemia is not improved by massive doses of riboflavine, although this vitamin suppresses the urinary excretion of an abnormal tryptophan metabolite, anthranilic acid, which is seen in this anemia (Altman and Miller, 1953).

(1b) *Histidine.* Deprivation of this amino acid causes only a moderate fall in hemoglobin in non-anemic rats normally fed previously (Fontès and Thivolle, 1930; Maun *et al.*, 1946; Fuller *et al.*, 1947; Bowles *et al.*, 1949; Nasset and Gatewood, 1954) but it prevents recovery from protein-deficiency anemia (Benditt *et al.*, 1947) or hemorrhagic anemia (Sebrell and McDaniel, 1952; Sós, 1964).

In dogs which are both anemic and hypoproteinemic, the addition of histidine to egg protein, which is short of histidine, favors the production of hemoglobin rather than of plasma proteins (Whipple and Robscheit-Robbins, 1951).

These results have been ascribed to the relatively high level of this amino acid in globin (8%) (Block and Bolling, 1947)—the rat, unlike man, being unable to synthesize iminazoles (Moore and Wilson, 1957).

(1c) *Phenylalanine and tyrosine.* A fall in hemoglobin has also been observed in young rats deprived of these two amino acids (Maun *et al.*, 1945a); on the other hand regeneration of hemoglobin after bleeding is enhanced by giving them in the dog (Whipple and Robscheit-Robbins, 1940), but not in the rat (Sós, 1964).

Cytological abnormalities of hematopoiesis (vacuolization of erythroblasts and myelocytes) have been seen in the bone marrow of premature infants fed for 24 or 48 hr on a casein hydrolysate poor in phenylalanine; the abnormalities disappeared as soon as the missing acid was added (Cockburn *et al.*, 1965).

In human pernicious anemia, there are often signs of abnormal metabolism of phenolic amino acids: an increase of phenols in urine (Swendseid *et al.*, 1943), and disorders of pigmentation (vitiligo and premature greyness of the hair) perhaps due to defective synthesis of melanin from tyrosine. All these disorders respond to vitamin B_{12}.

(1d) *Leucine.* Although globin is very rich in leucine (16 % according to Block and Bolling, 1947), lack of this amino acid causes no anemia (Maun *et al.*, 1945b, Bowles *et al.*, 1949). But a leucine-free diet given to rats prevents recovery from protein-deficiency anemia (Benditt *et al.*, 1947) or hemorrhagic anemia (Sebrell and McDaniel, 1952).

(1e) *Isoleucine.* The failure of bovine or human globin to promote hemoglobin formation in the rat is apparently due to their low content of isoleucine (Orten *et al.*, 1945).

Anemias due to protein deficiency (Benditt *et al.*, 1947), hemorrhage (Sebrell and McDaniel, 1952), or phenylhydrazine (Chandran and Damodaran, 1951) in the rat can be restored only if the diet provides isoleucine.

(1f) *Lysine, threonine, valine.* These three amino acids are all essential to recovery from anemias due to protein deficiency (Benditt *et al.*, 1947) or hemorrhage (Sebrell and McDaniel, 1952; Sós, 1964).

Diets of which the protein content is either gliadin or zein (with supplementary tryptophan), which thus lack only lysine, produce hypochromic anemia after a few weeks in young rats (Harris *et al.*, 1943; Gillespie *et al.*, 1945). Hexoserine, a lysine antagonist, likewise causes anemia (Gingras, 1953).

(1g) *Methionine.* The erythropoietic properties of this amino acid have received particular attention:

(1ga) *Selective lack of methionine.* Young rats given a mixture of essential amino acids lacking only methionine develop anemia with reticulocytosis (Glynn *et al.*, 1945).

Anemia has also been reported in rats given an oxidized hydrolysate of casein lacking sulfur-containing amino acids (Albanese *et al.*, 1946).

A mixture of amino acids without methionine does not cure protein-deficiency anemia (Benditt *et al.*, 1947).

(1gb) *Effect of methionine in protein deficiency.* Given alone to protein-deprived rats, methionine does not delay the anemia, though it does reduce the fall in plasma proteins, especially serum albumin (Aschkenasy *et al.*, 1949c).

It is only with a low-protein diet (7% of casein) that extra methionine exhibits a frank hematopoietic effect, mainly if such a diet is preceded by a prolonged nitrogen deprivation. Then the supplementary amino acid accelerates the restoration of hemoglobin and hematocrit without affecting the increase in erythrocyte count (Aschkenasy and Pariente, 1951) (Fig. 8).

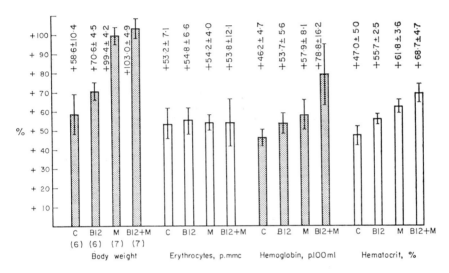

FIG. 8. Effects of addition to a recovery diet (7% casein) of vitamin B_{12}, methionine (M), or both factors together on the body weight, the erythrocyte counts and the levels of hemoglobin and hematocrit after 60 days of protein starvation. The columns represent the mean increases ($\pm$S.E.M.) after 40 days of the recovery diet, calculated as percentages of values found on the first day of restoration. C—Controls with a non-supplemented 7% casein diet. Numbers of rats in parentheses. Graph made from data of Aschkenasy, A. and Pariente, Ph., *Rev. Hématol.*, **6**: 166–83 (1951).

This represents an increase in mean corpuscular volume, which remains below normal without extra methionine (Fig. 9).

(1gc) *Effect of methionine in certain toxic anemias.* Methionine has an anti-anemic action in rats poisoned with carbon tetrachloride (Gajdos, 1947), sulfadiazine (Aschkenasy *et al.*, 1948), or phenylhydrazine (Bénard *et al.*, 1948).

K

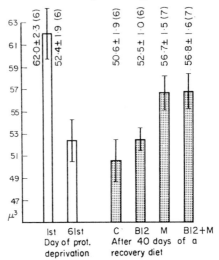

FIG. 9. Mean corpuscular volume ($\pm$S.E.M.) of erythrocytes before and after 60 days of protein deprivation and after 40 days of a recovery diet with 7% casein. Effects of supplementation with vitamin B_{12}, methionine (M) or their combination. C-Non-supplemented controls. Numbers of rats in parentheses. Graph constructed from data of Aschkenasy, A. and Pariente, Ph., *Rev. Hématol.*, **6**: 166–83 (1951).

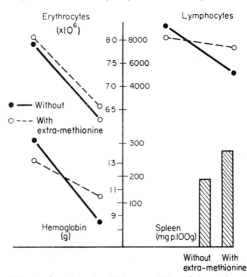

FIG. 10. Effects of methionine (0.3 g per 100 g of dry ration) on erythrocytes, hemoglobin and lymphocytes and on spleen weight in rats given a protein-poor diet (4 per cent) with added sulfadiazine (0.4 per cent) for 100 days. Reproduced from *Amer. J. Clin. Nutr.*, **5**: 14–25 (1957).

In sulfonamide poisoning, methionine is much more effective against the fall in hemoglobin than on red-cell count. But this is seen only if the diet is deficient in protein and consequently in methionine (Fig. 10). The protection against toxic effects of sulfonamides afforded by casein (Wright *et al.*, 1945; Shehata and Johnson, 1948) can probably be accounted for by the action of the methionine it contains.

The antitoxic action of methionine is perhaps explained by an increase of certain intracellular enzymes or peptides containing sulfhydryl groups, such as glutathione, of which the level in the blood and tissues is known to be lowered after deprivation of protein (Leaf and Neuberger, 1947); or else by the specific anabolic activity of methionine on the liver and the plasma proteins (Aschkenasy, 1965c), which could reinforce the detoxicating processes.

(1gd) *Effects of excess methionine.* An excess is as harmful, and as liable to cause anemia in rats without deficiency, as is lack of methionine.

Anemia from methionine excess is not due to reduced dietary intake caused by the excess, and in contrast with other toxic manifestations, it is apparently unrelated to over-production of homocysteine since it does not respond to serine, which is an antagonist of this amino acid (Klavins and Johansen, 1965).

(1gh) *Cystine and cysteine.* Lack of cystine alone does not cause anemia (Glynn *et al.*, 1945; Albanese *et al.*, 1946) since it can be replaced by methionine.

The high cystine content of serum albumin (Block and Bolling, 1947) must be involved in the remarkable anabolic activity of this amino acid on plasma proteins; in protein-deficient rats this action is more marked than the erythropoietic effect (Aschkenasy and Benhamou, 1950), and in bled dogs it is greater even than that of methionine (Madden and Whipple, 1940).

Cystine and cysteine are also reported to have a protective action against anemia and leucopenia due to X-rays (Patt *et al.*, 1950; Rosenthal *et al.*, 1951).

(2) *Recent results from this laboratory on the erythropoietic effect of incomplete mixtures of amino acids*

(2a) A synthetic diet lacking a single amino acid need be given to adult rats for only 7 days in order to produce a considerable fall in reticulocyte count and in the uptake by the red cells of ^{59}Fe given intravenously (Aschkenasy, 1962d) (Fig. 7).

This inhibition of erythropoiesis is greatest with diets lacking sulfur amino acids or isoleucine, which are almost as harmful as a completely nitrogen-free diet.

The duration of the deficiency is too short for tissue reserves of the amino acids to become depleted. And although these incomplete diets lead to a strong reduction of the total dietary intake, with the exception of a lysine-free diet they inhibit bone marrow to a much greater extent than a restricted but balanced diet given in doses corresponding with the amounts taken spontaneously with a nitrogen-free diet.

In nearly all these short-term amino acid deficiencies (except that of isoleucine) failure to utilize intravenous ^{59}Fe for erythropoiesis is accompanied by retention of the ositope in the bone marrow, especially if the deficiency is of histidine or of phenolic amino acids. The level of ^{59}Fe in

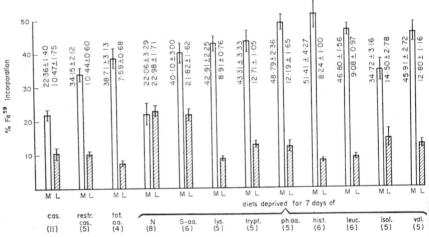

FIG. 11. Percentage incorporation of ^{59}Fe ($\pm$S.E.M.) into the bone marrow (M) and the liver (L) in rats fed for 7 days the following diets: *ad libitum* or restricted 18% casein diet, nitrogen (N)-deprived diet, or diet with a total amino acid mixture (tot.aa), or mixtures deprived of sulfur amino acids (S-aa.), lysine, tryptophan, phenolic amino acids (ph.aa.), histidine, leucine, isoleucine, or valine. Numbers of rats in parentheses. Reproduced from *C.R. Soc. Biol.*, **156**: 1971–6 (1962).

the liver is particularly high with deficiency of only sulfur amino acids, so that hepatic blockage of ^{59}Fe at the early stage of complete nitrogen starvation is apparently due mainly to the absence of methionine and cystine (Fig. 11).

(2b) If the diets with incomplete mixtures of amino acids are not given until after 7 weeks' nitrogen starvation, the release of reticulocytes which is typical of any recovery from protein-deficiency anemia is much less than with casein or a complete mixture of amino acids; if valine is lacking this response almost completely fails (Aschkenasy, 1966c).

The same applies to red-cell uptake of oral ^{59}Fe: if given on the 4th day of the recovery diet, 10–15% of it is found in the blood a week later when casein or a complete amino-acid mixture is used, as against 4.6%, 2.3%, and 3.7% on the average with mixtures lacking respectively tryptophan, histidine, and valine. Erythropoietic utilization is inhibited less by lack of sulfur amino acids (6.4%), lysine (7.0%), threonine (8.1%), or phenolic amino acids (5.7%).

(3) *Erythropoietic action of amino acids* in vitro. For maturation of reticulocytes *in vitro* (Nizet and Robscheit-Robbins, 1950; Nizet, 1955) the medium must contain not only the 9 essential amino acids, but also arginine and glycine, needed for the synthesis of heme which reticulocytes are able to carry out *in vitro* (Shemin and Rittenberg, 1945).

(4) *Critical analysis of the erythropoietic action of amino acids*

(4a) A complete mixture of amino acids has as much effect as casein on erythropoiesis, although it is decidedly less active as regards body weight, the condition of certain organs, especially the thymus, and leucopoiesis, as will be seen later.

(4b) All amino acids that are essential to the maintenance of weight and growth are equally so to erythropoiesis; but, because this function is given such high priority, deficiency of a single amino acid may cause serious tissue damage without leading to a real anemia, i.e. to a fall in cell count and hemoglobin with reduced blood volume.

(4c) In the rat, anemia due to lack of a single amino acid is nearly always microcytic and hypochromic, like that of complete nitrogen deprivation; in other words with all these deficiencies the synthesis of hemoglobin is more impaired than the multiplication of erythroblasts and their transformation into adult erythrocytes.

(4d) The erythropoietic effect of amino acids is to be explained not only by their direct involvement in the formation of red cells, but also by their effects on dietary intake and on oxygen consumption.

(4da) Most amino acids stimulate appetite provided that they are not given in excess, and lack of one of them causes loss of appetite, amounting almost to complete anorexia in the case of valine or isoleucine deficiency (Aschkenasy, 1963g).

A general restriction of diet is in itself enough to slow down erythro-poiesis (Aschkenasy, 1962d). However, if protein-deficient rats are given a recovery diet with 18 % of casein, in amounts not exceeding those taken spontaneously with a valine-free diet (which is highly anorexigenic), the bone marrow activity is not suppressed to the same extent as with the latter diet (Aschkenasy, 1966c).

(4db) Lack of any one essential amino acid also produces a rapid fall in oxygen consumption. This fall is relatively slight with some deficiencies (e.g. lysine), but with others (threonine, valine, isoleucine) it is almost as great as that which follows complete nitrogen starvation (Aschkenasy, 1963g).

Like hyperbaric hyperoxia (Linman and Pierre, 1964), hyperoxia due to relative oxygen excess from inhibition of oxidation tends to hold back erythropoiesis, and this may account for the early onset of this effect in amino-acid deficiency.

(4dc) The effect may well be exerted through blockage of erythropoietin release, as at the beginning of total nitrogen deprivation (Aschkenasy, 1962a,b).

B. LEUCOPOIETIC ACTION OF AMINO ACIDS

1. *Comparison of casein with "equivalent" mixtures of amino acids*

Kornberg (1946) found that very young rats deprived of nitrogen for 21 days, and then given a mixture of 10 essential amino acids for only 4 days, showed a considerable increase in the number of neutrophil granulocytes, provided that the diet also included folic acid.

In our own experiments with adult rats, the release of neutrophils, despite the presence of this vitamin, was much smaller with a mixture of 19 amino acids than with casein, after 10 days on a recovery diet preceded by 7 weeks of nitrogen starvation (Aschkenasy, 1966a).

The amino-acid mixture is also shown to be inferior to casein by a much smaller weight gain and much less regeneration of the spleen and, especially, the thymus (average 130 mg with the amino acids, against 215 mg with casein, after 10 days of recovery), and also by the fact that during the 10 days the eosinopenia of protein deficiency (less than 10 cells per mm^3) is still only slightly improved by the amino-acid mixture ($\sim$ 40 cells per mm^3), while it completely disappears with casein ($\sim$120 cells per mm^3) (Aschkenasy, 1966a).

Even after 30 days on a recovery diet, the eosinophils, like the other leucocytes, are much less numerous on an amino-acid regimen than with casein.

If adult rats, without previous starvation, are given the same mixture of amino acids for 21 days, they also show reduced weight gain and lower leucocyte counts (unpublished data), and also much greater reduction in the weight of the spleen and especially the thymus than controls on casein (Aschkenasy, 1964a); the same applies to the number of eosinophils in the blood and digestive tract (Aschkenasy, 1963h, 1965a).

All these observations, for which the racemic form of most constituents of the mixture used may account, show that leucopoiesis is much more sensitive than erythropoiesis to the quality of the dietary nitrogen.

2. *Deficiencies of particular amino acids*

(1) *Total leucocytes.* The diminished leucopoietic effect of a complete mixture of amino acids compared with casein is not of the same order as the virtually complete suppression of leucopoiesis by diets lacking one of the essential amino acids.

Thus, a general leucopenia has been described with deficiencies of histidine, leucine, lysine (Bowles *et al.*, 1949), methionine (Dinning *et al.*, 1950), tryptophan (Bowles *et al.*, 1949; Rigó *et al.*, 1959), or valine (Sebrell and McDaniel, 1952). On the other hand, if arginine is missing, a leucocytosis develops (Bowles *et al.*, 1949).

Though dissimilar effects on lymphocytes and eosinophils may be seen, e.g. with deficiency of sulfur amino acids, most cases of deficiency leucopenia affect all types of leucocytes; but many of the published reports deal only with one or other type.

(2) *Neutrophils.* Diets lacking any of the essential amino acids are unable to restore the neutropenia of protein-deficient rats, whether the rats are very young (Kornberg, 1946) or adult. Valine and lysine deficiencies are especially harmful, as opposed to lack of tryptophan or sulfur amino acids (Aschkenasy, 1966a).

(3) *Lymphocytes.* Methionine deficiency has received the most study. Deficiency causes lymphopenia (Dinning *et al.*, 1950), and methionine has a lymphopoietic effect when added to a low-protein diet containing benzene (Li and Freeman, 1947) or sulfadiazine (Aschkenasy *et al.*, 1948) (Fig. 10).

Lack of any other essential amino acid also causes lymphopenia, the degree of which depends on the particular deficiency.

Thus, after 7 weeks' nitrogen deprivation, a synthetic diet given for 10 days and lacking sulfur or phenolic amino acids, or lysine, tryptophan, histidine, valine, or threonine not only fails to increase the lymphocyte count but actually aggravates the existing lymphopenia.

The cellular and nuclear diameters of the lymphocytes, instead of increasing, remain unchanged or even decrease to less than their nitrogen-starvation values on some of these diets, particularly a valine-free diet (Aschkenasy, 1966b).

(4) *Lymphoid organs.* Amino-acid deficiencies always lead to involution of these organs, especially the thymus. Atrophy of the thymus has been described after deprivation of phenylalanine (Maun *et al.*, 1945a; Scott *et al.*, 1950), threonine (Scott and Schwartz, 1953; Sidransky and Verney, 1965), histidine (Maun *et al.*, 1946; Scott, 1954), tryptophan (Scott, 1955), isoleucine (Scott, 1956), and valine (Scott, 1964).

However, these studies, dealing separately with individual amino acids and made under differing conditions, do not lend themselves to quantitative comparison of the effects of various deficiencies; neither do they give generally any information about the condition of the spleen and lymph nodes.

However, if these effects are compared in young rats of the same litters subjected to deficiencies of various amino acids for 25 days (Aschkenasy, 1964a), the reduction in weight gain appears to be accompanied by a fall in the relative weight of the thymus but not of the spleen or lymph nodes.

Atrophy of the thymus differs considerably according to the deficiency. It is slight with arginine, lysine, or tryptophan deficiency, and greatest with isoleucine or valine deficiency (Table 2). The involution of the thymus is usually correlated with the reduction in circulating eosinophils and with the relative hypertrophy of the adrenals.

When protein-deficient rats are given recovery diets lacking particular amino acids, the regeneration of the lymphoid organs differs according to the diet, though it always lags behind the regeneration on a complete diet. The thymus is smallest after 10 days on diets lacking histidine, valine, threonine or phenolic amino acids; the spleen after a similar lack of sulfur amino acids, tryptophan or valine; and the lymph nodes, after lacking tryptophan or sulfur amino acids (Aschkenasy, unpublished).

(5) *Eosinophils.* These cells are particularly sensitive to dietary deficiency of some amino acids.

TABLE 2. RELATIVE WEIGHTS OF LYMPHOID ORGANS AND ADRENALS (mg/100 g terminal body weight) (±S.E.M.) IN MALE RATS DEPRIVED OF VARIOUS AMINO ACIDS OR OF ANY NITROGEN NUTRIENT. COMPARISON WITH CONTROLS GIVEN 18% CASEIN OR 17% COMPLETE AMINO ACID MIXTURE (TOTAL aa) [Reproduced from *C.R. Soc. Biol.* **158**: 479–83 (1964)].

	Diet		Diets deprived of										
	Casein	Tot. aa	Without N	Sulfur aa	Lysine	Trypto-phan	Phenol. aa	Histi-dine	Threo-nine	Leucine	Iso-leuc.	Valine	Argi-nine
Thymus	130.8 ±5.0	102.7 ±6.8	43.6 ±3.3	46.9 ±1.9	70.4 ±7.8	53.7 ±5.4	35.2 ±5.2	27.6 ±2.2	35.6 ±5.4	38.9 ±3.6	19.9 ±1.0	21.2 ±1.1	85.7 ±14.8
Spleen	164.6 ±4.6	182.0 ±6.3	161.1 ±4.6	170.0 ±3.6	178.5 ±15.7	168.6 ±7.3	149.4 ±8.1	162.2 ±9.1	188.6 ±12.8	173.8 ±6.1	152.3 ±10.1	153.3 ±7.2	183.8 ±11.0
Lymph nodes	22.4 ±2.2	28.5 ±0.7	29.5 ±2.3	35.7 ±4.0	43.8 ±4.4	26.7 ±3.1	30.6 ±1.5	28.6 ±4.6	34.0 ±3.0	27.5 ±2.7	33.4 ±2.7	36.7 ±3.4	24.7 ±0.7
Adrenals	12.2 ±0.7	13.4 ±0.8	17.5 ±0.7	21.1 ±0.4	18.3 ±0.8	16.4 ±1.0	21.4 ±0.8	20.2 ±0.6	20.4 ±0.7	20.9 ±0.8	25.6 ±1.4	21.2 ±0.8	16.6 ±0.7

K*

Deficiencies of isoleucine or valine are the most harmful and within 3 weeks produce almost complete disappearance of eosinophils from the blood and gastro-intestinal mucosa, together with arrest of medullary eosinopoiesis (Aschkenasy, 1963h, 1965a) (Fig. 12).

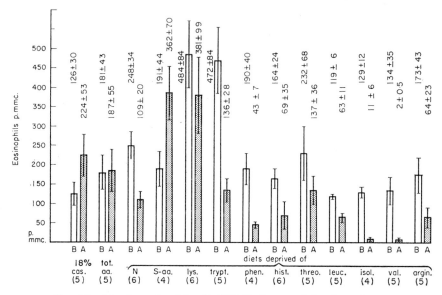

FIG. 12. Blood eosinophils (±S.E.M.) in non-infested male rats deprived for 21 days of various essential amino acids (aa.): sulfur amino acids (S-aa.), lysine, tryptophan, phenolic amino acids (phen.), histidine, threonine, leucine, isoleucine, valine or arginine. Controls were given either a 18% casein diet or a diet with 17% complete mixture of 19 amino acids (tot.aa.). Other rats were entirely deprived of alimentary nitrogen (N). B and A—Values found before and after the experimental period. Numbers of rats in parentheses. Graph made from data of *Rev. Fr. Et. clin. Biol.*, **10**: 299–307 (1965).

In attempts to restore protein-deficient rats with incomplete mixtures of amino acids, the eosinophils not only fail to recover but even disappear completely after some of these diets (lacking histidine, valine, or tryptophan), whereas they may undergo a slight increase on diets lacking lysine, threonine, or sulfur amino acids (Aschkenasy, 1966a).

(6) *Role played by general undernutrition in the effects of amino-acid deficiencies.* The leucopenic effect of amino-acid deficiencies, like the inhibition of erythropoiesis, is largely due to general underfeeding because of the anorexia which nearly all these deficiencies cause.

If, after prolonged nitrogen deprivation, rats are given a diet which, although complete (18 % of casein), is limited in quantity to the amount taken *ad libitum* of a diet lacking valine, the same general leucopenia develops as with the deficient diet. Yet the regeneration of eosinophils, and also that of the spleen and especially the thymus are greater on the restricted but balanced diet than on the valine-free diet (Aschkenasy, unpublished observations).

Furthermore, the proportion of medium and large lymphocytes is greater with the former diet than with the latter. Thus, even the very reduced supply of casein is sufficient to promote the increase in the size of lymphocytes which characterizes all protein restoration (Aschkenasy, 1966b).

3. *Effects of amino acids on leucocytes in the absence of deficiency*

(1) Against non-deficiency leucopenias caused by massive irradiation (Rosenthal *et al.*, 1951) or after treatment with nitrogen mustard, a protective action has so far been observed only with cysteine (Weisberger and Heinle, 1950).

(2) In normal rats, subcutaneous injections of methionine, cystine, or isoleucine produce only a transient leucocytosis with lymphopenia, of the alarm-reaction type, but injections of tryptophan are followed by lympho-cytosis and an increased platelet count.

Among the metabolites of this amino acid, those which most stimulate the bone marrow are serotonin and indoleacetic acid (Rigó *et al.*, 1959).

(3) Certain proteins such as casein (Vartiainen and Apajalahti, 1953) or meat proteins (Gromova, 1963), and also some amino acids such as tyrosine (Vartiainen and Apajalahti, 1953), leucine, and methionine (Góth *et al.*, 1955) cause eosinopenia for some hours after oral administration. But the eosinopenic action is greatest 4 hr after intraperitoneal injection of, for example, albumin, γ-globulin, or various amino acids, in particular tyrosine, lysine, cysteine, or histidine (Aschkenasy, 1957c, 1959a).

These eosinopenias are largely due to non-specific stimulation of the pituitary-adrenal system (Góth *et al.*, 1955; Aschkenasy, 1957c).

After feeding meat to dogs (Gromova, 1963), or leucine or methionine to rats (Munro *et al.*, 1963), the plasma corticoids are increased.

However, eosinopenia, though slighter, also follows intraperitoneal injection of amino acids in adrenalectomized rats, especially injection of tyrosine, valine, histidine, or phenylalanine (Aschkenasy, 1957c, 1959a).

In adrenalectomized rats the eosinopenic effect of an intraperitoneal injection of cortisone may be considerably enhanced if it is accompanied by injection of a mixture of amino acids (Aschkenasy, 1957b). It is perhaps because adrenalectomy is followed by a reduction in the plasma level of amino acids (Ingle *et al.*, 1948) that this operation lessens the eosinopenic response to cortisone in comparison with the response of normal rats (Aschkenasy, 1957b).

V. EFFECT OF CARBOHYDRATES ON THE HEMATOPOIETIC VALUE OF DIETARY PROTEINS

In the absence of vitamin B_{12}, protein-deficiency anemia and body-weight loss are restored only very slowly in the rat, if the amount of casein in the recovery diet does not exceed 7%, and the carbohydrate portion is represented by sucrose.

But if sucrose is replaced by potato starch, recovery of both weight and blood is considerably hastened. With 15% of casein, however, the two carbohydrates are equivalent (Aschkenasy *et al.*, 1949b).

The improvement by starch of the nutritive value of a low-protein diet may be due to stimulation of the intestinal microflora by starch, promoting the synthesis of some anabolic factors, e.g. amino acids or vitamins. Recovery is indeed stimulated by the addition of methionine or, to a lesser extent, vitamin B_{12}, to a diet containing 7% casein and sucrose (Aschkenasy and Pariente, 1951).

VI. EFFECT OF DIETARY FATS ON EXPERIMENTAL PROTEIN-DEFICIENCY ANEMIA

The hemolysis seen in prolonged nitrogen deprivation is affected by the level of fat in the diet: a level of 5% is more favourable to this hemolysis than a level of 10% (Aschkenasy and Blanpin, 1959).

In male rats on a diet with 7% of casein the severity of edema is proportional to the amount of fat in the diet. The level of hemoglobin remains normal for the first 15 weeks on this low-protein diet, provided that the fat content does not exceed 10%, but if it rises to 15–30% an apparent anemia develops from hemodilution (Alexander and Sauberlich, 1957).

This hemodilution might be due to defective inactivation of pitressin in the liver, as a result of fatty infiltration of this organ following the diet.

The liver damage is itself partly determined by lack of methyl groups, which explains a protective action of choline and betaine and also that of vitamin B_{12} and folic acid, both vitamins being involved in trans-methylation.

VII. INTERRELATIONS BETWEEN AMINO ACIDS AND VITAMINS IN HEMATOPOIESIS

1. *Amino acids and folic acid*

Because of its involvement in the synthesis of DNA* this vitamin is essential to the utilization of dietary proteins and amino acids for hematopoiesis.

Although folic acid is synthesized by the intestinal microflora (Mickel-sen, 1956), a dietary supply of it is still necessary in the rat particularly if the microflora is damaged, e.g. by sulfonamides or protein deficiency.

This is why recovery from protein-deficiency-induced anemia and leucopenia is delayed in the absence of folic acid from the diet. The delay is greater if the recovery diet is poor in protein, and the restoration of intestinal synthesis of the vitamin is retarded (Aschkenasy and Aschkenasy-Lelu, 1947; Aschkenasy *et al.*, 1949a).

Kornberg (1946) reported that protein-deficiency neutropenia could not be cured with a mixture of 10 amino acids unless folic acid was added, but his experimental study lasted only 4 days. In fact, even with this vitamin, mixtures of DL-forms of amino acids are much less leucopoietic than casein (Aschkenasy, 1966a).

Folic acid protects against the adverse effects of sulfonamides on the blood (Daft and Sebrell, 1943, 1945), as does methionine with a low-protein diet (Aschkenasy *et al.*, 1948). This amino acid may help the intestinal synthesis of the vitamin; but folic acid, like vitamin B_{12}, also takes part by way of N-methyltetrahydrofolate (Guest *et al.*, 1962) in the transfer of methyl groups, leading to the synthesis of methionine from homocysteine; this would explain a methionine-sparing effect of the vitamin (Schaefer *et al.*, 1951; Hutner *et al.*, 1959).

---

* A methylene derivative of tetrahydrofolic acid, itself a reduction product of folic acid, promotes the methylation of deoxyuridylic acid to thymidylic acid. This reaction is blocked in pernicious anemia (Waters and Mollin, 1963).

2. *Amino acids and vitamin* B_{12}

(a) Like folic acid, vitamin B_{12} takes part in the synthesis of thymidine and DNA (Dinning and Young, 1960; Williams *et al.*, 1963), and also of proteins, though here the mode of action is doubtful (Wagle *et al.*, 1958; Fraser and Holdsworth, 1959; Arnstein and Simkin, 1959). Vitamin B_{12} is also involved in transmethylation, which explains how it can partly replace methionine in hematopoiesis.

Thus, in leucopenia produced experimentally by deficiency of labile methyl groups, vitamin B_{12} and betaine given together can take the place of methionine and restore leucopoiesis, whereas betaine alone is ineffective (Dinning *et al.*, 1950).

Both methionine and vitamin B_{12} are erythropoietic in rats receiving a low protein recovery diet (7% casein) after two months of protein starvation, but they are not equivalent in this respect: the vitamin produces a higher reticulocytosis, but only methionine increases the mean corpuscular volume, thus suppressing the microcytosis of protein deficiency (Fig. 9). The level of hemoglobin is raised much more if vitamin B_{12} and methionine are given together than with either alone (Aschkenasy and Pariente, 1951) (Fig. 8).

In Addison's pernicious anemia the fall in the serum level of vitamin B_{12} corresponds to that of methionine (Karlin *et al.*, 1965). But methionine has no curative effect on this type of anemia.

(b) Not only does vitamin B_{32} take part in the synthesis of proteins, but conversely proteins and dietary amino acids affect the absorption (Deo and Ramalingaswami, 1964) as well as the distribution and tissue storage of the vitamin (Aschkenasy, 1963e; Aschkenasy and Wolff, 1963).

The reduced absorption of vitamin B_{12} in protein deficiency seems to be due mainly to lack of intrinsic factor (Armstead *et al.*, 1965).

After 24 days of protein deficiency, the amount of the vitamin in the liver and kidneys is diminished. But there is a still greater reduction of hepatic stores of vitamin B_{12} with a deficiency solely of sulfur amino acids, whereas nothing of the kind occurs with other amino-acid deficiencies.

Although greatly reducing the ability to store stable vitamin B_{12}, neither lack of sulfur amino acids nor total nitrogen deprivation reduces the uptake of ^{60}Co-labeled vitamin B_{12} by the liver after intraperitoneal injection.

Storage of vitamin B_{12} and uptake of labeled vitamin by the kidneys are decreased in histidine deficiency.

Most of all, however, deficiency of isoleucine or valine reduces the renal uptake of the labeled vitamin, while increasing the hepatic uptake; the ratio renal/hepatic radioactivity is 5 on a balanced diet but falls to 1.2, and to 1 with these two deficiencies (Aschkenasy, 1963e).

3. *Tryptophan and niacin*

Lack of tryptophan causes niacin deficiency; this vitamin, which is derived from tryptophan, participates via the pyridine coenzymes in the maturation and functional activity of blood cells.

Protein-deficiency anemia and leucopenia can in fact be considerably lessened by an excess of niacin (Aschkenasy, 1947).

Conversely, anemia due to the deficiency of this vitamin in the pig can be prevented by an increased protein intake (Cartwright *et al.*, 1948); and, in man, pellagra develops only if the diet is lacking in both tryptophan and niacin, as is the case when it consists predominantly of maize, which is not only deficient in both but also contains antagonists to them (Woolley, 1959).

4. *Tryptophan and pyridoxine*

Although the metabolic conversion of tryptophan to nicotinic acid is controlled by pyridoxine (Price, 1958), the anemias which follow deficiencies of tryptophan and pyridoxine are not similar, at least in the pig (Cartwright, 1947). Only pyridoxine deficiency causes hypersideremia and tissue siderosis, probably because pyridoxal 5-phosphate acts as a coenzyme in the first stage of the synthesis of heme (formation of δ-aminolevulinic acid by condensation of glycine and succinyl-coenzyme A) (Schulman and Richert, 1957), and blockage of this synthesis causes unutilized iron to accumulate.

In man, sideroblastic hypochromic anemia, which is often curable with pyridoxine, is commonly associated with disorders of tryptophan metabolism, with increased urinary excretion of xanthurenic acid (Harris and Horrigan, 1964).

5. *Methionine and pantothenic acid*

Some interaction has been shown in the lymphopoietic effect of these two factors (Dinning *et al.*, 1954). It has been attributed to the fact that in the synthesis of coenzyme A methionine may be a precursor of the thioethylamine moiety (Dinning *et al.*, 1955).

6. *Methionine, thiamine and niacin*

A further example of hematopoietic interaction between vitamins and amino acids is the antagonism between methionine and thiamine with a protein-free diet. In protein-deficient rats, a dietary excess of vitamin B_1 accentuates the fall in the number of erythrocytes (Aschkenasy, 1947), and also the decrease of proteins in the serum (Aschkenasy et al., 1948) and liver (Boissier and Aschkenasy, 1950). All these injurious effects are prevented by methionine.

VIII. EFFECTS OF DIETARY PROTEINS AND AMINO ACIDS ON INTESTINAL ABSORPTION OF IRON AND ERYTHROPOIETIC UTILIZATION OF THE LATTER AFTER ABSORPTION

As mentioned above, absorption of iron from the intestine may be inhibited by certain dietary proteins, for instance, by soya protein in the monkey (Fitch et al., 1964). On the other hand, absorption is favored by casein, and still more by maize flour (Higginson et al., 1963).

Absorption of iron decreases with a protein-deficient diet in the rat (Klavins et al., 1962; Higginson et al., 1963; Aschkenasy, 1965f), as well as in the monkey (Sood et al., 1965).

A suggested explanation of this phenomenon is the fact that chelation of iron by dietary amino acids improves absorption of the metal (Kroe et al., 1963). But absorption is still almost normal after a week of nitrogen deprivation, and is not much decreased until after very prolonged deficiency (Aschkenasy, 1965f) (Table 1).

Other possibilities must therefore be considered, such as a decrease in the intestinal cells of apoferritin, a protein which plays an important part in the absorption and storage of iron.

Transferrin is decreased in protein deficiency (Cartwright and Wintrobe, 1948; Ventura, 1953; Sood et al., 1965), but the level of this protein does not appear to affect intestinal absorption of iron (Pollack et al., 1963). Serum iron is either normal (Reissmann 1964b) or actually increased (Aschkenasy, unpublished observations) in protein-deficient rats, as in cases of human protein malnutrition (Berning, 1947).

The absorption of iron in rats deprived of protein is not controlled by the rate of erythropoiesis, for in the early stages of deficiency absorption remains almost normal although erythropoiesis practically stops, while the loss of absorption after prolonged nitrogen deficiency coincides with the resumption of some erythropoietic activity (Fig. 2, Table 1).

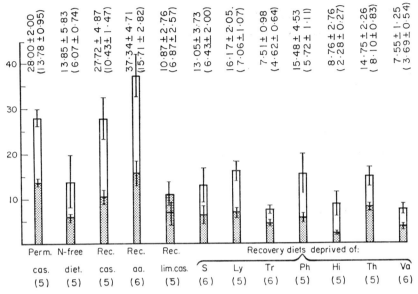

FIG. 13. Percentage (±S.E.M.) ^{59}Fe absorption (the entire columns) and red cell incorporation (the stippled segments of the columns and values in parentheses) one week after oral ^{59}Fe given on the 4th day of various recovery diets: with 18% casein given *ad libitum* (Rec. cas.), or in limited amounts (Rec. lim. cas.), with 17% total mixture of 19 amino acids (Rec. aa.); with mixtures deprived of: sulfur amino acids (S), lysine (Ly), tryptophan (Tr), phenolic amino acids (Ph), histidine (Hi), threonine (Th), or valine (Va). All the recovery diets have succeeded to 50 days of nitrogen deprivation. Controls have been maintained on a permanent 18% casein diet (first column) and other rats on a nitrogen-free diet (second column) for 60 days. Below: numbers of rats in parentheses.

Injections of erythropoietin, while preventing the blockage of erythropoiesis at the beginning of nitrogen deprivation, have no effect at all on the absorption of radio-iron (Aschkenasy, 1965f).

However, when a diet with casein or a complete mixture of amino acids is introduced after 7 weeks on a protein-free diet, there is a rapid increase of both absorption and erythropoietic utilization of ^{59}Fe.

On the other hand, if the recovery diet lacks one of the essential amino acids, absorption either remains at the level of prolonged nitrogen deprivation—this is the case with lack of lysine, sulfur or phenolic amino acids, or threonine—or it falls still lower than it was at the end of the protein deficiency, if the missing acid is tryptophan, histidine, or valine (Aschkenasy, 1966c) (Fig. 13).

Hematopoietic utilization of absorbed ^{59}Fe is also inhibited during these unsuccessful attempts at restitution with incomplete mixtures of amino acids.

IX. ACTION OF HORMONES IN THE DEVELOPMENT OF BLOOD DISORDERS OF PROTEIN DEFICIENCY

Certain hormones play a major part in the hematopoietic utilization of both dietary and tissue proteins.

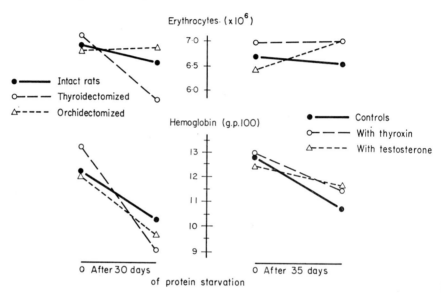

Fig. 14. Hormonal control of anemia induced by protein starvation. Graph constructed from data of Aschkenasy, A. and Pariente Ph. (*Acta Haematol.*, **9**: 29–46, (1953)), and Aschkenasy, A. (*Sang*, **25**: 15–30, (1954)).

1. *Thyroid hormones*

Thyroidectomy increases protein-deficiency anemia and (less regularly) leucopenia in male rats (Fig. 14), but not in females (Aschkenasy and Aschkenasy-Lelu, 1949; Aschkenasy and Puyo, 1952). The different response of the two sexes does not depend on the presence of androgens, for castrated male rats deprived of protein react to thyroidectomy in much the same way as intact rats (Aschkenasy and Pariente, 1953).

Thyroidectomy also delays recovery from protein-deficiency anemia and may prevent it completely—in females as well as males—if the recovery diet contains only 7% of casein (Aschkenasy and Aschkenasy-Lelu, 1949).

Conversely, thyroxine, injected during the first week of a protein-free diet, somewhat reduces the fall in reticulocytes and increases red-cell uptake of ^{59}Fe (Fig. 15), while preventing the sharp reduction in the basal metabolic rate which is typical of nitrogen deprivation (Aschkenasy, 1961b, 1963b).

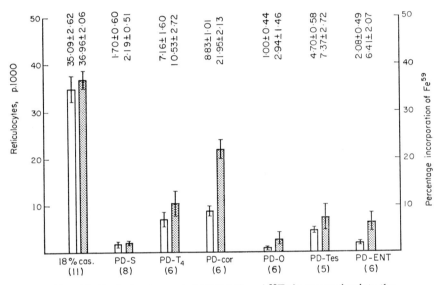

FIG. 15. Reticulocyte counts ($\pm$S.E.M.) and ^{59}Fe incorporation into the red cells ($\pm$S.E.M.) in rats given an 18% casein diet and in rats deprived of proteins for 7 days (PD). The latter group was injected either with saline (S), or DL-thyroxine (T$_4$) (30 mcg/day for 6 days), cortisone (Cor) (2 mg/day for 6 days), or, for one time only, the first day of the diet, with olive oil (O) (1 ml), testosterone oenanthate (Tes) (5 mg), or 17-ethyl, 19-nortestosterone propionate (ENT) (5 mg). The blank columns correspond to reticulocytes, the stippled columns to ^{59}Fe percentages. Numbers of rats in parentheses. Reproduced from *C.R. Soc. Biol.*, **157**: 91–5 (1963).

If these injections are continued daily from the beginning of the protein-free regimen, they delay the appearance of anemia (Fig. 14) and of leucopenia (Aschkenasy, 1954b, 1961b). Furthermore, they accelerate regeneration of all types of blood cells if they are given with a recovery diet containing only 7% of casein (Aschkenasy and Dray, 1953/4) (Fig. 16).

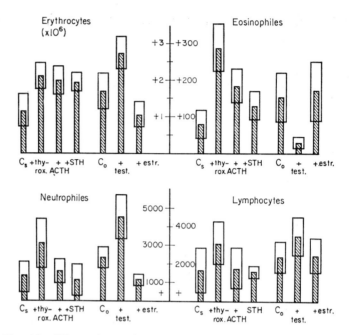

FIG. 16. Effects of several hormones (thyroxine, ACTH, STH, testosterone propionate, estradiol benzoate) on blood regeneration after prolonged protein starvation. Restoration is effected with a low-protein diet (7%) over 30 days. The hatched columns represent the mean quantitative increases p.mmc between the 1st and 31st day of restoration. The blank columns correspond to twice the standard errors of the means.

Dosages used: 10 mcg/d thyroxine; 1 mg/day ACTH; 2 Evans Units/day STH; twice a week 2.5 mg testosterone propionate; 3 times a week 12 rat Units estradiol benzoate. Cs—Controls injected with physiological saline; Co—Controls injected with olive oil. Reproduced from *Amer. J. Clin. Nutr.*, **5**: 14–25 (1957).

Stimulation of hematopoiesis in protein deficiency by thyroxine depends on at least three mechanisms: one is a *direct* action and involves specific activation of nitrogenous anabolism in the bone marrow and lymphoid tissues. Even *in vitro*, thyroxine stimulates the incorporation of amino acids into the polypeptide chains of hemoglobin (Krause and Sokoloff, 1965).

There are two *indirect* mechanisms the principal one of which is general stimulation of tissue oxidation, followed by release of erythropoietin and specific activation of erythropoiesis. This is what appears to happen when thyroxine is given at the beginning of a protein-free regimen.

The second indirect mechanism of thyroxine action in advanced protein deficiency is stimulation of intestinal absorption of vitamin B_{12}, which is otherwise reduced in this deficiency (Deo and Ramalingaswami, 1964).

The aggravation of anemia by thyroidectomy following a 2% casein diet can in fact be prevented by injections of vitamin B_{12}, although oral administration of the vitamin has no effect (Aschkenasy and Puyo, 1952).

It has been shown that thyroidectomy decreases absorption of vitamin B_{12} (Okuda and Chow, 1961), and conversely that thyroxine increases it, in protein-deficient rats (Armstead *et al.*, 1965), and also in thyroidectomized rats.

Despite histological evidence of hypofunction, the thyroid in protein-deficient rats retains for a long time a normal capacity for synthesizing hormones, as shown by biochemical and radiobiological tests (Aschkenasy *et al.*, 1962; Srebnik *et al.*, 1963; Ramalingaswami *et al.*, 1965). It may even be that the late onset and moderate degree of protein-deficiency anemia are due to this peculiarity.

2. *Androgens*

Although the inhibition of erythropoiesis seen at the beginning of a protein-free regimen is little affected by injection of androgens (testosterone or 17-ethyl 19-nortestosterone) (Aschkenasy, 1963b) (Fig. 15), true protein-deficiency anemia is almost wholly prevented by these hormones (Aschkenasy, 1954b; Blanpin and Aschkenasy, 1959; Reisert and Hunstein, 1963) (Fig. 14).

Testosterone propionate, given with a recovery diet containing 7% of casein, considerably accelerates the restitution of erythrocytes and also of neutrophils (Aschkenasy and Dray, 1953/4) (Fig. 16).

However, protein-deficiency anemia is no more severe (apart from a more obvious microcytosis) in orchidectomized rats than in intact rats (Aschkenasy and Pariente, 1953) (Fig. 14), perhaps because in the latter protein-deficiency causes an early decrease in the secretion of androgens (Aschkenasy, 1953), thus lessening the difference between controls and castrates.

While orchidectomy has little effect on anemia in protein-deficient rats, it does prevent the lymphopenia and involution of lymphoid tissue (Aschkenasy and Pariente, 1953).

Testosterone, on the other hand, is injurious to lymphopoiesis in these rats (Aschkenasy, 1954b); it also inhibits regeneration of the thymus (but not of circulating lymphocytes) and formation of eosinophils if it is injected during recovery on a 7% casein diet (Aschkenasy and Dray, 1953/4) (Fig. 16).

Under the same conditions, oestradiol benzoate has no significant effect on the restoration of hematopoiesis.

The erythropoietic effect of androgens in protein deficiency seems to be due principally to direct stimulation of protein anabolism in the erythropoietic tissues. In this way these hormones potentiate the action of erythropoietin (Naets and Wittek, 1964), though they are not able to replace the latter factor if it is completely missing (Aschkenasy, 1963b).

3. *Glucocorticoids*

(a) Cortisone, 2 mg daily, stimulates erythropoiesis at the beginning of protein deprivation (Fig. 15). If injections are continued for several weeks, protein-deficient anemia is at first improved, but later aggravated (Aschkenasy, 1954b, 1961b).

Small doses of corticotrophin (1 mg per day), injected from the first day of a recovery diet with 7% of casein, hasten recovery from the deficiency anemia (Fig. 16).

As with thyroxine, two explanations can be offered for the action of glucocorticoids on erythropoiesis in protein-deficient rats: firstly, stimulation of oxygen consumption followed by release of erythropoietin, which happens mainly at the beginning of protein deficiency (Aschkenasy, 1963b); and secondly, direct stimulation of erythropoiesis, with a supply of amino acids from the degradation of tissues such as muscle and lymphoid tissue caused by glucocorticoids. However, erythropoiesis gains by this degradation only for as long as the latter is moderate, and does not involve the proteins of the bone marrow itself, as seems to occur after prolonged excess of the hormones.

(b) In the absence of accessory adrenals it is impossible to keep adrenalectomized rats alive for more than 14 days on a diet with a very low protein content, even if excess salt is added (Aschkenasy, 1954a) or deoxycorticosterone is given (Leathem, 1957). Prolonged survival is possible only if cortisone and sodium chloride are given together (Aschkenasy, 1954a, 1955a), but the hormone is not needed for survival if adrenalectomized rats are given a diet with 18% of casein and salt in their drink. Thus the need for glucocorticoids appears to be increased in protein deficiency.

With advanced deficiency of protein or of certain amino acids (notably isoleucine, phenolic amino acids, or valine) there is a relative hyperadrenocorticism, indicated by increased amounts of corticosterone in the plasma, and especially in the adrenals, relative to body weight (Adam *et al.*, 1965), which probably contributes to the development of deficiency lymphopenia and eosinopenia.

It is in any case noteworthy that atrophy of the thymus and also eosinopenia are pronounced with almost all deficiencies of the amino acids which induce large increases in the relative weight (per 100 g body weight) of the adrenals (Aschkenasy, 1964a, 1965a) (Table 2), or in corticosterone production (valine or phenolic amino acid deficiency) (Aschkenasy *et al.*, 1965).

With early nitrogen deficiency, however, both eosinopenia and involution of the thymus might be determined not by a quantitative increase of endogenous glucocorticoids, but only by an abnormal sensitivity of the eosinophils and the thymus to the lytic action of these hormones: in fact, cortisone in doses as small as 100 mcg per 100 g per day is enough to provoke both disorders in adrenalectomized rats deprived of protein, whereas equivalent doses (per 100 g body weight) have no lytic action at all on eosinophils or thymus in adrenalectomized rats on normal diets (Aschkenasy, 1964b).

The abnormal sensitivity of eosinophils in protein deficiency is also shown by the fact that the eosinopenia following intraperitoneal injection of corticotrophin (4 mg per 100 g) or cortisone (0.4 mg per 100 mg body weight) is much more pronounced in protein-deficient rats (a fall of over 90 % after 4 hr) than in normally-fed rats ($\sim$ 60 %) (Aschkenasy, 1961a).

Although lymphopenia in protein-deficient rats also depends on the functional state of the adrenals (Aschkenasy, 1955a), its development apparently requires greater endogenous glucocorticoid activity than does that of eosinopenia.

In fact, as opposed to what has been described with eosinophils, rats without adrenals and lacking protein, given very small doses of cortisone (100 mcg per 100 g per day) for 21 days show a massive increase instead of a fall in the number of circulating lymphocytes. This hyperlymphocytosis is associated with hypertrophy of the lymph nodes, in contrast to the atrophy of the thymus and spleen (Aschkenasy, 1964b).

4. *Growth hormone*

Depletion of growth hormone (Srebnik *et al.*, 1959) may contribute to the development of deficiency anemia, since injections of the hormone stimulate recovery from the anemia if they are given in moderate doses

(1 or 2 Evans units daily) during the period of protein restoration (Asch-kenasy and Dray, 1954 (Fig. 16); Aschkenasy, 1959b).

Hypophysectomy and nitrogen deprivation are both followed in a few days by inhibition of erythropoiesis, together with gross reduction of general metabolism; in either case the inhibition can be prevented by injections of erythropoietin (Jacobson *et al.*, 1959), but the later progressive medullary hypoplasia of hypophysectomized animals (Crafts and Meineke, 1959) contrasts with the partial reactivation of the bone marrow in the later stages of protein deficiency—this reactivation coinciding exactly. with the development of a true anemia (Aschkenasy, 1946).

5. *Hypothalamic hormones and stimuli*

As regulator of adenohypophyseal activity and site of the appetite centers, the hypothalamus certainly plays a dominant part in the utiliza-tion of dietary proteins for hematopoiesis.

Indeed, the secretion of erythropoietin itself, like that of some pituitary hormones, may depend on the hypothalamus (Halvorsen, 1961). If this is so, then not only the sudden decrease in food intake caused by stopping the supply of protein or of one of the essential amino acids, but also the early (but temporary) failure of erythropoietin delivery, must be ascribed to inhibition of the hypothalamic centers.

However, it seems that the relations between the hypothalamus and nitrogen deprivation have not yet been studied experimentally.

6. *Erythropoietin*

The inhibition of erythropoiesis at the beginning of nitrogen starvation is wholly prevented by injections of rat plasma with a high erythropoietin content, while it is little affected by plasma from normal rats and still less by plasma from rats themselves deprived of protein for 7 days (Asch-kenasy, 1962a,b, 1963c,d) (Fig. 17). The inhibition is thus evidently due to disappearance of erythropoietin in the blood. This has been confirmed by Reissman (1964a,b).

However, intraperitoneal grafts of kidney, spleen and liver exhibit a significant erythropoietic potency in the protein-starved rats, even if these grafts are taken from protein-deprived donors (Aschkenasy, 1967d). It may be that there is retention of erythropoietin in these organs (especially in the kidneys) rather than failure of production in the initial stage of protein starvation. Release of this factor from the grafts might be con-ditioned by cellular breakdown.

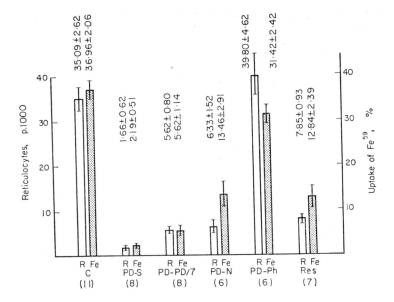

Fig. 17. Mean reticulocyte (R) levels p. 1000 red cells ($\pm$ S.E.M.) and percentage incorporation of ^{59}Fe ($\pm$ S.E.M.) into the red cells in control rats on a 18 % casein diet (C) and in protein-deprived rats (PD) injected between the 1st and the 7th day of a protein-free diet with either isotonic saline (S), or with plasma of rats deprived of proteins since 7 days (PD/7), normal rat plasma (N), phenylhydrazine anemic rat plasma (Ph), or plasma of rats restored with 18 % casein for 5 days after a protracted protein deprivation (Res). Numbers of rats in parentheses. Reproduced from *C.R. Soc. Biol.*, **156**: 1599–1605 (1962).

Inhibitory anti-erythropoietic factors could not be demonstrated in the plasma of protein-deprived rats (Aschkenasy, 1967a).

Surprisingly, but no doubt in association with the increasing hemolysis, the level of plasma erythropoietin rises again as the protein deficiency continues, as shown both by renewed erythropoietic activity in the marrow, and by the fact that exogenous erythropoietin has no effect if it is injected after more than 7 weeks of nitrogen deficiency (Aschkenasy, 1964c) (Fig. 18).

Furthermore, protein refeeding after 7 weeks' deficiency causes no significant release of erythropoietin in comparison with the amounts shown in the later stages of deficiency—plasma from rats during recovery is no more erythropoietic than plasma from normal rats (Aschkenasy, 1962a) (Fig. 17), despite the greatly enhanced erythropoiesis.

The ability of a low-protein recovery diet (7% casein) to stimulate erythropoiesis is not increased by injections of exogenous erythropoietin (Aschkenasy, 1964c) (Fig. 18).

Reissmann (1964b) reported a raised plasma level of erythropoietin at the beginning of a recovery diet, but this diet was given after only 10 days of

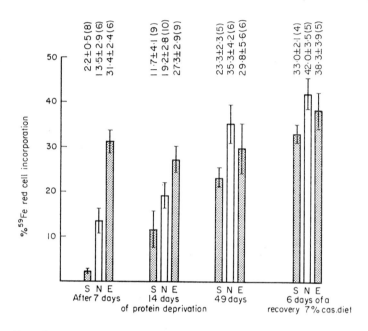

FIG. 18. Percentage (±S.E.M.) red cell incorporation of ^{59}Fe (24 hr after intravenous injection) in rats deprived of proteins for 7, 14, or 49 days and in rats fed with a 7% casein diet after 7 weeks of nitrogen starvation. Comparative effects of repeated injections of physiologics aline (S), normal rat plasma (N) and of erythropoietic plasma (E) taken from rats made anemic by phenylhydrazine. Numbers of rats in parentheses.

nitrogen starvation, and the levels of erythropoietin were thus compared with those at the early stage of a protein-free diet, when the release of the factor is completely suppressed.

In conclusion, while the absence of erythropoietin is responsible for the early inhibition of erythropoiesis, it cannot be held directly and exclusively responsible for the true protein-deficiency anemia, which appears later.

X. PATHOGENESIS OF BLOOD DISORDERS INDUCED BY PROTEIN DEFICIENCY

A. PATHOGENESIS OF PROTEIN-DEFICIENCY ANEMIA

Two anomalies seem to be responsible for protein-deficiency anemia: blockage of red-cell maturation, and excessive hemolysis.

1. *Blockage of maturation*

The blockage is especially severe at the beginning, but it persists to some extent until the final stages of nitrogen deprivation. Paradoxically, the stage of erythropoiesis affected becomes more advanced as the deficiency continues.

(a) At the beginning of the protein-free diet the division and hemoglobinization of the erythroblasts are blocked, as shown by the greatly reduced mitotic activity of these cells (Aschkenasy, 1963a), the abrupt fall in the reticulocyte count (Aschkenasy, 1946, 1961b), and in the uptake of ^{59}Fe by the red cells (Bethard *et al.*, 1958b; Aschkenasy, 1962a,b,c).

(b) At a later stage of deficiency the blockage affects mainly the conversion of erythroblasts to reticulocytes, as shown by the accumulation of erythroblasts in the bone marrow. However, this blockage is incomplete, since an increasing number of reticulocytes is found in the blood (Aschkenasy, 1946).

The massive transitory reticulocytosis following the introduction of a recovery diet is due to relief of the blockage of erythroblast–reticulocyte transformation.

(c) There is also blockage of the transformation of reticulocytes into adult erythrocytes.

This blockage, shown *in vitro* by Nizet (1950, 1955) is certainly involved in the increased reticulocytosis at the end of nitrogen starvation *in vivo*, but it is most apparent when the supply of protein is inadequate during the recovery period. In these circumstances only the transformation of erythroblasts to reticulocytes seems to be possible, the latter being incapable of maturation; hence the increasing reticulocytosis while the anemia deteriorates in rats during an unsuccessful attempt at restitution after prolonged protein starvation (Aschkenasy, 1957).

2. *Hemolysis*

Increased hemolysis may be responsible for the "shift to the right" of the blockage of maturation during nitrogen deficiency.

This hemolysis is suggested firstly by the increased sensitivity of protein-deficient erythrocytes to the hemolytic action of digitonin (Aschkenasy *et al.*, 1956a), and of saponin (Aschkenasy and Blanpin, 1959; Delmonte *et al.*, 1964) (Fig. 19), and by the increased resistance to mechanical trauma (Table 3) and alkalis (Fig 20) Delmonte *et al.*, 1964); and secondly by the short life of deficient erythrocytes compared with that of normal erythrocytes in the rat (Aschkenasy *et al.*, 1956b) and in the dog (Mariani and Migliaccio, 1964).

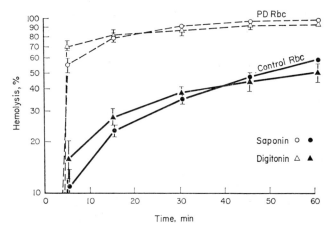

FIG. 19. Percentage hemolysis as a function of time of contact, of saponin (20 mcg/ml) and digitonin (2 mcg/ml) with erythrocytes of rats on balanced and protein-deficient (PD) diets (hemocytometric method) (Means ±S.E.M.). Reproduced from Delmonte, L. *et al.*, *Blood*, **24**: 49–68 (1964).

Ito and Reissmann (1966) reported that ^{59}Fe-labeled red cells of protein-starved rats injected with ^{59}Fe five days before the bleeding showed the same survival time as red cells taken from non-starved donors, if they were transfused into normal recipients. These results (confirmed in our laboratory) may be interpreted as due to the immaturity of the transfused cells (reticulocytes) which still contained enough RNA for protein synthesis from amino acids present in the plasma of the normal recipients. On the other hand, if the protein-starved donors were injected with ^{59}Fe

TABLE 3. MECHANICAL FRAGILITY, IN PRESENCE AND ABSENCE OF ANTI-
SPHERING FACTOR (ASF), OF ERYTHROCYTES OF RATS ON BALANCED AND
PROTEIN-DEFICIENT (PD) DIETS, FOLLOWING TRAUMATIZATION AT 90 RPM FOR
60 MIN (MEANS ± S.E.M.) (Reproduced from DELMONTE, L. *et al.*, *Blood*, **24**:
49–68 (1964))

Anticoagulant Method	ASF	No. of Rats	Hemolysis (%)	
			Control RBC	PD RBC
Mechanical defibrinization		9	31.1 ± 2.7	
	−	9		52.3 ± 3.3
Heparinization	+[a]	4	17.7 ± 3.0	
		5		27.6 ± 3.1
	−	4	13.2 ± 3.0	

[a]ASF adsorption from erythrocytes prevented by siliconation of glassware.

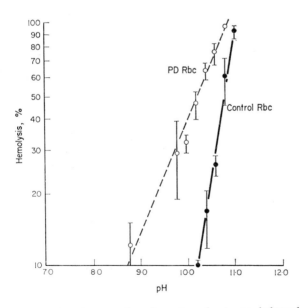

FIG. 20. Alkali resistance of erythrocytes of rats on balanced and
protein-deficient (PD) diets (Means ± S.E.M.). Reproduced from
Delmonte, L. *et al.*, *Blood*, **24**: 49–68 (1964).

two weeks before the bleeding, the labeled (almost all adult) red cells were found to have a much shorter lifespan in the blood of the recipients than red cells of the same age taken from normal donors (Aschkenasy, 1967b).

3. *Factors responsible for blockage of maturation and for hemolysis*

(a) The blockage of maturation of erythroblasts reaches its maximum at a very early stage of deficiency. It cannot be ascribed, at any rate at this stage, to depletion of protein stores, nor to the absence of transferrin which is needed for the transport of iron to the bone marrow.

This blockage can be relieved by injections of erythropoietin, and also to some extent by injecting adenosine triphosphate or monophosphate (Aschkenasy, 1963f). These metabolites may act by stimulating the secretion or utilization of erythropoietin, or by taking part in the synthesis of the ribonucleic acid and proteins of the erythroblasts.

The actual delivery of erythropoietin is apparently prevented by an abrupt decrease in oxygen consumption; the limited protective action of thyroxine and cortisone could be explained simply by the calorigenic effect of these hormones (Aschkenasy, 1961b).

The mechanism of *late* blockage (erythroblast–reticulocyte) is more complex.

A first factor is still the general reduction of the metabolic rate, which might explain the anti-anemic effect (which is, however, only temporary) of 2,4-dinitrophenol in protein-deficient rats (Aschkenasy, 1959c).

However, as distinct from what is seen with early blockage, lack of erythropoietin does not appear to be involved, since injections of this factor lose their effect completely in the later stages of nitrogen deprivation (Fig. 18), and they increase neither the uptake of ^{59}Fe by the red cells nor the release of reticulocytes at the beginning of recovery (Aschkenasy, 1964c).

A priori, the late blockage of erythropoiesis might be partly attributed to disturbance of the transport of iron in the blood, and its uptake by erythroblasts in the marrow through deficiency of transferrin. But serum iron levels are not lowered in protein-deficient rats, and in all probability the primary cause of the blockage is not inadequate iron uptake by the erythroblasts, but lack of amino acids, which can no longer be mobilized from the tissues in sufficient amounts for the synthesis of hemoglobin. It is possible that involution of the gonads in male rats or inactivation of the thyroid may be involved in the late blockage of erythropoiesis.

(b) Hemolysis seems to arise from disturbances in both plasma and erythrocytes in the deficient animals.

A disorder of the plasma is shown by the fact that mechanical or chemical hemolysis can be reduced by the addition *in vitro* of serum from a normal rat to a suspension of erythrocytes, while serum from protein-deficient rats is less effective. The efficiency of the latter can be increased by lecithin (Delmonte *et al.*, 1964).

Besides, if one transfuses to protein deprived recipients adult erythrocytes tagged *in vivo* with ^{59}Fe taken from normal rats, the survival of these cells is much shorter than the survival of the same cells transfused to non deprived rats (Aschkenasy, 1967c).

But hemolysis is also a consequence of a structural defect of protein-deficient erythrocytes, as proved by the shorter life-span of these cells in comparison with normal erythrocytes.

No abnormality of the electrophoretic mobility or of the alkali resistance of hemoglobin has been found. On the other hand, the stroma of the erythrocytes has a higher nitrogen content in protein-deficient rats than in normally fed rats. The amounts of total lipids, cholesterol, and phospholipids seem to be about normal (Aschkenasy *et al.*, 1959), but more detailed analysis of these constituents would perhaps show some difference.

In any case, the permeability of the erythrocyte membrane is deeply altered as shown by the abnormalities of the electrolyte levels in the erythrocytes: from the very first week of nitrogen deprivation there is a strong loss of the intracellular potassium and magnesium and a rise in the sodium content. These changes may favour hemolysis. Opposite changes are noticed after one week of protein refeeding following a prolonged protein free diet (Spach and Aschkenasy, 1969). On the other hand, the levels of electrolytes remain almost the same as during protein starvation if the recovery diet lacks only one essential amino acid (Spach and Aschkenasy, 1970).

Protein deprivation also induces but only at a late stage a significant fall in the erythrocyte level of ATP which increases again soon after the start of a protein recovery diet (Aschkenasy *et al.*, 1969). The loss of ATP does not seem to be responsible for the failure of the cation pump because the electrolyte abnormalities appear at an earlier stage than the ATP depletion. Besides, recovery diets deprived of only one essential amino acid do not prevent the increase in the erythrocyte ATP levels (Gajdos-Török *et al.*, 1969) whereas the same diets oppose the return of the electrolyte levels to the normal.

It may be that a primary alteration of the membrane due to the protein deficiency stimulates the hydrolysis of ATP by ATPase in an attempt to compensate the failure of the cation pump. In rats given incomplete amino acid diets the paradoxical increase in ATP is possibly due to a deficiency of ATPase. Experiments are under way to control this hypothesis.

Certain enzymatic disorders have been found in the erythrocytes from the very first days of nitrogenous malnutrition, e.g. a reduction of transaminases (Sabry *et al.*, 1965), lactic dehydrogenase, aldolase (Bisiani, 1965) and also of methemoglobin reductase, glutathione reductase and glucose 6-phosphate-dehydrogenase (Sanchez de Jimenez *et al.*, 1965a,b; Bisiani, 1965). The three last-named enzymes are known to be involved in the protection of red cells against hemolysis.

(c) It must be borne in mind that the two mechanisms of blockage and hemolysis, far from being independent, are intimately associated.

In the first place, hemolysis and blockage occur together in the late stages of deficiency, although the blockage is much less complete that in the early stage. In the second place, in view of the enzymatic disorders of the erythrocytes already reported in short-term nitrogen deficiency, it may be regarded that some such disorders likely to favour hemolysis appear in the first few days of protein deficiency. It is even possible that the temporary failure of erythropoietin production causes pathological red cells to be produced and so is partly to blame for later hemolysis.

B. PATHOGENESIS OF PROTEIN-DEFICIENCY LEUCOPENIA

A priori, this leucopenia might be due to migration of leucocytes into certain tissues, or to intravascular lysis, or last but not least to blockage of maturation.

1. The first possibility has not been demonstrated, and as regards the eosinophils a quantitative reduction has been shown not only in the blood but also in the spleen, lungs, and particularly the gastro-intestinal mucosa (Aschkenasy and Jobard, 1961; Aschkenasy, 1965a).

2. Intravascular lysis might play some part in lymphopenia in view of the increasing proportion of degenerate lymphocytes found in rats after protracted protein deficiency (Aschkenasy, 1946).

The abnormal sensitivity of eosinophils to glucocorticoids during a protein-free regimen has already been mentioned.

3. However, the principal cause of protein-deficiency leucopenia appears to be failure to produce white cells, as shown by the decrease in the neutrophil and eosinophil series in the bone marrow (Aschkenasy, 1946;

Aschkenasy and Jobard, 1961), and by the involution of the lymphoid organs.

Since medium and large lymphocytes are regarded as being metabolically the most active forms of lymphocyte (cf. Yoffey, 1964), the selective disappearance of these cells in nitrogen deprivation might be explained by the failure of processes of protein synthesis in which these lymphocytes are involved.

As already shown, the early involution of the thymus seen in nitrogen deprivation, as in other forms of malnutrition, plays a significant part in the disappearance of these lymphocytes. It may thus be that involution of the thymus arises from reduced utilization of the cells produced under its control.

This kind of negative feedback from lymphocytes to thymus could be transmitted, at least in part, by the thymolytic action of glucocorticoid hormones. Indeed, prolonged nitrogen deprivation tends on the one hand to increase the production of these hormones (Adam *et al.*, 1965), and on the other to render the thymus abnormally sensitive to their action (Aschkenasy, 1964b).

XI. GENERAL CONCLUSIONS

The hematopoietic effect of proteins is due to their paramount importance in the chemical constitution of the blood cells, and to the enzymatic reactions involved in the formation of these cells.

This effect, which is greatest in proteins of animal origin, depends primarily on their content of various essential amino acids, but also on the extent to which the organism is able to liberate the amino acids and to apply them to its metabolic needs.

The action of proteins and amino acids on the hematopoietic tissues is clearly not only a direct one; it is also carried out by way of various intermediate processes: firstly, the action of vitamins derived from certain amino acids, e.g. niacin, or synthesized in the digestive tract by virtue of the supply of dietary proteins, e.g. vitamin B_{12} and folic acid; secondly, the stimulation of oxygen consumption, promoting release of erythropoietin; thirdly, the effects of various hormones, especially thyroid hormones, androgens, glucocorticoids, and growth hormone.

These hormones act on hematopoiesis either synergestically or, on the contrary, as antagonists, e.g. thyroxine and glucocorticoids in relation to lymphocytes and eosinophils.

L

Further, the same hormone may have opposite effects on different cell-types, as in the case of the androgens which stimulate the erythrocytic and neutrophil series, but also inhibit the production of lymphocytes and eosinophils.

Deficiency solely of dietary protein produces only a delayed and moderate anemia, which is generally microcytic and hypochromic.

The mildness of this anemia is explained by the priority given to erythropoiesis and this priority depends largely on thyroid activity.

Protein-deficiency anemia is a result both of blockage of erythroblast maturation and of hemolysis.

The blockage is more complete in the early stage than in the late stages of protein deficiency. In the early stage it is due to failure of erythropoietin production or excretion, but later this factor again becomes available under the stimulating influence of hemolysis.

Protein-deficiency leucopenia involves at first the eosinophils and later the lymphocytes and neutrophils.

Lack of protein causes selective disappearance of large and medium lymphocytes, perhaps as a result of failure of the protein synthesis at the site of these cells.

Early involution of the thymus plays a part in the reduction in the number and size of the lymphocytes in protein deficiency.

REFERENCES

(a). BOOKS, REVIEWS AND MONOGRAPHS

BLOCK, R. J. and BOLLING, D. (1947). *The Amino Acid Composition of Proteins and Foods*, Ch. C. Thomas, Springfield, Ill., 1st. ed.
GOUNELLE, H. (1953). Étude clinique de la dénutrition azotée, pp. 609–30. In: *29e Congrès fr. de Médecine*, éd. Masson, Paris.
SÓS, J. (1964). *Die Pathologie der Eiweissernährung*, ed. Ung. Akad. der Wissensch., Budapest.
WOOLLEY, D. W. (1959). *A study of antimetabolites*, ed. Wiley, New York.

(b). ORIGINAL PAPERS

ADAM, Y., JOLY, P. and ASCHKENASY, A. (1965). Teneurs du plasma et des surrénales en corticostérone chez des rats carencés en protéines ou en certains acides aminés. *C.R. Soc. Biol.*, **159**: 294–8.
ALBANESE, A. A., HOLT, L. E. JR., IRBY, V. and BRUMBACK, J. E. JR. (1946). Observations on sulfur amino acid deficiencies in rats. Chemical and morphological changes in the blood. *J. Biol. Chem.*, **165**: 179–86.

ALBANESE, A. A., HOLT, L. E., KAJDI, C. and FRANKSTON, J. E. (1943). Observations in tryptophan deficiency in rats. Chemical and morphological charges in the blood. *J. Biol. Chem.*, **148**: 299–309.
ALEXANDER, H. D. and SAUBERLICH, H. E. (1957). The influence of lipotropic factors on the prevention of nutritional edema in the rat. *J. Nutr.*, **61**: 329–41.
ALTMAN, K. I. and MILLER, G. (1953). A disturbance of tryptophan metabolism in congenital hypoplastic anemia. *Nature*, **172**: 868.
ALTMANN, A. and MURRAY, J. F. (1948). The anaemia of malignant malnutrition (Infantile Pellagra, Kwashiorkor): protein deficiency as a possible aetiological factor. *S. Afr. J. Med. Sc.*, **13**: 91–113.
ARMSTEAD, E. E., HSU, J. M. and CHOW, B. F. (1965). Malabsorption of vitamin B_{12}-Co^{60} in protein depleted rats. *Fed. Proc.*, **24**: 499.
ARNSTEIN, H. R. V. and SIMKIN, J. L. (1959). Vitamin B_{12} and biosynthesis in rat liver. *Nature*, **183**: 523–5.
ASCHKENASY, A. (1946). Étude sur l'anémie expérimentale par inanition protéique chez le Rat. Les altérations du sang, de la moelle osseuse et de la rate. Les relations avec l'évolution du cycle oestral. *Sang*, **17**: 34–61.
ASCHKENASY, A. (1947). Nouvelles études sur l'intervention de quelques vitamines B dans l'hématopoïèse. *Ann. Biol. Clin.*, **5**: 262–72.
ASCHKENASY, A. (1953). Action de la testostérone, de la thyroxine et de la cortisone sur l'ingestion alimentaire. la chute de poids et l'état des organes chez le rat carencé en protéines. *Ann. Endocrinol.*, **14**: 353–56.
ASCHKENASY, A. (1954a). Action des protéines et de certains acides aminés alimentaires sur la survie de rats surrénalectomisés. Protection de ces rats contre l'effet léthal de l'inanition protéique par la cortisone. *C.R. Acad. Sc.*, **239**: 1000–2.
ASCHKENASY, A. (1954b). Action de la testostérone, de la thyroxine et de la cortisone sur l'évolution de l'anémie et de la leucopénie protéiprives. *Sang*, **25**: 15–30.
ASCHKENASY, A. (1955a). Influence des protéines alimentaires sur la survie ainsi que sur la lymphopoïèse et sur l'éosinopoïèse de rats surrénalectomisés. *Rev. Belge de Pathol.*, **24**: 365–76.
ASCHKENASY, A. (1957a). On the pathogenesis of anemias and leukopenias induced by dietary protein deficiency. *Amer. J. Clin. Nutr.*, **5**: 14–25.
ASCHKENASY, A. (1957b). Pourquoi la cortisone est-elle moins éosinopéniante chez le Rat surrénalectomisé que chez le Rat normal? *C.R. Soc. Biol.*, **151**: 521–4.
ASCHKENASY, A. (1957c). Sur le rôle joué par certains métabolites organiques et minéraux dans l'éosinopénie provoquée par la cortisone. *Rev. Fr. Et. clin. Biol.*, **2**: 1013–24.
ASCHKENASY, A. (1958). Recherches expérimentales sur le rôle de la thyroïde dans la régulation de la leucopoïèse. *Path. Biol. (Paris)*, **34**: 683–97.
ASCHKENASY, A. (1959a). Some new experimental data on the role of the adrenals in the regulation of blood eosinophilia. *Ann. N.Y. Acad. Sc.*, **77**: 574–88.
ASCHKENASY, A. (1959b). Effets de l'insuline et de l'hormone somatotrope sur la réparation de l'anémie protéiprove du Rat. *Sang*, **30**: 168–75.
ASCHKENASY, A. (1959c). Effet anti-anémique du 2,4-dinitrophénol chez des rats carencés en protéines. *J. de Physiol. (Paris)*, **51**: 390–1.
ASCHKENASY, A. (1961a). Influence de la privation de protéines alimentaires sur l'action éosinopéniante de l'ACTH et de la cortisone chez le rat. *Nouv. Rev. Fr. d'Hematol.*, **1**: 213–8.
ASCHKENASY, A. (1961b). Recherches sur le rôle joué par la réduction des besoins tissulaires en oxygène dans la genèse de l'anémie par carence protidique. *Rev. Fr. Et. clin. Biol.*, **6**: 756–65.
ASCHKENASY, A. (1961c). Les aspects hématologiques de l'ostéolathyrisme expérimental. *Thérapie*, **16**: 192–205.

L*

ASCHKENASY, A. (1962a). Teneurs en érythropoïétine du plasma sanguin du rat, au cours de la carence protidique et de sa réparation. *C.R. Soc. Biol.*, **156**: 226–30; *J. de Physiol.* (*Paris*), **54**: 279.

ASCHKENASY, A. (1962b). Nouvelles recherches sur le tarissement de la production d'érythropoïétine au cours de l'inanition protidique du rat. *C.R. Soc. Biol.*, **156**: 1599–1605.

ASCHKENASY, A. (1962c). Incorporation du ^{59}Fe dans les globules rouges, la moelle osseuse et certains autres tissus au cours de l'inanition protidique expérimentale. *C.R. Soc. Biol.*, **156**: 1786–90.

ASCHKENASY, A. (1962d). Inhibition précoce de l'érythropoïèse après privation de divers acides aminés essentiels chez le rat mâle. *C.R. Soc. Biol.*, **156**: 1971–6.

ASHKENASY, A. (1963a). Activité mitotique de la moelle osseuse chez le rat privé de protéines alimentaires. *C.R. Acad. Sc.*, **256**: 1155–7.

ASCHKENASY, A. (1963b). Effets de la thyroxine, de la cortisone et des androgènes sur la réticulocytose sanguine et sur l'incorporation du ^{59}Fe dans les érythrocytes et dans certains organes chez des rats carencés en protéines. *C.R. Soc. Biol.*, **157**: 91–5; *J. de Physiol.* (*Paris*), **55**: 187–8.

ASCHKENASY, A. (1963c). Réactivation par l'érythropoïétine des mitoses érythroblastiques inhibées par la privation de protéines alimentaires. *C.R. Soc. Biol.*, **157**: 275–80.

ASCHKENASY, A. (1963d). Études sur la production d'érythropoïétine chez le rat carencé en protéines. *Rev. Fr. Et. clin. Biol.*, **8**: 985–99.

ASCHKENASY, A. (1963e). Effets exercés par la privation de protéines ou de certains acides aminés essentiels sur le métabolisme de la vitamine ^{60}Co-B_{12} chez le rat mâle. *C.R. Soc. Biol.*, **157**: 1740–6.

ASCHKENASY, A. (1963f). Mise en évidence d'une action érythropoïétique modérée des acides adénosine-5-monophosphorique (AMP) et adénosine-triphosphorique (ATP) ainsi que de l'adénosine chez le rat carencé en protéines. *C.R. Soc. Biol.*, **157**: 1893–7.

ASCHKENASY, A. (1963g). Effets comparés de la privation de divers acides aminés essentiels sur le métabolisme de base chez le rat mâle. *C.R. Soc. Biol.*, **157**: 1950–4.

ASCHKENASY, A. (1963h). Effets comparés de la privation de divers acides aminés essentiels sur les taux des éosinophiles sanguins et médullaires chez le rat mâle. *C.R. Soc. Biol.*, **157**: 2169–73.

ASCHKENASY, A. (1964a). Poids des organes lymphoïdes et des surrénales dans diverses carences en acides aminés essentiels chez le rat mâle. *C.R. Soc. Biol.*, **158**: 479–83.

ASCHKENASY, A. (1964b). Nouvelles données sur le rôle joué par les surrénales dans l'éosinopénie sanguine et dans l'atrophie des organes lymphoïdes chez le rat carencé en protéines. *C.R. Soc. Biol.*, **158**: 708–11.

ASCHKENASY, A. (1964c). Recherches complémentaires sur le rôle joué par l'érythropoïétine dans l'anémie de l'inanition azotée expérimentale. *C.R. Soc. Biol.*, **158**: 1226–9.

ASCHKENASY, A. (1964d). Influence des protéines alimentaires sur le volume cellulaire et nucléaire des lymphocytes sanguins chez le rat mâle. *C.R. Soc. Biol.*, **158**: 1293–7.

ASCHKENASY, A. (1965a). Effets des carences en divers acides aminés sur la production des éosinophiles et sur la répartition de ces cellules dans le sang et dans la muqueuse gastrointestinale. Rôle des corticosurrénales dans la genèse de l'éosinopénie carentielle. *Rev. Fr. Et. clin. Biol.*, **10**: 299–307.

ASCHKENASY, A. (1965b). Sur le rôle joué par l'atrophie du thymus dans l'inhibition de la lymphopoïèse provoquée par la carence alimentaire en protéines chez le rat mâle. *Experientia*, **21**: 225.

ASCHKENASY, A. (1965c). Effets comparés de la privation de protéines alimentaires ou de certains acides aminés essentiels sur les protéines sériques et sur leur répartition électrophorétique sur papier chez le rat. *C.R. Soc. Biol.*, **159**: 800–4.

ASCHKENASY, A. (1965d). Influence of alimentary proteins on the size of blood lymphocytes in the rat. The role of the thymus in this effect. *Israel J. Med. Sc.*, 1: 552–62.

ASCHKENASY, A. (1965e). Effets hématologiques de la thymectomie chez des rats recevant un régime équilibré ou un régime dépourvu de protéines. *Rev. Fr. Et. clin. Biol.*, 10: 709–23.

ASCHKENASY, A. (1965f). Effet de la carence expérimentale en protéines sur l'absorption digestive du ^{59}Fe et sur la répartition tissulaire du fer absorbé. *Proc. 10th Congr. europ. Soc. Haemat., Strasbourg 1965, II*, 71–5. Karger, Basel, 1967.

ASCHKENASY, A. (1966a). Effets de divers mélanges d'acides aminés sur la régénération des leucocytes chez des rats carencés en protéines. I. Neutrophiles et éosinophiles. *C.R. Soc. Biol.*, 160: 933–7. (1966b); II. Lymphocytes. *Ibid.*, 160: 1787–92.

ASCHKENASY, A. (1966c). Effets comparés de la caséine et de divers mélanges d'acides aminés sur l'absorption intestinale du ^{59}Fe et sur l'utilisation érythropoïétique du radio-fer absorbé chez des rats carencés en protéines. *C.R. Soc. Biol.*, 160: 1383–7.

ASCHKENASY, A. (1967a). Recherche d'un facteur inhibiteur de l'érythropoïèse dans le plasma de rats carencés en proteines. *C.R. Soc. Biol.*, 161: 2377–80.

ASCHKENASY, A. (1967b). Nouvelles études sur la durée de vie des érythrocytes dans la carence prolongée en protéines. I. Confirmation de l'existence d'une fragilité anormale *in vivo* des érythrocytes de rats privés de protéines alimentaires. *C.R. Soc. Biol.*, 161: 1860–3. (1967c); II. Démonstration d'une intervention de facteurs extra-érythrocytaires dans l'hémolyse *in vivo* chez des rats carences en protéines. *Ibid.*, 161: 1925–8.

ASCHENKASY, A. (1967d). Données nouvelles sur le mécanisme de l'inhibition de l'érythropoïèse au début de l'inanition azotée. Probabilité d'une rétention rénale, splénique et hépatique de l'érythropoïétine chez des rats carencés en protéines. *Arch. Sc. Physiol.*, 22: 357–74.

ASCHKENASY, A., ADAM, Y. and JOLY, P. (1965). Quelques données sur l'état fonctionnel des corticosurrénales chez le rat carencé en protéines ou en certains acides aminés. *Ann. d'Endocrinol.*, 27: 27–36.

ASCHKENASY, A. and ASCHKENASY-LELU, P. (1947). Étude sur la réparation pondérale et sanguine de l'inanition protéique. *Arch. Sc. Physiol.*, 1: 225–55.

ASCHKENASY, A. and ASCHKENASY-LELU, P. (1949). Influence de la thyroïdectomie sur l'évolution et sur la réparation de l'anémie protéiprive expérimentale. *Sang*, 20: 77–89.

ASCHKENASY, A., ASCHKENASY-LELU, P. and ROLLAND, G. J. (1949a). Nouvelles études sur l'action anabolisante de l'acide ptéroylglutamique et des extraits antipernicieux dans la réparation de rats carencés en protéines. *Bull. Soc. Chim. Biol.*, 31: 1451–65.

ASCHKENASY, A., ASCHKENASY-LELU, P. and ROLLAND, G. J. (1949b). Influence de la nature de l'apport hydrocarboné de la ration sur la réparation du rat carencé en protéines. *C.R. Soc. Biol.*, 143: 382–4.

ASCHKENASY, A., BOISSIER J. and ROLLAND, G. J. (1949c). Comparaison des effets exercés par la méthionine, la thiamine et le glycocolle sur le poids, les éléments figurés du sang et les protéines sériques du rat carencé en protéines. *Bull. Soc. Chim. Biol.*, 31: 1019–28.

ASCHKENASY, A. and BENHAMOU, J. P. (1950). Étude comparée de l'action anabolisante de la méthionine et de la cystine en régime pauvre en protéines. Répartition anatomique de l'augmentation de poids réalisée par les deux acides aminés soufrés. *Bull. Soc. Chim. Biol.*, 32: 657–71.

ASCHKENASY, A. and BENHAMOU, J. P. (1952). Recherches sur l'existence d'un relais thyroïdien ou testiculaire dans la croissance de rats normaux, thyroïdectomisés ou castrés. *Ann. Endocrinol.*, 13: 143–63.

ASCHKENASY, A. and BLANPIN, O. (1959). Influence de la teneur du régime en graisses sur l'anémie et l'hémolyse ainsi que sur les taux des protéines, du cholestérol et des phospholipides sériques chez des rats carencés en protéines. *Sang*, 30: 574–82.

ASCHKENASY, A., BLANPIN, O. and COQUELET, M. L. (1959). Étude des protéines et lipides stromatiques et de l'hémoglobine chez des rats carencés en protéines. *Sang*, 30: 566–73.

ASCHKENASY, A., DELMONTE, L. and EYQUEM, A. (1956a). Mise en évidence d'une hémolyse anormale dans la carence expérimentale en protéines. *C.R. Soc. Biol.*, 150: 474–6.

ASCHKENASY, A., DELMONTE, L., GUÉRIN, R. and GUÉRIN, M. T. (1956b). Réduction de la survie des globules rouges chez des rats carencés en protéines, démontrée par le marquage au Cr^{51}. *C.R. Acad. Sc.*, 242: 2174–6.

ASCHKENASY, A. and DRAY, F. (1953). Action de la thyroxine, des hormones corti-cotrope et somatotrope et des hormones génitales sur la régénération sanguine après inanition protéique. *C.R. Soc. Biol.*, 147: 1781–5; (1954). *Sang*, 25: 461–89.

ASCHKENASY, A., GAJDOS-TÖRÖK, M., SPACH, C. and GAJDOS, A. (1969). Effets de la privation de protéines alimentaires sur les teneurs érythrocytaires en ATP chez le rat. *C.R. Soc. Biol.*, 163: 1275–9.

ASCHKENASY, A. and JOBARD, P. (1961). Répartition tissulaire des granulocytes éosino-philes chez le rat rendu éosinopénique par une carence prolongée en protéines. *Nouv. Rev. Fr. d'Hématol.*, 1: 202–12.

ASCHKENASY, A., NATAF, B., PIETTE, C. and SFEZ, M. (1962). Le fonctionnement thyroïd-ien chez le rat carencé en protéines. *Ann. Endocrinol.*, 23: 311–32.

ASCHKENASY, A. and PARIENTE, PH. (1951). Comparaison des actions anabolisante set hématopoïétiques de la vitamine B_{12}, de la méthionine et d'un extrait hépatique anti-pernicieux sur la réparation de l'inanition protéique. *Rev. Hématol.*, 6: 166–83.

ASCHKENASY, A. and PARIENTE, PH. (1953). Recherches sur la régulation hormonale de l'utilisation hématopoïétique des protéines. *Acta Haematol.*, 9: 29–46.

ASCHKENASY, A., ROLLAND, G. J. and POLONOVSKI, C. (1948). Action de la méthionine sur l'anemie sulfamidique du rat. *Sang*, 19: 675–83.

ASCHKENASY, A. and PUYO, G. (1952). Effet aggravant de la thyroïdectomie sur l'anémie hypoprotidique du rat. Neutralisation de cet effet par des injections de vitamine B_{12}. *C.R. Soc. Biol.*, 146: 352–4.

ASCHKENASY, A. and WOLFF, R. (1963). Teneurs du foie et des reins en vitamine B_{12} et excrétion urinaire de cette vitamine chez des rats carencés en certains acides aminés essentiels (acides aminés soufrés ou phénoliques, lysine, tryptophane, histidine). *C.R. Soc. Biol.*, 157: 1746–50.

BÉNARD, H., GAJDOS, A., GAJDOS-TÖRÖK, M. and POLONOVSKI, M. (1948). Étude de l'action sur l'érythropoïèse, de la méthionine et de deux de ses dérivés d'oxydation. *Sang*, 19: 264–8.

BENDITT, E. D., HUMPHREYS, E. M., STRAUBE, R. L., WISSLER, R. W. and STEFFEE, C. H. (1947). Studies on amino acids utilization. II. Essential amino acids as a source of plasma proteins and erythrocytes in the hypoproteinemic rat. *J. Nutr.*, 33: 85–94.

BENDITT, E. P., STRAUBE, R. L. and HUMPHREYS, E. M. (1946). The determination of total circulating serum protein and erythrocyte volumes in normal and protein-depleted rats. *Proc. Soc. Exp. Biol. Med.*, 62: 189–92.

BENDITT, E. P., WISSLER, R. W., WOOLRIDGE, R. L., ROWLEY, D. A. and STEFFEE, C. H. (1949). Loss of body protein and antibody production by rats on low-protein diets. *Proc. Soc. Exp. Biol. Med.*, 70: 240–3.

BERNING, H. (1947). Die Eiweissmangelanämie. *Klin. Wchsch.*, 24/5: 585–90.

BETHARD, W. F., WISSLER, R. W., THOMPSON, J. S., SCHROEDER, M. A. and ROBSON, M. J. (1958a). The effects of acute protein depletion on the distribution of radio-iron in rat tissues. *Blood*, 13: 146–55.

BETHARD, W. F., WISSLER, R. W., THOMPSON, J. S., SCHROEDER, M. A. and ROBSON, M. J. (1958b). The effect of acute protein deprivation upon erythropoiesis in rats. *Blood*, 13: 216–25.

BETHELL, F. H., BLECHA, E. and VAN SANT, J. H. (1943). Nutritional inadequacies in pregnancy correlated with the incidence of anemia. *J. Amer. Diet. Ass.*, **19**: 165–72.

BEVAN, W. JR., LEWIS, G. T., BLOOM, W. L. and ABESS, A. T. (1950). Spontaneous activity in rats fed on amino acid-deficient diet. *Amer. J. Physiol.*, **163**: 104–10.

BISIANI, M. (1965). Influenza della dieta A-proteica su alcune attivita enzimatiche degli eritrociti dell'animale. *Haematol. Arch.*, **50**: 12 suppl., 1351–60.

BLANPIN, O. and ASCHKENASY, A. (1959). Action du propionate de testostérone sur les protéines sériques ainsi que sur le cholestérol et les phospholipides sériques et érythrocytaires chez des rats carencés en protéines. Rapports avec l'évolution de l'anémie et de l'hémolyse. *C.R. Soc. Biol.*, **153**: 997–9.

BOISSIER, J. and ASCHKENASY, A. (1950). Effets comparés de l'administration de glycocolle, de thiamine et de méthionine sur les organes des rats privés de protéines alimentaires. II. Comparaison de la richesse des organes en azote. *Bull. Soc. Chim. Biol.*, **32**: 942–6.

BORCHERS, J. (1961). Counteraction of the growth depression of raw soybean oil meal by amino-acid supplements in weanling rats. *J. Nutr.*, **75**: 330–4.

BOURGEAT, J. and ASCHKENASY, A. (1948). Efficacité comparée de la caséine et de ses acides aminés constitutifs pour la restauration physiologique du rat blanc protéiprive: Hématopoïèse. *C.R. Acad. Sc.*, **226**: 962–4.

BOWLES, L. L., HALL, W. K. and SYDENSTRICKER, V. P. (1949). Blood changes in the rat with acute deficiency of amino acids. *Anat. Rec.*, **103**: 113 (Abstr.).

BUECHLER, E. and GUGGENHEIM, K. (1949). The effect of quantitative and qualitative protein deficiency on blood regeneration. II. Hemoglobin. *Blood*, **4**: 964–9.

CANNON, P. R., CHASE, W. E. and WISSLER, R. W. (1943). The relationship of the protein-reserves to antibody-production. I. The effects of a low-protein diet and of plasmapheresis upon the formation of agglutinins. *J. Immunol.*, **47**: 133–47.

CARTWRIGHT, G. E. (1947). Dietary factors concerned in erythropoiesis. *Blood*, **2**: 111–53; 256–98.

CARTWRIGHT, G. E., TATTING, B. and WINTROBE, M. M. (1948). Niacin deficiency anemia in swine. *Arch. Biochem.*, **19**: 109–18.

CARTWRIGHT, G. E. and WINTROBE, M. M. (1948). Studies on free erythrocyte protoporphyrin, plasma copper, and plasma iron in protein-deficient and iron-deficient swine. *J. biol. Chem.*, **176**: 571–83.

CHANDRAN, K. and DAMODARAN, M. (1951). Amino acids and proteins in hemoglobin formation. II. Isoleucine. *Biochem. J.*, **49**: 393–8.

CHITRE, R. G. and VALLURY, S. M. (1956). Studies on protein value of cereals and pulses; effect of feeding on growth blood heemoglobin and plasma protein in young rats. *Indian J. Med. Res.*, **44**: 555–63.

COCKBURN, F., SHERMAN, J. D., INGALL, D. and KLEIN, R. (1965). Effect of phenylalanine deficient diet on bone marrow and amino acid metabolism. *Proc. Soc. Exp. Biol. Med.*, **118**: 238–45.

CRAFTS, R. C. and MEINEKE, H. A. (1959). The anemia of hypophysectomized animals. *Ann. N.Y. Acad. Sc.*, **77**: 501–17.

DAFT, F. S. and SEBRELL, W. H. (1943). The successful treatment of granulocytopenia and leukopenia in rats with crystalline folic acid. *Pub. Health. Rep.*, **58**: 1542; (1945). Sulfonamides and vitamine deficiencies. *Vitamins and Hormones*, **3**: 49–72.

DELMONTE, L., ASCHKENASY, A. and EYQUEM, A. (1964). Studies on the hemolytic nature of protein-deficiency anemia in the rat. *Blood*, **24**: 49–68.

DELMONTE, L., EYQUEM, A. and ASCHKENASY, A. (1962). Recherches sur le comportement immunologique du rat carencé en protéines. *Ann. Inst. Pasteur*, **102**: 420–36.

DEO, M. G. and RAMALINGASWAMI, V. (1964). Absorption of Co[58] labeled cyanocobalamin in protein deficiency. An experimental study in the rhesus monkey. *Gastroenterology*, **46**: 167–74.

316   *Hematopoietic Agents*

DINNING, J. S., NEATROUR, R. and DAY, P. L. (1954). Interrelationship of pantothenic acid and methionine in lymphocyte production by rats. *J. Nutr.*, **43**: 557–62.

DINNING, J. S., NEATROUR, R. and DAY, P. L. (1955). A biochemical basis for the inter-relationship of pantothenic acid and methionine. *J. Nutr.*, **56**: 430–5.

DINNING, J. S., PAYNE, L. D. and DAY, P. L. (1950). The requirements of rats for methyl groups and vitamin B_{12} in the production of leucocytes. *Arch. Biochem.*, **27**: 467–9.

DINNING, J. S. and YOUNG, (1960). Some effects of folic and vitamin B_{12} on nucleic acid metabolism in lactobacillus leichmannii. *J. biol. Chem.*, **235**: 3008–10.

DRABKIN, D. L. (1951). Metabolism of hemin chromoproteins. *Physiol. Rev.*, **31**: 345–431.

FITCH, C. D., HARVILLE, W. E., DINNING, J. S. and PORTER, F. S. (1964). Iron deficiency in monkeys fed diets containing soybean protein. *Proc. Soc. Exp. Biol. Med.*, **116**: 130–3.

FONTÈS, G. and THIVOLLE, L. (1930). Recherches expérimentales sur les processus chimiques de l'hématopoïèse et sur la pathogénie des anémies. *Sang*, **4**: 658–730.

FRASER, M. J. and HOLDSWORTH, E. S. (1959). Vitamin B_{12} and biosynthesis in chick liver. *Nature*, **183**: 519–23.

FULLER, A. T., NEUBERGER, A. and WEBSTER, T. A. (1947). Histidine deficiency in the rat and its effect on the carnosine and anserine content of muscle. *Biochem. J.*, **41**: 11–19.

GAJDOS, A. (1947). L'action de la méthionine sur l'érythropoïèse chez le rat. *Sang*, **18**: 114–21.

GAJDOS-TÖRÖK, M., SPACH, C., GAJDOS, A. and ASCHKENASY, A. (1969). Effets de régimes dépourvus de certains acides aminés sur l'ATP érythrocytaire chez des rats préablement carencés en protéines. *C.R. Soc. Biol.*, **163**: 1317–20.

GILLESPIE, M., NEUBERGER, A. and WEBSTER, T. A. (1945). Further studies on lysine deficiency in rats. *Biochem. J.*, **39**: 203–8.

GINGRAS, R. (1953). Contribution à l'étude du métabolisme de quelques acides aminés. *Leval méd.*, **18**: 727–44.

GLYNN, L. E., HIMSWORTH, H. P. and NEUBERGER, A. (1945). Pathological states due to deficiency of the sulphur-containing amino-acids. *Brit. J. Exp. Path.*, **26**: 326–37.

GONTZEA, I., SUTZESCO, P., COCORA, D. and LUNGU, D. (1964). Importance de l'apport de protéines sur la résistance de l'organisme à l'intoxication par le plomb. *Arch. Sc. Physiol.*, **18**: 211–24.

GÓTH, A., LENGYEL, L., BENCZE, E., SÁVELY, C. and MAJSAY, A. (1955). The role of amino-acids in inducing hormone secretion. *Experientia*, **11**: 27–9.

GRAY, I. (1964). Effect of protein nutrition on leukocyte mobilization. *Proc. Soc. Exp. Biol. Med.*, **116**: 414–6.

GROMOVA, E. G. (1963). Functional state of the pituitary-adrenal system in the process of digestion. *Bjull. Eksp. Biol. Med.*, **55**: 21–5.

GUEST, G. R., FRIEDMAN, S., WOODS, D. D. and SMITH, E. L. (1962). A methyl analogue of cobamide coenzyme in relation to methionine synthesis by bacteria. *Nature*, **195**: 340–2.

GUGGENHEIM, K. (1964). The role of zinc, copper and calcium in the etiology of the "Meat Anemia". *Blood*, **23**: 786–94.

GUGGENHEIM, K. and BUECHLER, E. (1948). Nutrition and resistance to infection. The effect of quantitative and qualitative protein deficiency on the bactericidal properties and phagocytic activity of the peritoneal fluid of rats. *J. Immunol.*, **58**: 133–9.

GUGGENHEIM, K. and BUECHLER, E. (1949). The effect of quantitative and qualitative protein deficiency on blood regeneration. I. White blood cells. *Blood*, **4**: 958–63.

HAHN, P. F. and WHIPPLE, G. H. (1939). Hemoglobin production in anemia limited by low protein intake. Influence of iron intake, protein supplements and fasting. *J. Exp. Med.*, **69**: 315–26.

HALLGREN, B. (1954). Haemoglobin formation and storage iron in protein deficiency. *Acta Soc. Med. Upsal.*, **59**: 79–208.

HALVORSEN, S. (1961). Plasma erythropoietin levels following hypothalamic stimulation in the rabbit. *J. clin. lab. Invest.*, **13**: 564–75.

HARRIS, H. A., NEUBERGER, A. and SANGER, F. (1943). Lysine deficiency in young rats. *Biochem. J.*, **37**: 508–13.

HARRIS, J. W. and HORRIGAN, D. L. (1964). Pyridoxine-responsive anemia-prototype and variations on the theme. *Vitamins and Hormones*, **22**: 722–53.

HIGGINSON, J., GRADY, H. and HUNTLEY, C. (1963). The effects of different diets on iron absorption. *Lab. Invest.*, **12**: 1260–9.

HUTNER, S. H., NATHAN, H. A. and BAKER, H. (1959). Metabolism of folic acid and other pterin-pteridine. *Vitamins and Hormones*, **17**: 2–52.

INGLE, D. J., PRESTRUD, M. C. and NEZAMIS, J. E. (1948). Effect of adrenalectomy on level of blood amino acids in the eviscerated rat. *Proc. Soc. Exp. Biol. Med.*, **67**: 321–2.

ITO, K. and REISSMANN, K. R. (1966). Quantitative and qualitative aspects of steady state erythropoiesis induced in protein-starved rats by long-term erythropoietin injection. *Blood*, **27**: 343–51.

ITO, K., SCHMAUS, J. W. and REISSMANN, K. R. (1964). Protein metabolism and erythropoiesis. III. The erythroid marrow in protein-starved rats and its response is erythropoietin. *Acta Haematol.*, **32**: 257–64.

JACOBSON, L. O., GOLDWASSER, E., GURNEY, C. W., FRIED, W. and PLZAK, L. (1959). Studies of erythropoïetin: the hormone regulating red cell production. *Ann. N.Y Acad. Sc.*, **77**: 551–73.

KARLIN, R., CREYSSEL, R., CREYSSEL, H. and CROIZAT, P. (1965). Teneur du sérum sanguin en méthionine et en vitamine B_{12} au cours de l'anémie de Biermer. *Nouv. Rev. Fr. d'Hématol.*, **5**: 721–8.

KHO, L. K., ODANG, O., THAJEB, S. and MARKUM, A. H. (1962). Erythroblastopenia (pure red cell aplasia) in childhood in Djakarta. *Blood*, **19**: 168–80.

KLAVINS, J. V. and JOHANSEN, P. V. (1965). Pathology of amino acid excess. IV. Effects and interactions of excessive amounts of dietary methionine, homocystine, and serine. *Arch. Path.*, **79**: 600–14.

KLAVINS, J. V., KINNEY, T. P. and KAUFMAN, N. (1962). The influence of dietary protein on iron absorption. *Brit. J. Exp. Path.*, **43**: 172–80.

KORNBERG, A. (1946). Amino acids in the production of granulocytes in rats. *J. biol. Chem.*, **164**: 203–12.

KRAUSE, R. L. and SOKOLOFF, L. (1965). Thyroxin stimulation of amino acid incorporation into protein chains of hemoglobin *in vitro*. *Bioch. Biophys. Acta*, **108**: 165–8.

KROE, D., KINNEY, TH. D., KAUFMAN, N. and KLAVINS, J. V. (1963). The influence of amino acids on iron absorption. *Blood*, **21**: 546–52.

LAYANI, F., ASCHKENASY, A., LEGRAIN, M. and MALVEZIN, J. (1949). Guérison d'une anémie hypochrome protéiprive par des extraits hépatiques antipernicieux et par la méthionine. *Bull. Mém. Soc. Méd. Hôp. Paris*, **65**: 734–9.

LEAF, G. and NEUBERGER, A. (1947). The effect of diet on the glutathione content of the liver. *Biochem. J.*, **41**: 280–7.

LEATHEM, J. H. (1957). The adrenal and dietary protein. *Arch. Int. Pharm. Thér.*, **110**: 103–13.

LEATHEM, J. H. (1958). Hormones and protein nutrition. *Rec. Progress in Horm. Research*, **14**: 141–76.

LI, T. W. and FREEMAN, S. (1947). The effect of methionine on protein-deficient rats exposed to benzene. *Amer. J. Physiol.*, **148**: 358–64.

LINMAN, J. W. and PIERRE, R. V. (1964). The effect of hyperbaric hyperoxia on erythropoiesis. *Abst. Xth Congr. Intern. Soc. Haematol.*, M: 14.

MADDEN, S. C. and WHIPPLE, G. H. (1940). Plasma proteins: their source, production and utilization. *Physiol. Rev.*, 20: 194–217.

MADDEN, S. C., KATTUS, A. A., CARTER, J. R., MILLER, L. L. and WHIPPLE, G. H. (1945). Plasma protein production as influenced by parenteral protein digests, very high protein feeding, and red blood cell catabolism. *J. Exp. Med.*, 82: 181–91.

MARIANI, A. and MIGLIACCIO, P. A. (1964). Influenza della deplezione proteica sulla sopravvivenza eritrocitaria. *Quad. Nutrizione*, 24: 89–98.

MAUN, M. E., CAHILL, W. M. and DAVIS, R. M. (1945a). Morphologic studies of rats deprived of essential amino-acids. I. Phenylalanine. *Arch. Path.*, 39: 294–300.

MAUN, M. E., CAHILL, W. M. and DAVIS, R. M. (1945b). Morphologic studies of rats deprived of essential amino-acids. II. Leucine. *Arch. Path.*, 40: 173 8.

MAUN, M. E., CAHILL, W. M. and DAVIS, R. M. (1946). Morphologic studies of rats deprived of essential amino-acids. III. Histidine. *Arch. Path.*, 41: 25–31.

MEHTA, G. and GOPALAN, C. (1956). Haematological changes in nutritional oedema syndrome (Kwashiorkor). *Ind. J. Med. Res.*, 44: 727–36.

METCOFF, J., DARLING, B., SCANLON, M. H. and STARE, F. J. (1948). Nutritional status and infection response. I. Electrophoretic circulating plasma protein, hematologic, hematopoietic and immunologic responses to Salmonella typhimurium infection in the protein-deficient rat. *J. lab. clin. Med.*, 33: 47–66.

METCOFF, J., FAVOUR, C. B. and STARE, F. J. (1945). Plasma protein and hemoglobin in the protein-deficient rat. *J. clin. Invest.*, 24: 82–91.

MICKELSEN, O. (1956). Intestinal synthesis of vitamins in the nonruminant. *Vitamins Hormones*, 14: 1–95.

MILLS, C. A. and COTTINGHAM, E. (1943). Phagocytic activity as affected by protein intake in heat and cold. *J. Immunol.*, 47: 503–4.

MOORE, T. B. and WILSON, J. E. (1957). Histidine as an essential nutrient for the adult rat. *J. Nutr.*, 62: 357–65.

MOORE, T., SHARMAN, J. M., CONSTABLE, B. J., SYMONDS, K. R., MARTIN, P. E. N. and COLLINSON, E. (1962). Meat diets: effect of supplements of calcium and ferrous carbonates on rats fed meat. *J. Nutr.*, 77: 415–27.

MUNRO, H. N., STEELE, M. H. and HUTCHINSON, W. C. (1963). Blood corticosterone levels in the rat after administration of amino-acids. *Nature*, 199: 1182–3.

NAETS, J. P. and WITTEK, M. (1964). Étude du mécanisme d'action des androgènes sur l'érythropoièse. *C.R. Acad. Sc.*, 259: 3371–4.

NASSET, E. S. and GATEWOOD, V. H. (1954). Nitrogen balance and hemoglobin of adult rats fed amino acid diets low in L- and D-histidine. *J. Nutr.*, 53: 163–76.

NIZET, A. (1955). Erythropoïèse et métabolisme protéique. Rapport à la 23e Réun. de l'Assoc. Physiol. de langue franç. *J. de Physiol. (Paris)*, 47: 7–60.

NIZET, A. and ROBSCHEIT-ROBBINS, F. S. (1950). Reticulocyte ripening in experimental anemia and hypoproteinemia. Effect of amino acids *in vitro*. *Blood*, 5: 648–59.

OKUDA, K. and CHOW, B. F. (1961). The thyroid and absorption of vitamin B_{12} in rats. *Endocrinology*, 68: 607–15.

ORTEN, J. M., BOURQUE, J. E. and ORTEN, A. U. (1945). Inability of human or beef globin to support normal hematopoiesis in the rat without added isoleucine. *J. biol. Chem.*, 160: 435–40.

ORTEN, A. U. and ORTEN, J. M. (1943). The rôle of dietary protein in hemoglobin formation. *J. Nutr.*, 26: 21–31.

ORTEN, J. M. and ORTEN, A. U. (1945). The production of polycythemia by cobalt in rats made anemic by a diet low in protein. *Amer. J. Physiol.*, 144: 464–7.

ORTEN, J. M. and ORTEN, A. U. (1946). The comparative value of certain dietary proteins for hemopoiesis in the rat. *J. Nutr.*, 31: 765–75.

PATT, H. M., SMITH, D. E. and JACKSON, E. (1950). Effect of cysteine on peripheral blood of the irradiated rat. *Blood*, 5: 758–63.

PEARSON, P. B., ELVEHJEM, C. A. and HART, E. B. (1937). The relation of protein to hemoglobin building. *J. biol. Chem.*, 119: 749–63.

PIHA, R. S. (1954). The effect of repeated bleedings on free amino acids in rabbit plasma and red cells. *Acta Physiol. Scand.*, 31: suppl. 114, *Abstr. VIIth Scand. Physiol. Congress*, 46–7.

POLLACK, S., BALCERZAK, S. P. and CROSBY, W. H. (1963). Transferrin and the absorption of iron. *Blood*, 21: 33–8.

PRICE, J. M. (1958). *Univ. Mich. Med. Bull.*, 24: 461–85; cited by HARRIS and HORRIGAN (1964).

RAMALINGASWAMI, V., VICKERY, A. L. JR., STANBURY, J. B. and HEGSTED, D. M. (1965). Some effects of protein deficiency on the rat thyroid. *Endocrinology*, 77: 87–95.

REISERT, P. and HUNSTEIN, W. (1963). Die Wirkung anaboler Steroide auf die proteinoprive Anämie der Ratte. *Klin. Wchsch.*, 41: 339.

REISSMANN, K. R. (1964a). Protein metabolism and erythropoiesis. I. The anemia of protein deprivation. *Blood*, 23: 137–45.

REISSMANN, K. R. (1964b). Protein metabolism and erythropoiesis. II. Erythropoietin formation and erythroid responsiveness in protein-deprived rats. *Blood*, 23: 146–53.

RIGÓ, J., TAKÁCS, F. and SÓS, J. (1959). Die Wirkung von Tryptophan auf die Leukozytenzahl. *Acta Physiol. Hung.*, 15: 83–8.

ROBSCHEIT-ROBBINS, F. S., MILLER, L. L. and WHIPPLE, G. H. (1943). Hemoglobin and plasma protein. Simultaneous production during continued bleeding as influenced by amino-acids, plasma, hemoglobin and digests of serum, hemoglobin and casein. *J. Exp. Med.*, 77: 375–96.

ROBSCHEIT-ROBBINS, F. S., MILLER, L. L. and WHIPPLE, G. H. (1945). Maximal hemoglobin and plasma protein production under the stimulus of depletion. *J. Exp. Med.*, 82: 311–6.

ROBSCHEIT-ROBBINS, F. S. and WHIPPLE, G. H. (1937). Globin utilization by the anemic dog to form new hemoglobin. *J. Exp. Med.*, 66: 565–78.

ROBSCHEIT-ROBBINS, F. S. and WHIPPLE, G. H. (1949). Dietary effects on anemia plus hypoproteinemia in dogs. I. Some proteins further the production of hemoglobin and others plasma protein production. *J. Exp. Med.*, 89: 339–58.

ROSE, W. C., OESTERLING, M. J. and WOMACK, M. (1948). Comparative growth on diets containing ten and nineteen amino-acids, with further observations upon the rôle of glutamic and aspartic acids. *J. biol. Chem.*, 176: 753–62.

ROSENTHAL, R. L., GOLDSCHMIDT, L. and PICKERING, B. J. (1951). Hematologic changes in rats protected by cysteine against total body X-irradiation. *Amer. J. Physiol.*, 166: 15–9.

SABRY, Z. I., CHENEY, M. C., MILNE, H., FOLEY, A., GERRIE, E. A., YEUNG, D. L. and BEATON, G. H. (1965). Effect of dietary protein on erythrocyte and hepatic transaminases. *Fed. Proc.*, 24: 499.

SANCHEZ DE JIMENEZ, E., TORRES, J., VALLES, V. E., SOLIS, J. and SOBERON, G. (1965a). Studies on the oxidation-reduction systems of the erythrocyte. *Biochem. J.*, 97: 887–91.

SANCHEZ DE JIMENEZ, E., VALLES, V. E., DE LA PAZ DE LEON, M. and SOBERON, G. (1965). Active transport and enzymes of the erythrocyte membrane under protein deprivation. *Biochem. J.*, 97: 892–6.

SANCHEZ-MEDAL, L., LABARDINI, J. and LORIA, A. (1963). Hemolysis and erythropoiesis. I. Influence of intraperitoneal administration of whole hemolysates on the recovery of bled dogs, as measured by changes in the total erythrocytic volume. *Blood*, 21: 586–93.

320   *Hematopoietic Agents*

SCHAEFER, A. E., KNOWLES, J. L. and SALMON, W. D. (1951). Influence of vitamin B_{12} and folacin on synthesis of choline and methionine by the rat *in vivo* and *in vitro*. *Fed. Proc.*, 10: 393.

SCHULMAN, M. P. and RICHERT, D. A. (1957). Heme synthesis in vitamin B_6 and pantothenic acid deficiencies. *J. biol. Chem.*, 226: 181–9.

SCOTT, E. B. (1954). Histopathology of amino acid deficiencies. III. Histidine. *Arch. Path.*, 58: 129–41.

SCOTT, E. B. (1955). Histopathology of amino acid deficiencies. *Amer. J. Path.*, 31: 1111–29.

SCOTT, E. B. (1956). Histopathology of amino acid deficiencies. V. Isoleucine. *Proc. Soc. Exp. Biol. Med.*, 92: 134–40.

SCOTT, E. B. (1964). Histopathology of amino acid deficiencies. VII. Valine. *Exp. Molecular Pathol.*, 3: 610–21.

SCOTT, E. B. and SCHWARTZ, C. (1953). Histopathology of amino acid deficiencies. II. Threonine. *Proc. Soc. Exp. Biol. Med.*, 84: 271–6.

SCOTT, E. B., SCHWARTZ, C. and FERGUSON, R. (1950). Some effects of phenylalanine and tyrosine deficient diets on the rat. *Anat. Rec.* 108: 528.

SEBRELL, W. H. JR. and McDANIEL, E. G. (1952). Amino acids in the production of blood constituents in rats. *J. Nutr.*, 47: 477–86.

SHEHATA, O. and JOHNSON, B. C. (1948). Protein level and pteroylglutamic acid intake on growth rate and hemoglobin level in rat. *Proc. Soc. Exp. Biol. Med.*, 67: 332–5.

SHEMIN, D. (1954/5). The biosynthesis of porphyrins. *The Harvey Lectures*, 50: 258–84.

SHEMIN, D. and RITTENBERG, D. (1945). The utilization of glycine for the synthesis of porphyrin. *J. biol. Chem.*, 159: 567–8.

SIDRANSKY, H. and VERNEY, E. (1965). Chemical pathology of acute amino acid deficiencies. 8. Influence of amino acid intake on the morphologic and biochemical changes in young rats force-fed a threonine-devoid diet. *J. Nutr.*, 86: 73–81.

SOOD, S. K., DEO, M. G. and RAMALINGASWAMI, V. (1965). Anemia in experimental protein deficiency in the Rhesus monkey with special reference to iron metabolism. *Blood*, 26: 421–32.

SPACH, C. and ASCHKENASY, A. (1969). Teneurs plasmatiques et érythrocytaires en eau, en sodium, potassium et magnésium chez des rats carencés en protéines et des rats restaurés aprés cette carence. *C.R. Soc. Biol.*, 163: 834–8.

SPACH, C. and ASCHKENASY, A. (1970). Effets de la privation alimentaire de certains acides aminés essentiels sur les électrolytes et plasmatiques chez le Rat. I. Teneurs en eau, en sodium, potassium et magnésium des érythrocytes. *C.R. Soc. Biol.* (in press).

SREBNIK, H. H., EVANS, E. S. and ROSENBERG, L. L. (1963). Thyroid function in female rats maintained on a protein-free diet. *Endocrinology*, 73: 267–70.

SREBNIK, H. H., NELSON, M. M. and SIMPSON, M. E. (1959). Reduced growth hormone content in anterior pituitaries of rats on protein-free diets. *Proc. Soc. Exp. Biol. Med.*, 101: 97–9.

SWENDSEID, M. E., BURTON, I. F. and BETHELL, F. H. (1943). Excretion of keto-acids and hydroxyphenyl compounds in pernicious anemia. *Proc. Soc. Exp. Biol. Med.*, 52: 202–3.

TASKER, P. K., JOSEPH, K., RAO, D. R., RAO, M. N., INDIRAMMA, K., SWAMINATHAN, M., SREENIVASAN, A. and SUBRAHMANYAN, V. (1963). Effect of feeding groundnut protein fortified with limiting essential amino-acids on growth and composition of liver, blood, carcass and certain liver enzymes in albino rats. *Ann. Biochem. Exp. Med.*, 23: 279–84.

VARTIAINEN, I. and APAJALAHTI, J. (1953). Effect of ingested protein and tyrosine on circulating eosinophils. *J. Clin. Endoctrinol.*, 13: 1502–6.

VENTURA, S. (1953). La transferrina. *Haematologica Arch.*, **37**: 749–54.

WAGLE, S. R., MEHTA, R. and JOHNSON, B. C. (1958). Vitamin B_{12} and protein biosynthesis. VI. Relation of vitamin B_{12} to amino acid activation. *J. biol. Chem.*, **233**: 619–24.

WATERS, A. H. and MOLLIN, D. L. (1963). Observations on the metabolism of folic acid in pernicious anemia. *Brit. J. Haemat.*, **9**: 319–27.

WEECH, A. A., WOLLSTEIN, M. and GOETTSCH, E. (1937). Nutritional edema in dog; development of deficits in erythrocytes and hemoglobin on diet deficient in protein. *J. clin. Invest.*, **16**: 719–28.

WEIMER, H. E. (1961). The effects of protein depletion and repletion on the concentration and distribution of serum proteins and protein-bound carbohydrates of the adult rat. *Ann. N.Y. Acad. Sc.*, **94**: 225–49.

WEISBERGER, A. S. and HEINLE, R. W. (1950). Protective effect of cystine on leucopenia induced by nitrogen mustard. *J. lab. clin. Med.*, **36**: 872–6.

WHIPPLE, G. H. and ROBSCHEIT-ROBBINS, F. S. (1940). Amino-acids and hemoglobin production in anemia. *J. exp. Med.*, **71**: 569–83.

WHIPPLE, G. H. and ROBSCHEIT-ROBBINS, F. S. (1951). Anemia plus hypoproteinemia in dogs. Various proteins in diet show various patterns in blood protein production. Beef muscle, egg, lactalbumin, fibrin, viscera and supplements. *J. exp. Med.*, **94**: 223–42.

WILLIAMS, A. M., CHOSY, J. J. and SCHILLING, R. F. (1963). Effect of vitamin B_{12} *in vitro* on incorporation of nucleic acid precursors by pernicious anemia bone marrow. *J. clin. Invest.*, **42**: 670–4.

WISSLER, R. W. (1947). The effects of protein depletion and subsequent immunization upon the response of animals to pneumococcal infection. 1. Experiments with rabbits. *J. Inf. Dis.*, **80**: 250–63.

WRIGHT, L. D., SKEGGS, H. R. and SPRAGUE, K. L. (1945). Effect of feeding succinylsulfathiazole to rats receiving purified diets high in carbohydrate, protein, fat or protein and fat. *J. Nutr.*, **29**: 431–9.

YESHODA, K. M. and DAMODARAN, M. (1947). Aminoacids and proteins in hemoglobin formation. I. Tryptophan. *Biochem. J.*, **41**: 382–8.

YOFFEY, J. M. (1964). Further problems of lymphocyte production. *Ann. N.Y. Acad. Sc.*, **113**: 867–86.

YUILE, C. L. (1949). Hemoglobin synthesis and turnover in dogs measured with radioactive lysine. *Science*, **110**: 441.

CHAPTER 6

DRUG TREATMENT OF CHRONIC
BONE-MARROW FAILURE

Bernard Dreyfus, Claude Sultan, and Henri Rochant

Unité de Recherche sur les Anemies (I.N.S.E.R.M.),
UER de Creteil 94, France

CHRONIC bone-marrow failure is defined as a persistent reduction, of a moderate or severe nature, in the formation of the three types of myeloid cells (erythrocytic, granulocytic, thrombocytic).

1. PANCYTOPENIA FROM CHRONIC
BONE-MARROW APLASIA

The clinical signs correspond with the decrease of the three cell-types. The symptoms associated with anemia depend on its severity and on the age of the patient. The level of granulopenia determines the incidence and severity of infections. Thrombopenia is responsible for cutaneous, mucosal, or visceral bleeding which is often difficult to control. On examination there is neither adenopathy nor enlargement of liver or spleen. The anemia is normocytic or macrocytic. The reticulocyte count is very low, seldom exceeding 10 or 15 thousand per mm^3. There are cases in which the percentage of reticulocytes is slightly raised, but the absolute number is still low. Some workers maintain that anisocytosis and even poikilocytosis are common, and schistocytes may be found (Lewis, 1962, 1965).

Electrophoresis and studies of resistance of hemoglobin to alkali denaturation show an increase in the amount of alkali-resistant hemoglobin to some 3–5% (Shahidi *et al.*, 1962).

Neutropenia is pronounced. The granulocyte count is generally below 2000 per mm^3. More than one third of cases show anomalies of the neutrophils, of which the cytoplasm contains evenly distributed granules, stained dark red (Lewis, 1965).

The platelet count is below 100,000 per mm^3; in most cases below 50,000.

The bone marrow is examined by taking several specimens from different sites, but the information is purely qualitative. The marrow is deficient, containing mainly lymphocytes and some plasma cells and macrophages, but very few cells of the three myeloid types. Sometimes the lymphocytes are so profuse as to suggest lymphoid leukemic infiltration (Waitz *et al.*, 1964). In a few cases, however, the marrow is normocellular, with a normal erythrocyte/granulocyte ratio; but no megakaryocytes are found.

No precise picture of the marrow cells can be obtained without a biopsy, which should be routine. It confirms the diagnosis and allows the efficacy of treatment to be assessed. The marrow is replaced by fatty cells. It contains few if any islets of active cells (Lewis, 1965; Najean *et al.*, 1965; Shahidi and Diamond, 1959). Perls staining may show an excess of iron in the reticulum cells and sometimes in the erythroblasts. The quantitative results of marrow biopsy are in general roughly equivalent to those of isotope studies of erythropoiesis in a stabilized patient (Najean and Bernard, 1964). *Isotope studies* with ^{59}Fe show the precise extent of medullary erythropoiesis (Harris, 1963; Movitt *et al.*, 1963; Najean *et al.*, 1963). The plasma iron is increased as a result of its reduced clearance. Uptake of iron by the red cells is reduced but within normal time limits. There is a moderate increase of iron storage, especially in the liver.

Some cases of chronic bone-marrow failure with pancytopenia show a characteristic marrow picture. The smears are highly cellular. The proportion of erythroblasts is increased, sometimes to 50% or more. The cytoplasm of these cells is rich in iron granules, which are often arranged as a ring around the nucleus. These hypersideroblastic anemias show a peculiar state of iron balance. Serum iron is raised, and siderophilin often saturated. Ineffective erythropoiesis has already been indicated by the contrast between the profusion of erythroblasts in the marrow and the scarcity of reticulocytes in the blood. Radio-iron studies show that iron clearance is increased. Labeled iron enters the marrow, but its uptake by the red cells is very reduced and retarded. Storage is greatly increased (Bernard *et al.*, 1963).

Classification of marrow failure

Aplastic anemias may arise at any age. Some are congenital; they are associated with other defects and form part of the Fanconi syndrome. They are an affliction of childhood, but they may appear in adolescents, and even in young adults. Chromosomal anomalies have been described (Bloom *et al.*, 1966). Others are acquired; numerous aetiologies are known.

Ionizing radiation; benzene and its derivatives; alkylating agents such as nitrogen mustards, ethylenimines, sulphoxylic esters, and epoxides; vegetable alkaloids such as colchicine and its derivatives, and the periwinkle alkaloids, vincaleucoblastine and vincristine; urethane; certain antibiotics such as actinomycin-D; antipurines, folic acid antagonists, and antipyrimidines—in general terms, all the antimitotic substances used against cancer regularly cause medullary aplasia if they are given long enough.

In certain subjects, the bone marrow is especially sensitive to drugs which most people would tolerate well in the same doses. These are chloramphenicol, sulfonamides, arsenicals, hydantoins, phenylbutazone, gold salts, and insecticides such as DDT. Many other substances have been blamed for causing medullary aplasia. Proof of their toxicity is often unobtainable.

When no cause can be found, the following have to be considered before a diagnosis of idiopathic marrow failure can be made.

The Marchiafava-Micheli syndrome occasionally presents as "idiopathic' marrow failure (Hartmann and Jenkins, 1965). A thymoma can similarly cause medullary aplasia with pancytopenia (Dreyfus *et al.*, 1962; Harvard, 1965; Roland, 1964).

Reversible marrow failure associated with pregnancy has been reported, at confinement or termination of the pregnancy (Wintrobe, 1962). Finally, medullary aplasia may arise during acute hepatitis (Levy *et al.*, 1965).

The course of the disease

This varies: some types are rapidly fatal, regardless of the treatment given. The cause of death is more often from hemorrhage than from infection. Of the 116 cases described by Najean *et al.* (1965), 61 survived for less than a year. Half of Lewis's (1965) patients died within 15 months of the onset of the illness. Histologically, the marrow in these cases shows a depleted architecture, with no foci of active cells, and fatty infiltration. The pancytopenia is severe, with a very low platelet count. In other cases, the disease is protracted beyond 15 months. The pancytopenia is less pronounced. Marrow biopsy and isotope studies show that erythropoiesis, while definitely reduced, is not abolished. Some of these idiopathic or toxic aplasias have recovered after a course of several months or even years (Dreyfus, 1959; Israëls and Wilkinson, 1961; Loeb *et al.*, 1953; Mohler and Leavell, 1958; Scott *et al.*, 1959). These recoveries have followed symptomatic treatment, alone or with corticosteroid therapy; there have been some after splenectomy. But failure is usual. The cure-rate in these treated does not exceed 3% (Wolff, 1957).

Differential diagnosis

Before the diagnosis of marrow failure is established certain other conditions have to be excluded by means of bone-marrow aspiration and biopsy.

These include: acute leukemia and myeloma; bony metastases of carcinoma and neuroblastoma; the malignant form of myelosclerosis, the hematological signs of which are pancytopenia without palpable enlargement of the spleen (Lewis and Szur, 1962); tuberculosis of the blood-forming organs; medullary histiocytosis, in which peripheral pancytopenia is accompanied by enlargement of liver, spleen, and lymph nodes, and by invasion of bone marrow by dystrophic histiocytes (Friedman and Steigbigel, 1965); splenomegaly is usual, reticulum cells are sometimes found in the blood, and marrow biopsy shows a characteristic picture (Schrek and Donnely, 1966).

Treatment of bone-marrow failure

(a) *Corticosteroids.* Corticotrophin and corticosteroids are known to have a stimulating effect on myelopoiesis (Wintrobe, 1950), and since their introduction these drugs have been used in various types of anemia and hemopathy (Loeb *et al.*, 1953, Wintrobe 1950). However, they have not improved prognosis of marrow failure.

It is true that Mohler and Leavell (1958) and Israëls and Wilkinson (1961) have reported remissions and even cures with doses of the order of 1 mg per kg of prednisone; but most authors have observed no useful effect (Dreyfus, 1959; Lewis, 1965; Najean *et al.*, 1965).

Any effect that prednisone may have seems to be due to its action on hemolysis, which it reduces, and not on marrow activity (Lewis, 1962). It also appears to lessen vascular fragility, which could be a reason for using it. The initial dose can be from 0.5 to 1 mg per kg daily. After a few weeks this can be reduced to a smaller, intermittent maintenance dosage.

(b) *Androgens.* Androgens have given promising results in the treatment of acquired and congenital medullary aplasia. MacGullagh and Jones (1942) have shown that androgen replacement therapy corrects the anemia of male hypogonadism. Kennedy and Gilbersten (1957) treated women in advanced stage of breast cancer with large doses of male hormones. In some cases, polycythemia with an increase of circulating hemoglobin appeared. This stimulating effect of androgens on erythropoiesis has been confirmed in animals (Fried *et al.*, 1964; Kennedy, 1962). In view of these findings, Shahidi and Diamond (1959) suggested treatment with a combination of large doses of androgens and moderate doses of steroids. The initial results were encouraging in both acquired and congenital forms, and a long series of cases (Shahidi and Diamond, 1962) seems to confirm the beneficial effect.

Opinions differ on this subject. Some workers have obtained good results (Kennedy, 1962; Bjorntorp *et al.*, 1965; Desposito *et al.*, 1964; Gardner and Pringle, 1961; Huguley, 1960; Kennedy and Gilbersten, 1957; Khall, 1962; Sanchez-Medal *et al.*, 1964; Seip, 1961; Seligmann, 1966), but others maintain that the treatment has no effect, suggesting spontaneous remissions (Lewis, 1965, Najean *et al.*, 1965, Seligmann, 1966).

From a recent survey (Seligmann, 1966), it appears that the authors who have reported no beneficial effect have used either fairly low doses or large doses for too short a time. When large doses have been given over a long period, good results have been achieved in 25–40% of cases.

Erythropoiesis can be stimulated with numerous hormone derivatives, provided that large doses are given. The compounds which have been given successfully are: *intramuscular administration* in adults of testosterone propionate (75–100 mg three times a week), stanolone (100 mg three times a week), testosterone oenanthate (400–800 mg weekly) and cyclopentyl testosterone propionate (200 mg weekly); *oral administration* of fluoxymesterone (20 mg daily), methyl testosterone (50 mg daily), and testosterone (given sublingually, 200 mg daily). But according to Dameshek (see Seligmann, 1966), the only active compound is oxymetholone, an anabolic agent with few side-effects. It is given in daily doses of 1–2 mg per kg. Oral administration is preferable in cases of thrombopenia to avoid the risk of hematoma formation.

Whichever drug is used, it is essential to give it for several months. In most cases showing a good response to treatment, remission was achieved after about six months. The criteria of remission are a hemoglobin level above 11 g per 100 ml, a neutrophil count of 3000 or more per mm^3, and a platelet count above 100,000 per mm^3.

These figures are not always reached, but the patients are stabilized and their marrow remains sufficiently active.

A. COURSE OF ACQUIRED APLASTIC ANEMIA UNDER TREATMENT

Several of the patients do not receive treatment at once and have had numerous transfusions and corticosteroids without effect. Before starting treatment a complete, hematological examination and marrow biopsy were carried out in all of 47 cases of marrow failure, of which 16 were idiopathic and 21 showed a toxic effect. Of the former, 4 (25%) showed good results, and of the total 25 (53%) showed good results.

There are acute, rapidly fatal cases in which for unknown reasons the treatment has insufficient time to succeed. In other cases the course is unaffected by treatment.

When hormone therapy is effective, the first sign is a reticulocytosis of 5–10% (Desposito *et al.*, 1965; Sanchez-Medal *et al.*, 1964; Shahadi and Diamond, 1961), frequently followed by a sufficient increase of hemoglobin for transfusions to be spread out or stopped. The above authors, and Bellanti and Pinkel (1961), and Bjorntorp *et al.* (1965), report intervals of 1–7 months before the appearance of reticulocytosis.

The increase of the granulocyte count runs parallel with that of hemoglobin, whereas the effect on erythropoiesis is prompt (Desposito *et al.*, Shahidi and Diamond, 1961).

The effect of treatment on platelet formation is less marked, and appears later, between the 5th and 17th months. However, even at the end of treatment the platelet count is seldom normal: figures around 100,000 per mm^3 are commonest.

Repeated marrow puncture and biopsy show progressive regeneration of hematopoietic foci. These seem to arise from the division of large cells that look like reticulum cells and are the earliest sign of a therapeutic effect. The first differentiated cell-types to be recognizable are of the erythroid series; in different cases they appear between the 1st and 4th months (Shahidi and Diamond, 1961). From this time the number of cellular foci increases, while the fat which has infiltrated the marrow recedes. The first megakaryocytes are not seen until much later.

This biological improvement is accompanied by obvious improvement of the clinical picture. Stopping the treatment can be considered when the hemoglobin level is between 12 and 14 g per 100 ml (Desposito *et al.*, 1964; Sanchez-Medal *et al.*, 1964; Shahidi and Diamond, 1961). The neutrophil and platelet counts are also satisfactory; and continued treatment does not improve the result already achieved.

All authors (Desposito *et al.*, 1964; Kennedy, 1962; Sanchez-Medal *et al.*, 1964; Shahidi and Diamond, 1961) have observed the same phenomenon when treatment is stopped—a slow fall of reticulocyte and hemoglobin levels for 2 months, followed by a spontaneous recovery towards the previous levels from the 3rd month. The neutrophils and platelets

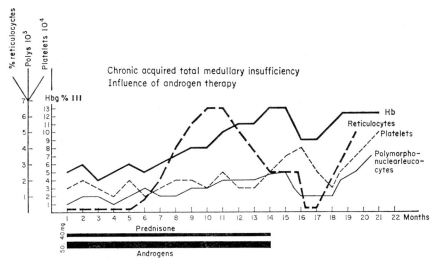

show a similar rebound. Shahidi and Diamond (1961) suggest that the duration of this rebound is proportional to the rapidity of recovery.

Changes in the serum iron are seen during treatment (Kennedy, 1962; Shahidi and Diamond, 1961). In patients who respond favourably, the serum iron falls and the siderophilin becomes less saturated. The reduced corpuscular hemoglobin concentration leads to hypochromia. In patients whose iron reserves have not been built up by previous transfusions, it may be necessary to give iron by mouth.

The free protoporphyrins in the red cells is increased, whereas the amount of coproporphyrin is little changed (Bjorntorp *et al.*, 1965). The amount of alkali-resistant hemoglobin decreases in patients who are recovering (Shahidi *et al.*, 1962).

M

B. EFFECT OF ANDROGENS ON CONGENITAL APLASTIC ANEMIA

The hematological findings before treatment are slightly different (Desposito *et al.*, 1964; Shahidi and Diamond, 1961). The anemia is clearly macrocytic, and the anisocytosis is more marked. The reticulocyte count is lower than in the acquired forms. The granulocyte count is not so low, but there are the same cytoplasmic anomalies (Lewis, 1965). Marrow biopsy shows a few remaining centres of erythropoiesis (Shahidi and Diamond, 1961).

The proportion of patients responding to treatment appears to be higher than with acquired marrow failure. Androgens were given to 11 patients. In 7 cases the treatment was beneficial provided that a maintenance dosage was kept up. The general course is much the same as that of acquired aplastic anemias. The platelets are less increased; a definite thrombocytopenia persists.

The marrow undergoes the same changes, but the megaloblastic appearance of some of its elements is unaffected.

When treatment is stopped, most patients relapse without rebound. Further hormone treatment brings a further remission. It is thus best to reduce the doses of androgens and steroids progressively, to discover the least dose that will keep the patient in a satisfactory hematological state (Desposito *et al.*, 1964; Shahidi and Diamond, 1961).

C. SIDE-EFFECTS OF TREATMENT

The ill effects of an excess of androgens are seen in all patients who receive large doses of the hormones for long enough (Desposito *et al.*, 1964; Kennedy, 1962; Kennedy and Gilbersten, 1957; Sanchez-Medal, 1964; Shahidi and Diamond, 1961).

The signs of virilization vary in severity. They include hirsutism, voice changes, hyperpigmentation, and increased size of the external genitalia with male type of hair-growth. These symptoms arise from the second month, and are the slowest to disappear after treatment is stopped.

Added to these signs of virilization are the effects of long-term corticosteroid therapy. Increased weight is associated with fluid retention. Headache is not constant. No effect on bone has been reported, in particular no effect on epiphyseal cartilages. Five cases of jaundice have been reported among 52 cases of various blood disorders treated with androgens (Kennedy, 1962). But in other series there has been no clinical sign of liver damage (Sanchez-Medal, 1964; Shahidi and Diamond, 1961), though BSP retention is slightly increased in some cases, transaminase levels remaining within normal limits. In patients who have died, no lesions of the liver cells or bile passages have been found (Kennedy, 1962).

D. MODE OF ACTION OF ANDROGENS

Several workers have attempted to establish the mechanism whereby androgens affect erythropoiesis.

One suggestion (Fried *et al.*, 1964; Gurney and Fried, 1965) is that the kidney is the site of action of the hormones or their intermediate metabolites, where they increase production of erythropoietin. In nephrectomized animals, injection of androgens in fact produces no erythropoietic response, and the amount of erythropoietin formed is considerably greater in animals receiving androgens than in controls subjected to the same stimulus. Androgens also act on the stem cells in the bone marrow to make them more sensitive to erythropoietin, or to the stimulus to erythropoiesis. The effects of androgens and of anabolic hormones are identical.

Naets and Wittek (1964) regard erythropoietin as essential, but their experimental studies suggest either a potentiation of the action of erythropoietin on stem cells, or a hormonal effect on a later stage of erythropoiesis rather than cellular differentiation.

The hopes raised by androgen treatment of idiopathic medullary aplasia have encouraged its use in other types of bone-marrow failure.

E. ANDROGENS AND MARROW FAILURE IN MARCHIAFAVA-MICHELI SYNDROME

Paroxysmal nocturnal hemoglobinuria is known to be a cause of bone-marrow failure (Hartmann and Jenkins, 1965). Gardner and Pringle (1961) have treated 3 patients for periods from 8 to 12 months. In one, treatment failed completely. A second relapsed when treatment was stopped. In the third, the anemia was partially corrected, and small doses of hormones sufficed to keep the patient in good condition.

Hartmann and Jenkins (1965) have treated 6 patients with fluoxymesterone in doses of 15–60 mg daily, together with iron by mouth. They have recorded 4 good results, with raised hemoglobin levels, decreased hemolysis, and less severe hemosiderinuria. In two cases, profuse hemoglobinuria followed abrupt withdrawal of androgen therapy. These

M*

encouraging results suggest that androgens should be given in serious, unstabilized cases of the syndrome.

F. TREATMENT OF PRIMARY MYELOFIBROSIS WITH ANDROGENS

Deficient erythropoiesis usually accounts for the anemia of primary myelofibrosis. Several authors have reported good results with large doses of hormones.

Gardner and Pringle (1961) have treated 9 patients. In all cases there was increased erythropoiesis with a less frequent need of transfusions, which can be regarded as the first sign that the treatment was efficacious; 3 patients actually became polycythemic.

In a later study, Gardner and Nathan (1966) investigated erythropoiesis in 28 patients, of whom 8 were anemic. The effect of androgens can be predicted from the dynamics of labeled iron. One group of patients had a very fibrous marrow and almost no splenic erythropoiesis: androgens had no effect on them. In a second group, with anemia from inadequate erythropoiesis, androgens were useless or even dangerous. In the third group, who responded well to treatment, the anemia was due to relative incompetence of the marrow, but with enough remaining presursors of the erythroid series to respond to androgen therapy.

Kennedy (1962) has met with less success; but 3 of the 8 patients showed definite improvement for several months.

West (1965) has reported 4 successes among 7 patients. The best results achieved by Silver *et al.* (1964) were in women, either after splenectomy or with little enlargement of the spleen.

Thus, hormone therapy can be given in those cases of myelofibrosis where there is little splenomegaly and the anemia is due to marrow failure. The hemolytic factor must be assessed before treatment begins.

G. HORMONE TREATMENT OF MARROW FAILURE IN CHRONIC LYMPHOID LEUKEMIA

Some cases of chronic lymphatic leukemia in which the anemia is not hemolytic or appears to have been caused by chemotherapy are improved by androgens. In one series (Kennedy, 1964), 7 patients were treated continuously for at least 6 months. Erythropoiesis increased without other treatment, and the hemoglobin level rose significantly. Thrombopoiesis was stimulated in 3 of the cases. West (1965) was successful with 10 of 18 patients.

H. TREATMENT OF MARROW FAILURE IN MYELOMA

Androgens have also been suggested for the treatment of myeloma (Brodsky *et al.*, 1965a). The subjective symptoms are often improved, but the other effects of the plasmacytic dyscrasia are little changed. Nitrogen mustards such as melphalan often have an effect on the neoplastic proliferation, but their toxicity to bone marrow prevents any prolonged cure. Brodsky and his colleagues believe that erythropoiesis can be stimulated with male hormones, and that they allow the maximum benefit to be obtained from chemotherapy by the use of effective doses.

I. HYPOPLASIA OF MARROW WITH PANCREATIC FAILURE

This is a new syndrome, described by Shwachman and his colleagues (1964). There is pancreatic failure without broncho-pulmonary involvement. The degree of pancytopenia varies, but the granulocytic series is more affected than the other cell-types. Marrow specimens show the usual appearances of medullary aplasia. All forms of treatment attempted by the authors failed.

3. SELECTIVE CHRONIC BONE-MARROW FAILURE

A. PURE ERYTHROBLASTOPENIA

There are both congenital and acquired forms. *Congenital erythroblastopenia* (Diamond-Blackfan syndrome) has an early onset in the first few weeks of life. There is a reticulocytopenia in the blood and bone marrow, together with a general and severe reduction of erythroblastic elements. Corticosteroid therapy has often proved efficacious (Gasser, 1951). Initially, large doses of prednisone should be given, of the order of 3 mg per kg daily. It takes some 4–6 weeks to correct the anemia; after this the dosage is reduced to the smallest dose required to keep the hemoglobin level above 10 g per 100 ml without transfusions (Bernard *et al.*, 1962).

Chronic acquired erythroblastopenia may be isolated, but more often it is associated with a tumour of the thymus. In most cases only the erythroid series is affected, but sometimes pancytopenia develops later (Dreyfus *et al.*, 1962, Harvard, 1965; Roland, 1964).

The thymic tumour is generally benign with few symptoms evident; often it is discovered only in the course of full investigation. The time-relationship between tumour induction and the anemia is difficult to establish. In some cases the tumour is discovered as a result of the anemia; in others it has been present for a long time with or without myasthenia.

It is not easy to lay down rules for treating erythroblastopenia associated with thymic tumour. Thymectomy is sometimes beneficial (8 out of 24 cases).

Steroid therapy may not work until after thymectomy. Prednisone is given in a daily dosage of 0.5–0.7 mg per kg. If the first course is ineffective, splenectomy may be needed. However, failure of steroid therapy may be only apparent: in one patient massive doses led to definite remission after moderate doses had been ineffective (Dreyfus *et al.*, 1963).

Large doses of androgens can produce a remission when other treatment has failed (Lehnoff 1960).

Treatment could be introduced in the following order: large doses of corticosteroids, thymectomy, corticosteroids, splenectomy, corticosteroids, androgens (Dreyfus *et al.*, 1963).

In chronic erythroblastopenia without thymic tumour, some authors (Fountain and Dales, 1955; Seaman and Koler, 1953, Voyce 1963) claim good results with cobalt chloride. It is given in daily doses of 100 mg in courses of 6–8 weeks separated by intervals of 4 weeks.

B. PURE NEUTROPENIA

Brodsky and his colleagues (1965b) have studied androgen therapy of cyclic neutropenia. The course of the disease was changed: it remained cyclic, but there were no symptoms during exacerbations and the agranulocytosis was not complete.

There is no effective medication for severe chronic pure neutropenia (Dreyfus, 1957).

C. PURE THROMBOCYTOPENIA

Congenital amegakaryocytic thrombopenia is rare: fewer than 35 cases have been reported (Masliah, 1965). Thrombocytopenia develops within a few days or months of birth. The severity of the purpura varies greatly; the more serious manifestations of the syndrome include mucosal and visceral hemorrhages. The degree of thrombocytopenia varies from case to case, and from time to time in the same patient.

As a rule megakaryocytes are totally or almost totally absent from the marrow. The other cell-types are normal or hyperplastic. In addition to the blood disorder, 75% of cases show other anomalies, of which the commonest is complete bilateral aplasia of the radius.

The outlook with these purpuras is poor, and treatment is disappointing. The usual doses of corticosteroids produce only occasional and transient increase of platelets (Masliah, 1965).

No improvement followed androgen therapy in 3 cases. Splenectomy, suggested by some workers, failed apart from the appearance of a few megakaryocytes in the marrow and a slight increase of platelets in one case (Masliah, 1965).

The chronic acquired form of pure amegakaryocytic thrombocytopenia is also rare. The same kinds of treatment have been tried without success.

Drugs under trial

(1) *Phytohemagglutinin.* Acting on Yoffey's theories of the stem-cell potential of lymphocytes, Humble (1964) suggested the treatment of bone-marrow failure with injections of phytohemagglutinin. This plant extract has little toxicity for man.

Six patients with toxic marrow failure were given repeated injections of lyophilized extracts. In four there was no effect despite intensive treatment. There was admittedly a reticulocyte response, and some suggestion of lymphocyte transformation, but the pancytopenia was not affected. In two other patients Humble (1964) considered that the natural course of the disease would have been favourable. Following Humble (1964), others have attempted the same treatment. Retief *et al.* (1964) reported failure in all of 6 cases; he observed transformed lymphocytes in the peripheral blood. Fleming (1964), Baker and Oliver (1965), and Gruenwald *et al.* (1969) recorded similar results. Astaldi *et al.* (1965) suggested injections of a marrow culture stimulated *in vitro* with phytohemagglutinin, and found some increased cellularity of the marrow, but no significant effect on the blood.

(2) *Cobaltous chloride.* Several workers have used this compound in the treatment of acquired erythroblastopenia in adults (Fountain and Dales, 1955; Seaman and Koler, 1953; Voyce, 1963). It has no effect when used for treating pancytopenia (Harvard, 1965; Roland, 1964).

(3) *Batyl alcohol.* This is an ester extracted from yellow bone marrow, which according to Wysocky *et al.* (1962) stimulates myelopoiesis in

animals. With it, they successfully treated a case of toxic aplasia which had resisted treatment for 11 weeks with steroids and androgens. Since this is the minimum period needed for these drugs to work, the result is difficult to interpret.

Clifford (1964) was impressed by the effect of batyl alcohol on normal subjects and in various types of anemia. However, there was no effect on patients with marrow failure. The reports are still too few to allow any clear picture to be formed of the therapeutic value of this substance.

REFERENCES

(a.) BOOKS, REVIEWS AND MONOGRAPHS

HARRIS, J. W. (1963). *The red cell.* Harvard University Press.
WINTROBE, M. (1962). *Clinical hematology.* Lea and Febiger, Philadelphia.

(b.) ORIGINAL PAPERS

ASTALDI, G., AIRO, R., SAULI, S. and COSTA, G. (1965). Phytohaemagglutinin in the treatment of aplastic anemia. *Lancet,* 1: 1070.
BAKER, G. P. and OLIVIER, R. A. (1965). Phytohaemagglutinin in the treatment of aplastic anemia. *Lancet,* 1: 438.
BELLANTI, J. A. and PINKEL, O. (1961). Idiopathic aplastic anemia treated with methyl-testosterone and fresh platelets. *J.A.M.A.,* 178: 70.
BERNARD, J., SELIGMANN, M., CHASSIGNEUX, J. and DRESCH, C. (1962). Anémie de Blackfan-Diamond. *N.R.F. Hemat.,* 2: 721.
BERNARD, J., LORTHOLARY, P., LEVY, J. P., BOIRON, M., NAJEAN, Y. and TANZER, J. (1963). Les anémies normochromes sidéroblastiques primitives. *N.R.F. Hemat.,* 3: 723.
BJÖRNTORP, P., WEINFELD, A., and LUNDIN, P. (1965). A case of aplastic anemia success-fully treated with androgens. *Acta. Med. Scand.,* 177: 275.
BLOOM, G. E., WARNER, S., GERALD, P. S. and DIAMOND, L. K. (1966). Chromosomes abnormalities in constitutional aplastic anemia. *New Eng. J. Med.,* 274: 8.
BRODSKY, I., DENNIS, L. H., DE CASTRO, N. A., BRADY, L. and KAHN, S. B. (1965a). Effect of testosterone enanthate and alkylating agents on multiple myeloma. *J.A.M.A.,* 193: 874.
BRODSKY, I., REIMANN, H. A. and DENNIS, L. H. (1965b). Treatment of cyclic neutro-penia with testostérone. *Amer. J. Med.,* 38: 802.
CLIFFORD, G. O. (1964). The hematopoietic effects of batyl alcohol in man subjects. In: *Xth congress of Internal Society of Haematology. Abstracts.* Stockholm.
DESPOSITO, F., AKATSUKA, J., THATCHER, L. G. and SMITH, M. J. (1964). Bone marrow failure in pediatric patients. I. Cortisone and testosterone treatment. *J. Pediat.,* 64: 683.
DREYFUS, B. (1957). Les agranulocytoses ou neutropénies chroniques primitives sans splénomégalie notable. *Rev. Hemat.,* 12: 250.
DREYFUS, B. (1959). A propos de 81 observations de pancytopénies idiopathiques chro-niques sans splenomégalie. *Rev. Hemat.,* 14: 62.

DREYFUS, B., AUBERT, P., PATTE, D., FRAY, A. and LE BOLLOCH-COMBRISSON, A. (1962). Erythroblastopénies chroniques avec tumeur du thymus, analyse de 43 observations. *N.R.F. Hemat.*, **2**: 739.

DREYFUS, B., AUBERT, P., PATTE, D., LE BOLLOCH-COMBRISSON, A. (1963). Erythroblastopénie chronique découverte après une thymectomie. Heureux effets de la corticotherérapie à fortes doses après échec de doses moyennes. *N.R.F. Hemat.*, **3**: 765.

FLEMING, A. F. (1964). Phytohaemagglutinin. *Lancet*, **11**: 647.

FOUNTAIN, J. R. and DALES, M. (1955). Pure red cell aplasia treated with cobalt. *Lancet*, **1**: 541.

FRIED, W., DE GOWIN, R., FORDE, R. and GURNEY, C. W. (1964). The erythropoïetic effect of androgens. *J. lab. clin. Med.*, **64**: 858.

FRIEDMAN, R. M. and STEIGBIGEL, N. H. (1965). Histiocytic medullary reticulosis. *Am. J. Med.*, **38**: 130.

GARDNER, F. H. and PRINGLE, J. C., Jr. (1961). Androgens and erythropoiesis. I. Preliminary clinical observations. *Arch. int. Med.*, **107**: 846.

GARDNER, F. H. and NATHAN, D. G. (1966). Androgens and erythropoiesis. 3. Further evaluation of testosterone treatment of myelofibrosis. *New Eng. J. Med.*, **274**: 420.

GASSER, C. (1951). Aplastische anamie (chronische erythroblastophtisie) und cortison. *Schweiz. Med. Wschnschr.*, **81**: 1241.

GRUENWALD, H., TAUB, R. N., WONG, F. M., KIOSSOGLU, K. A. and DAMESHEK, W. (1969). Phytohaemagglutinin in treatment of aplastic anaemia. *Lancet*, **1**: 962.

GURNEY, C. W. and FRIED, W. (1965). The mechanism of action of androgens on erythropoïesis. *J. clin. Invest.*, **44**: 1057.

HARTMANN, R. C. and JENKINS, D. E., JR. (1965). Paroxysmal nocturnal hemoglobinuria: Current concepts of certain pathophysiologic features. *Blood*, **25**: 850.

HARVARD, C. W. H. (1965). Thymic tumours and refractory anemia. *Series haematologica*, **5**: 18.

HUGULEY, C. H. M. (1960). Aplastic anemia treated with prednisone, thyroid testosterone and growth hormone. *Blood*, **15**: 246.

HUMBLE, J. G. (1964). The treatment of aplastic anemia with phytohaemagglutinin. *Lancet*, **1**: 1345.

ISRAËLS, M. C. G. and WILKINSON, J. F. (1961). Idiopathic aplastic anemia. Incidence and management. *Lancet*, **1**: 63.

KENNEDY, B. J. (1962). Stimulation of erythropoiesis by androgenic hormones. *Ann. int. Med.*, **57**: 917.

KENNEDY, B. J. Androgenic hormone therapy in lymphatic eukemia. *J.A.M.A.*, **190**: 1130.

KENNEDY, B. J. and GILBERSTEN, A. S. (1957). Increased erythropoiesis induced by androgenic hormone therapy. *New Eng. J. Med.*, **256**: 719.

KHALL, M. (1962). Treatment of aplastic anemia with anabolic steroids. *Acta Pediatrica*, **51**: 201.

LEHNOFF, H. J. (1960). Androgen therapy for the refractory anemia, report of a case associated with thymoma. *Ann. int. Med.*, **53**: 1059.

LEVY, R. N., SAWITSKY, A., FLORMAN, A. L. and RUBIN, E. (1965). Fatal aplastic anemia after hepatitis. Report of five cases. *New Eng. J. Med.*, **273**: 1118.

LEWIS, S. M. (1962). Red cell abnormalities and haemolysis in aplastic anemia. *Brit. Med. J.*, **8**: 322.

LEWIS, S. M. (1965). Course and prognosis in aplastic anemia. *Brit. Med. J.*, **1**: 1027.

LEWIS, S. M. and SZUR, L. (1962). Malignant myelosclerosis. *Brit. Med. J.*, **II**: 472.

LOEB, V., JR., MOORE, C. V. and DUBACH, R. (1953). The physiologic evaluation and management of chronic bone marrow failure. *Amer. J. Med.*, **15**: 499.

MACGULLAGH, E. P. and JONES, T. R. (1942). Effect of androgens on blood count of men. *J. clin. Endocrin.* **2**: 243.

MASLIAH, A. (1965). Le purpura thrombopénique amégacaryocytaire congénital. Thèse, Paris.

MOHLER, D. H. and LEAVELL, B. S. (1958). Aplastic anemia, an analysis of 50 cases. *Ann. int. Med.,* **49**: 326.

MOVITT, E. R., MANGUM, J. F. and PORTER, W. R. (1963). Idiopathic true bone marrow failure. *Amer. J. Med.,* **34**: 500.

NAETS, J. P. and WITTEK, M. (1964). Étude du mécanisme d'action des androgènes sur l'érythropoïèse. *C.R. Acad. Sci., Paris,* **259**: 3371.

NAJEAN, Y., ARDAILLOU, N. and BERNARD, J. (1963). Études des compartiments non héminiques du fer. Explorations faites *in vivo. N.R.F. Hemat.,* **3**: 17.

NAJEAN, Y. and BERNARD, J. (1964). Modes d'exploration et surveillance d'une in- suffisance médullaire. *Rev. Prat.,* **14**: 3993.

NAJEAN, Y., BERNARD, J., WAINBERGER, M., DRESCH, C., BOIRON, M. and SELIGMANN, M. (1965). Evolution et pronostic des pancytopénies idiopathiques. Étude de 116 observations. *N.R.F. Hemat.,* **5**: 639.

NAJEAN, Y., DRESCH, C., SCHAISON, G., CHASSIGNEUX, J., JACQUILLAT, C. and BERNARD, J. (1966). Étude de l'effet de l'androgénothérapie au cours des insuffisances médul- laires. *Presse Méd.,* **74**: 2537–40.

RETIEF, F. P., WASSERMANN, H. P. and HOFMEYER, N. G. (1964). Phytohaemagglutinin in aplastic anemia. *Lancet,* **2**: 1343.

ROLAND, A. S. (1964). The syndrome of benign thymoma and primary aregenerative anemia; an analysis of 43 cases. *Amer. J. med. Sci.,* **247**: 719.

SANCHEZ-MEDAL, L., PIZZUTO, J., TORRE-LOPEZ, E. and DERBEZ, R. (1964). Effect of oxymetholone in refractory anemia. *Arch. int. Med.,* **113**: 721.

SCHMID, J. R., KIELY, J. M., HARRISON, E. G., JR., BAYRD, E. D. and PEASE, G. L. (1965). Thymoma associated with pure red-cell agenesis. Review of literature and report of 4 cases. *Cancer,* **18**: 216.

SCHREK, R. and DONNELY, W. J. (1966). "Hairy" cells in blood in lympho-reticular neoplastic disease and "flagellated" cells of normal lymph nodes. *Blood,* **27**: 199.

SCOTT, S., CARTWRIGHT, G. E. and WINTROBE, M. (1959). Acquired aplastic anemia: analysis of thirty nine cases and review of the pertinent literature. *Medicine,* **38**: 119.

SEAMAN, A. J. and KOLER, R. D. (1953). Acquired erythrocyte hypoplasia. Recovery during cobalt therapy. Report of two cases with review of literature. *Acta Haemat.,* **9**: 153.

SEIP, (1961). Aplastic anemia treated with steroids and corticoïds. *Acta Pediat.,* **50**: 561.

SELIGMANN, M. (1966). Confrontations thérapeutiques. *N.R.F. Hamat.,* **6**: 407.

SHAHIDI, N. T. and DIAMOND, L. K. (1961). Testosterone induced remission in aplastic anemia of both acquired and congenital types. Further observations in 24 cases. *New Eng. J. Med.,* **264**: 953.

SHAHIDI, N. T. and DIAMOND, L. K. (1959). Testosterone induced remission in aplastic anemia. *A.M.A.D. Dis. Child.,* **98**: 293.

SHAHIDI, N. T., GERALD, P. S. and DIAMOND, L. K. (1962). Alkaki resistant hemo- globine in aplastic anemia of both acquired and congenital types. *New Eng. J. Med.,* **266**: 117.

SHAHIDI, N. T. (1963). Morphologic and biochemical characteristics of erythrocytes in testerone-induced remission in patients with acquired and constitutional aplastic anemia. *J. lab. clin. Med.,* **62**: 294.

SHWACHMAN, H., DIAMOND, L. K., OSKI, F. A. and KHAW, K. T. (1964). The syndrome of pancreatic insufficiency and bone marrow dysfunction. *J. Pediat.,* **65**: 645.

SILVER, R. T., JENKINS, D. E., JR. and ENGLE, R. L., JR. (1964). Use of testosterone and bisulfan in the treatment of myelofibrosis with myeloid metaplasia. *Blood,* **23**: 341.

Voyce, M. A. (1963). A case of pure red cell. Aplasia successfully treated with cobalt. *Brit. J. Hemat.*, **9**: 412.

Waitz, R., Mayer, S. and Mayer, G. (1964). Les aplasies médullaires de l'adulte: leur étude anatomo-clinique. *Sem. Hôp.*, **40**: 163.

West, W. O. (1965). The treatment of bone marrow failure with massive androgen therapy. *Ohio M.J.*, **61**: 347.

Wintrobe, M. (1950). A.C.T.H. and cortisone in hemopathic disorders. *Amer. J. Med.*, **9**: 715.

Wolff, J. A. (1957). Anemia caused by infection and toxic idiopathic aplastic anemia caused by renal disease. *Pedat. Clin. North America*, **4**: 499.

Wysocky, D. J., Antonelli, J. N. and Kenoyer, W. L. (1962). Aplastic anemia treated with batyl alcohol, a case report. *Clin. Research*, **10**: 20.

CHAPTER 7

ERYTHROPOIETIN

J. P. Naets

Laboratoire de Médicine Experimentale,
Bruxelles, Belgium

I. DEFINITION

ERYTHROPOIETIN—hematopoietin, erythropoietic stimulating factor (ESF), erythropoietic factor—is a substance able to stimulate erythropoiesis in normal animals. This definition distinguishes this substance from factors taking part in erythropoiesis, without being able to stimulate it in normal animals, such as vitamin B_{12}, vitamin B_6, folic acid, iron, and proteins. Now that the mode of action of erythropoietin is better understood the definition can be restricted to a substance able to promote the differentiation of stem cells into erythroblasts.

II. HISTORICAL BACKGROUND

At the end of the last century, Bert (1882) showed that mammals adapted themselves to low partial pressure of oxygen at high altitude by increasing their red-cell mass. Miescher (1893) suggested that hypoxia of the bone marrow, resulting from the low oxygen pressure, was responsible for the increased production of red cells. In 1906 Carnot and Deflandre advanced the theory of the humoral control of erythropoiesis by a hormone that they called hematopoietin. These authors showed that 9 ml of plasma from rabbits rendered anemic by bleeding, given for 2 consecutive days to normal rabbits, caused their red-cell count to rise considerably in 2 days. A few years later Müller (1912) suggested that the humoral factor appeared also in the blood of animals subjected to hypoxia. Unfortunately these results were not reproducible, and were followed by numerous contradictory reports. Consequently the theory of humoral control of erythropoiesis was not accepted until recently.

In 1950 Reissman was the first to demonstrate this hypothesis unequivocally. He found that if only one member of a pair of paraboitic

N

rats was submitted to hypoxia erythropoiesis was stimulated in both animals. In these conditions the blood of the hypoxic rat only, was desaturated in oxygen. The erythroblastic hyperplasia found in the bone marrow of the normally oxygenated partner must be due to the action of an erythropoiesis-stimulating factor produced by the rat subjected to hypoxia. Furthermore, Grant (1955) reported that young rats in a normal atmosphere, but suckled by a mother intermittently exposed to reduced oxygen tension, develop polycythemia.

These experimental findings have been confirmed by clinical observations. Stohlman *et al.* (1954) have reported the case of a patient with a patent ductus arteriosus complicated by a reversed shunt. Although this patient's sternal marrow was supplied by normally oxygenated blood, it showed a similar degree of erythroblastic hyperplasia to that of the iliac crest where oxygenation was deficient. Schmid and Gilbertsen (1955) have published a similar observation. These findings argue against a direct effect of hypoxia on the marrow, and suggest a humoral factor produced by an organ situated below the diaphragm.

The presence of a factor stimulating erythropoiesis was definitely proved by Toha *et al.* (1952) and by Erslev (1953). These authors showed that large amounts of plasma (50 ml/day) from anemic rabbits induced reticulocytosis, and stimulated erythropoiesis in bone marrow, in normal recipient rabbits. Borsook *et al.* (1954) showed that the ability to stimulate erythropoiesis was retained in the filtrate obtained after boiling plasma from a rabbit rendered anemic with phenylhydrazine.

III. METHODS OF ASSAY

Since the chemical nature of erythropoietin has not been established, biological assay is required. Small animals, rats or mice, are generally used. At first variations in hematocrit and hemoglobin level were recorded, but these measurements were soon abandoned in favour of the red-cell mass, which is independent of changes in plasma volume. The usual current practice is to measure the variation in reticulocytosis and in ^{59}Fe uptake by the red blood-cells.

A. *Assay of erythropoietic factor from increase in red-cell mass* (Garcia and Van Dyke, 1959)

The material to be assayed is injected subcutaneously into normal rats or mice, daily for 10–14 days. The red-cell mass is then measured either with ^{51}Cr (Read, 1954) or by means of red cells labeled with ^{59}Fe taken from an animal previously injected with radio-iron (Garcia, 1957). Figure 1, from Garcia and Van Dyke (1959), shows that the increase in red-cell mass is proportional to the dose given. This kind of method obviously requires a large amount of material, which restricts its use. Secondly, erythropoietin given in repeated small doses does not increase

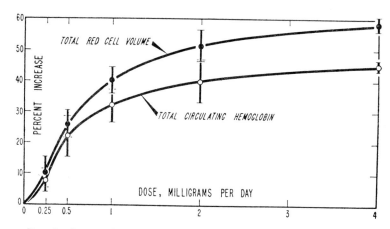

FIG. 1. Increase in total red cell volume and total circulating hemoglobin of normal adult rats after 14 days of injection with urinary erythropoietin. Limits of one S.E. of the mean are given for each observation. (Reproduced by courtesy of *J. Appl. Physiol.*, Garcia and Van Dyke, 1959).

the red-cell mass, for the blood level of the hormone must be increased beyond the recipient animal's endogenous production, in order to exert an effect. Thirdly, repeated injections of material may lead to abscess formation, which depresses erythropoiesis. Fourthly, repeated injection of foreign protein may in time induce reactions of immunity (Lowy *et al.*, 1959). In spite of these troubles and difficulties, this laborious method gives the best measure of the erythropoietic activity of a substance, since the production of red cells is measured directly.

B. *Assay of erythropoietic factor from uptake of iron-59 in the rat*

Rats are given 2 ml of the material to be tested by subcutaneous injection on 3 successive days; then ^{59}Fe is injected intraperitoneally or intravenously and the uptake by the red cells is measured 18–20 hr later (Plzak *et al.*, 1955). The response is a function of the stimulation of erythropoiesis. But the percentage of radio-iron incorporated into the red cells in control rats, injected with saline, is high—about 30%—and the relative increase following injection of the active material is fairly small. Individual variation within a group of animals is great enough to reduce the sensitivity of the test.

Fried *et al.* (1956) have suggested the use of hypophysectomized rats instead of normal rats. After hypophysectomy, there is a rapid fall in erythropoiesis, and consequently in iron uptake (Fig. 2), reaching a

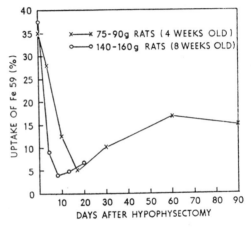

FIG. 2.   Iron-59 incorporation in erythrocytes of rats hypophysectomized at 4 and 8 weeks of age. (Reproduced by courtesy of *Proc. Soc. exp. Biol. Med.* Fried *et al.*, 1957).

minimum 8–14 days after the operation. The reduced erythropoiesis is explained by the fact that after removal of the pituitary, metabolic requirements decrease while the red-cell mass remains normal. The rats are comparable with normal animals rendered polycythemic by transfusions whose erythropoiesis is depressed. Sixteen hours after injection of ^{59}Fe the hypophysectomized rats have an iron uptake of only 4–5%. After injection of material containing erythropoietin the uptake may increase up to 30 or 40% (Garcia and Van Dyke, 1959). Fried *et al.* (1957) later suggested an assay of erythropoietin in fasted rats. In these animals uptake of ^{59}Fe falls and reaches a minimum on the fourth day of fasting (Fig. 3). The method has been widely adopted because of its simplicity.

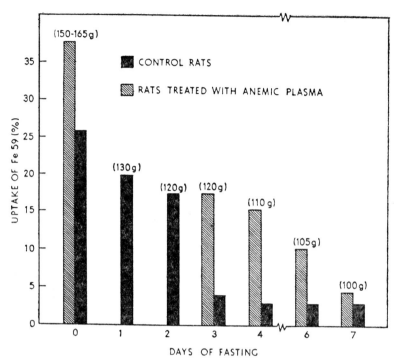

FIG. 3. Effect of duration of starvation on ^{59}Fe incorporation and on response to erythropoietin in 8-week-old rats. (Reproduced by courtesy of *Proc. Soc. exp. Biol. Med.*, Fried *et al.* (1957)).

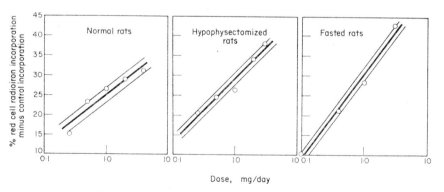

FIG. 4. Correlation between dose of urinary erythropoietin and red cell incorporation of ^{59}Fe in various assay animals. Limits of one S.E. of the estimate are given. (Reproduced by courtesy of *J. Appl. Physiol.*, Garcia and Van Dyke (1959)).

The usual technique is as follows. Fasting is begun on day 0. On days 1 and 2 the rats are given subcutaneous injections of the material, and 24 hr later (day 3) ^{59}Fe is injected either intravenously or intraperitoneally. The simplicity of the latter route is offset by the disadvantage that the iron is sometimes injected erroneously into the bladder or intestine, giving a falsely low uptake. 16–20 hours after giving ^{59}Fe a count is made on blood from the aorta or the heart. In calculating the total ^{59}Fe incorporation the blood volume is assumed as 5% of body weight. The result is expressed as the percentage of the injected radioactivity. Figure 4, from Garcia and Van Dyke (1959), shows the relation of ^{59}Fe uptake to increasing doses of erythropoietin in normal, hypophysectomized, and fasted rats.

It must be pointed out that methods utilizing ^{59}Fe uptake in hypophysectomized of fasted animals are liable to error. The injected plasma or crude extracts of organs might contain hormones able to affect erythropoiesis in hypophysectomized animals, which are very sensitive to corticotrophin, adrenal hormones, and thyroid hormone (Crafts, 1954). Furthermore, erythropoiesis is stimulated in fasted animals by protein or caloric intake. Thus, if cannibalism occurs before ^{59}Fe is injected the results in the animals surviving in the cage are invalidated. Lastly, the labile iron pool, of which the serum iron is an index, affects the uptake of ^{59}Fe (Hodgson *et al.*, 1957). Lowering the serum iron increases uptake by the red cells and *vice versa*. It is important to check the hematocrit of the treated animals, as the tested material could induce hemolysis in the recipient, the resulting anemia stimulating endogenous production of erythropoietin, and as a result the erythropoiesis is misleadingly increased. Results from animals with low hematocrit must be discarded. Hodgson *et al.* (1960) have suggested to measure turnover rather than uptake of iron, but this method, requiring estimation of serum iron in each rat, is impracticable when numerous assays are to be done.

C. *Assay of erythropoietic factor from uptake of iron-59 in polycythemic mice*

As Jacobson and Goldwasser (1957) have suggested, the production of erythropoietin seems to depend on an autoregulatory mechanism involving the supply and demand of oxygen in the tissues. When the supply of oxygen to the tissues increases the output of erythropoietin falls, and the erythropoietic activity of the bone marrow is accordingly reduced. In mice after transfusion, reticulocytes completely disappear from the blood (Jacobson *et al.*, 1957b). Injection of erythropoietic factor in these animals is followed by a wave of differentiation of *stem cells* into erythroblasts (Filmanowicz and Gurney, 1961). If ^{59}Fe is injected when the normoblasts in the marrow reach their peak, 50 hr after the injection of erythropoietic factor, the induced differentiation can be assessed by the uptake of ^{59}Fe in the red cells during the next few days. De Gowin *et al.* (1962a) have described the following technique. The mice are given 1 ml of washed red cells with a hematocrit of 75–80 %, on 2 consecutive days. 1 ml of the material to be tested is injected subcutaneously 6 days after the second transfusion when erythropoiesis is suppressed. Fifty hours later, 0.5 mcli of ^{59}Fe are injected into a caudal vein, and 72 hr later blood radioactivity is measured. Incorporation is calculated assuming the blood volume represents 7 % of the body weight. Results from animals in which hematocrit is below 55 % are discarded. This method is time-consuming and expensive. For each assay sample 6 mice have to be treated, and each mouse requires blood from 4 donors.

The use of mice rendered polycythaemic by prolonged hypoxia is a more convenient method. Devised by Cotes and Bangham (1961) and employed with various modifications by several workers (De Gowin *et al.*, 1962b; Weintraub *et al.*, 1963). The use of polyeythaemic mice for estimating erythropoiesis has the following advantages:

1. The definition of erythropoietin is confined to substances able to induce differentiation of stem cells into normoblasts.

2. In contrast with hypophysectomized or fasted rats, polycythemic mice do not respond to other hormones, protein, or caloric intake.

3. These mice are highly sensitive to erythropoietin, so that small amounts of the hormone (0.05 standard A units) can be detected (Fig. 5).

D. *Standardization*

Goldwasser and White (1959) suggested an erythropoietin standard based on the use of cobalt. They defined a cobalt unit as the erythropoietic response (expressed as ^{59}Fe uptake) to a dose of 5 mcMol of $CoCl_2$ per 100 g of body weight. Unfortunately it seems that cobalt in this dosage is active only in male Sprague-Dawley rats, which limits its use (Keighley, 1962); consequently a standard of erythropoietin has been proposed (Bangham, 1962). The first to be used, "standard A", was distributed by the Department of Biological Standards of the National Institute of

Medical Research, London. It was a partially purified extract of erythropoietin from the plasma of anemic sheep (Armour Laboratories, Chicago).
The present standard, "standard B", also obtainable from the Department
of Biological Standards, is prepared from the urine of a patient with
paroxysmal nocturnal hemoglobinuria.

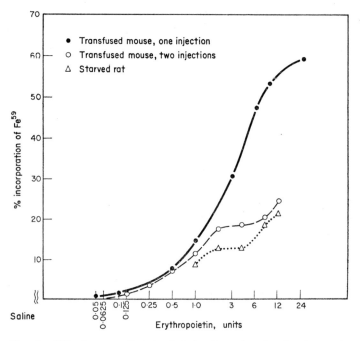

FIG. 5. ^{59}Fe incorporation in fasted rats and polycythemic mouse
following administration of erythropoietin. (Reproduced by courtesy of
Proc. Soc. exp. Biol. Med., De Gowin *et al.* (1962a)).

IV. PRODUCTION OF ERYTHROPOIETIN AND REGULATION OF ERYTHROPOIESIS

Hypoxia and anemia are the primary stimuli to the production of erythropoietin. After exposure to reduced atmospheric pressure for 2–48 hr,
erythropoietin can be detected in the plasma (Stohlman and Brecher,
1957b; Erslev, 1957; Mirand and Prentice, 1957). In the rat, if stimulation
is continued beyond 24 hr, the level of erythropoietin falls, and can no
longer be measured (Mirand and Prentice, 1957). Stohlman (1959) has

suggested that prolonged hypoxia induces a hyperplasia of the erythroid marrow which increases the consumption of erythropoietin. This relationship between erythropoietin utilization and marrow hyperplasia has not been confirmed by our studies. In the dog the utilization of erythropoietin is the same whether the normoblast content of the marrow is high or normal (Naets and Wittek, 1965). It could be that an eventual store of

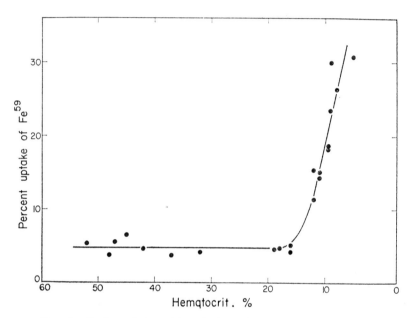

FIG. 6. Erythropoietic activity of plasma from bled dogs in regard to hematocrit measurements, expressed in ^{59}Fe uptake into red cells of starved rats. (Reproduced by courtesy of *Proc. Soc. exp. Biol. Med.* Naets (1959a)).

erythropoietin is released in the first hours of hypoxia. However, this hypothesis is unlikely, as the level of erythropoietin is not found to decrease after prolonged bleeding in the rabbit (Erslev, 1957) or dog (Naets, 1959a). It is more likely that in response to hypoxia compensatory mechanisms intervene, such as increased pulmonary ventilation and cardiac output, which reduce the stimulus by improving tissue oxygenation. Anemia due to bleeding or to administration of phenylhydrazine also produces a rise in the plasma level of erythropoietin, provided that the hemoglobin is below 7 g per 100 ml (Erslev, 1957; Stohlman and Brecher, 1956; Borsook *et al.*,

N*

1954). Already three hours after bleeding erythropoietin is detectable in the plasma (Erslev and Boissevain, 1961). The erythropoietin plasma titer rises in proportion to the severity of the anemia (Naets, 1959a; White and Josh, 1959), as shown in Fig. 6. At first sight phenylhydrazine anemia appears to produce a greater increase of erythropoietin than a similar anemia resulting from bleeding. In fact, the hematocrit in animals treated

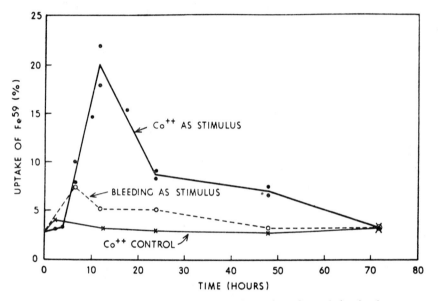

FIG. 7. Time course of erythropoietin formation after cobalt stimulation. Each point represents the average of values obtained from a group of 5 assay rats. (Reproduced by courtesy of *Blood*, Goldwasser *et al.*, (1958b)).

with phenylhydrazine gives a false notion of the amount of hemoglobin available for tissue oxygenation, since a considerable part of the blood pigment is in the form of methemoglobin (Jacobsen *et al.*, 1956).

A. *Effect of cobalt on erythropoietin production*

Cobalt ions have been known for some years to produce polycythemia in man and animals (Barron and Barron, 1936; Berk *et al.*, 1949). Goldwasser *et al.* (1958b) have shown that cobalt affects erythropoiesis by the way of erythropoietin. As shown in Fig. 7, after injection of a single dose of 25 mcMol of $CoCl_2$ per 100 g in the rat the plasma level of erythropoietin rises, attaining its maximum at 12 hr. The precise mechanism by which cobalt increases erythropoietin production is as little understood as the mechanism involved in anemia or hypoxia. It may be that cobalt produces tissue asphyxia by inhibiting certain oxidative enzymes (Levy *et al.*, 1950; Daniel *et al.*, 1963).

B. *Role of erythropoietin in the regulation of erythropoiesis*

Since the life-span of a human red blood-cell is 120 days, it follows that 1/120 of the red-cell mass is destroyed every day. Yet the number of red cells remain constant, for at precisely the rate at which they are destroyed new cells are formed to replace them. The question is whether this perfectly adjusted homoeostatic mechanism depends on erythropoietin. While humoral regulation of erythropoiesis seems to have been clearly demonstrated in conditions where the oxygen supply of the tissues is defective, there is only indirect experimental evidence for humoral control of the day-to-day physiological production of erythrocytes. Indeed, the presence of erythropoietin in the plasma of normal subjects has not yet been definitely proved. This does not necessarily mean that there is no erythropoietin in normal plasma. The present methods of biological assay are probably not sensitive enough, and detect only increased levels of the hormone. The following arguments are in favour of a humoral control of physiological erythropoiesis:

1. By injecting human erythropoietin into rabbits, Schooley and Garcia (1962) have obtained an antibody against erythropoietin; injected into normal mice it reduces erythropoiesis in the same way as transfusion. It may be inferred that the neutralizing effect of this antibody inactivates erythropoietin normally present in the plasma, by which erythropoiesis is maintained.

2. There are several reasons for thinking that the kidney is essential to the formation of erythropoietin (Jacobson *et al.*, 1957a; Naets, 1960c). In the dog, normal erythropoiesis is suppressed by bilateral nephrectomy, whereas it is only slightly modified by ligation of the ureters, although the uremic intoxication is similar in either condition. It is consequently possible that the physiological production of red cells depends on a factor which disappears from the plasma as a result of bilateral nephrectomy (Naets, 1958b).

3. The level of erythropoietin in the plasma rises after bleeding; it would be expected to decrease after transfusion of red cells. In fact erythropoiesis is depressed by transfusion (Gurney and Chao Pan, 1958), and it is possible that erythropoietin titer in the plasma decreases accordingly to a level at which normal erythropoiesis is no longer maintained.

Jacobson and Goldwasser (1957) have advanced the hypothesis that the regulation of erythropoiesis is dependant on the amount of erythropoietin in the plasma, and that the production of the hormone is determined by the relation between requirement and supply of oxygen in the tissues.

TABLE 1. RELATIONSHIP OF OXYGEN SUPPLY AND DEMAND TO ERYTHROPOIESIS

Condition	O_2 supply	O_2 demand	Rate of erythropoiesis	Sensitivity to erythropoietin
Hypophysectomy	Normal	Decreased	Reduced	Increased
Hyperoxia	Increased	Normal	Reduced	Increased
Starvation	Normal	Decreased	Reduced	Increased
Polycythemia[1]	Increased	Normal	Reduced	Increased
Anemia due to				
Phlebotomy	Reduced	Normal	Increased	Decreased
Phenylhydrazine	Reduced	Normal	Increased	Decreased
Dinitrophenol	Normal	Increased	Increased	Decreased
Triiodothyronine	Normal	Increased	Increased	Decreased

[1] Induced by red cell injection.

From Homeostatic mechanisms—Brookhaven Symposia in Biology, Jacobson and Goldwasser, 1957.

Table 1 shows that when the oxygen supply to the tissues is reduced (anemia, hypoxia), the blood level of erythropoietin rises and becomes measurable. On the other hand, in the case of reduced requirements (after hypophysectomy or prolonged fasting) whereas the oxygen supply to the tissues remains normal, erythropoiesis decreases. It may be inferred that in these conditions the production of erythropoietin decreases, increasing consequently the sensitivity to erythropoietin. If, however, oxygen requirements are increased by giving dinitrophenol or triiodothyronine, erythropoiesis is stimulated and the animal becomes less sensitive to exogenous erythropoietin. Although it is impossible to demonstrate a fall in the plasma concentration of erythropoietin below the normal (undetectable) level, it might be suggested that the production of erythropoietin in response to hypoxia is less in an organism with reduced oxygen demand than in a normal subject. Accordingly we have observed in rats whose oxygen demand had been reduced by hypophysectomy or prolonged fasting that after a hypoxic stimulation the plasma level of erythropoietin rises distinctly less in these animals than in normal controls (Naets, 1963).

The tissue sensitive to this balance between supply and requirement of oxygen is unknown. Is it the organ producing erythropoietin, or is the latter dependent on another, "erythrostatic" organ? Is this sensitive organ unique, and does it respond to changes of oxygen tension or to metabolites resulting from variations in the ratio between oxygen supply and demand? None of these questions has yet been answered. The hypothalamus has been suggested as the organ responding to hypoxia and regulating the production of erythropoietin. Chronic electrical stimulation of certain regions of the hypothalamus provokes polycythemia and a reticulocyte response (Seip *et al.*, 1961), while their destruction suppresses the response to hypoxia (Halvorsen, 1964). However, it cannot be concluded from these experiments that the hypothalamus has a specific influence on erythropoiesis, as the effects of stimulation or injury in this part of the nervous system might be secondary to changes of pituitary function.

The autoregulatory mechanism suggested for maintaining erythropoiesis is shown schematically in Fig. 8 (Erslev, 1962). Tissue hypoxia increases erythropoietin secretion, resulting in the differentiation of more stem cells into erythroid cells, increased synthesis of hemoglobin and, by an autoregulatory mechanism, reduced production of erythropoietin.

All authors accept this unitary view of the control of erythropoiesis. Brecher and Stohlman (1959) suggest that erythropoietin intervenes only in cases of acute oxygen demand, and that normal control of erythropoiesis is independent of the hormone. They do not accept that trivial changes of red-cell mass occurring after insignificant loss of blood, or in the course of compensated hemolytic disease can reduce the oxygen supply of a sensitive organ, enough to affect its metabolism. Obviously the same argument holds for maintaining the normal number of red cells, bringing up the whole problem of homeostasis. The fact that the variations of tissue oxygenation seem insignificant does not completely rule out an autoregulatory mechanism based on the relation of oxygen supply to erythropoietin. Similar mechanisms are known to allow adjustment to infinitesimal changes.

Brecher and Stohlman (1958) have advanced an alternative hypothesis of an erythropoietin inhibitor, formed in the aging red cells and released into the circulation when they are destroyed. Thus lowering the number

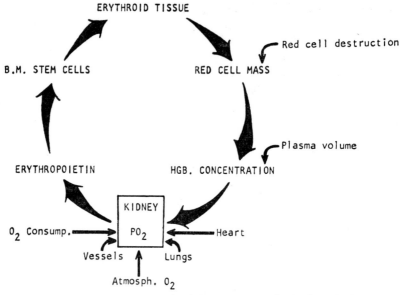

F<small>IG</small>. 8. Proposed feedback circuit for the control of red cell production.
(Reproduced by courtesy of *Trans. N.Y. Acad. Sci.*, Erslev (1961)).

of red cells by hemorrhage would reduce the inhibitor, and accordingly increase erythropoiesis. In compensated hemolytic disease, the red cells, being destroyed before reaching maturity, would not release the inhibitor. This concept has no experimental support, for the hypothetical erythropoietin inhibitor in red cells has never been demonstrated. It is furthermore open to the following objections. In polycythemic animals there should be increased production of the inhibitor, yet erythropoiesis does not appear to be inhibited in them for they are especially sensitive to erythropoietin. Nor can it explain the intense stimulation of erythropoiesis which follows sudden hemolysis, e.g. after giving phenylhydrazine, in spite of the expected sudden release of the inhibitor in the plasma.

V. RELATION OF ENDOCRINE GLANDS TO ERYTHROPOIETIN

Anemia after removal of various endocrine glands (pituitary, adrenals, thyroid, testes) can be corrected by administration of the lacking hormone (Van Dyke *et al.*, 1954, Gordon, 1954). It has been suggested that the anemia is due to the reduced oxygen demand that follows removal of endocrine glands (Crafts and Meineke, 1957), and consequently reduced erythropoiesis. The various hormones restore erythropoiesis in the hypophysectomized animal by stimulating metabolism (Evans *et al.*, 1961). However, it seems that a rise in caloric requirements does not by itself explain the restitution to normal erythropoiesis in the hypophysectomized rat. Growth hormone, thyroid-stimulating hormone, and thyroxine, increase metabolism in animals to the same extent as corticotrophin and hydrocortisone, but do not elicit a comparable increase in red cell production (Evans *et al.*, 1964). Moreover testosterone (Naets and Wittek, 1964) and prolactin (Jepson and Lowenstein, 1964) stimulate erythropoiesis in the mouse without raising metabolism. Testosterone may act by potentiating the effect of erythropoietin on bone marrow (Naets and Wittek, 1966), or by stimulating production of the hormone (Mirand *et al.*, 1965). Polactin probably acts in this latter way (Jepson and Lowenstein, 1965).

VI. MECHANISM OF ACTION

A model of the erythron has been described by Lajtha and Oliver (1960). The bone marrow contains a pool of stem cells which are differentiated to pronormoblasts. The synthesis of hemoglobin begins in these cells and is continued through maturation and the four successive divisions leading to the orthochromic normoblast. Secondary to this model, several sites of action of erythropoietin can be suggested (Fig. 9):

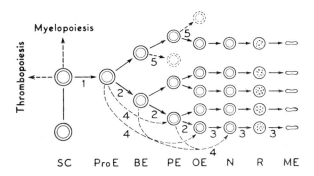

FIG. 9. Possible mechanisms of action of erythropoietin. (Reproduced by courtesy of Grune & Stratton, New York, from *Erythropoiesis*, Fischer (1962)).

(1)   increased differentiation of stem cells into pronormoblasts;
(2)   reduction of the intermitotic generation time;
(3)   reduction of the maturation time of polychromatophilic-normo-blasts;
(4)   reduction of the number of divisions;
(5)   reduction of ineffective erythropoiesis.

Only (1) and (5) could account for a continued increase in the red-cell mass. As recent studies (Robinson and Schmid, 1964; Cronkite, 1964) seem to demonstrate the absence of ineffective erythropoiesis in normal animals, only the effect on cellular differentiation could explain the stimulation of bone marrow by erythropoietin.

Various experimental observations support this hypothesis. Steele (1933) and Huff *et al.* (1951) have found that the proportion of pronormoblasts and normoblasts in the bone marrow is the same whether erythropoiesis is normal or hyperactive. Alpen and Cranmore (1959) have shown in the dog by autoradiography of bone marrow that the intermitotic generation time was the same in normal animals and in animals in which erythropoiesis had been stimulated by bleeding. In addition, the percentage of labeled pronormoblasts decreases much more rapidly in dogs with hyperactive than with normal erythropoiesis, which suggests that this pool is fed by unlabeled stem cells. Furthermore, Filmanowicz and Gurney (1961) have shown that after injection of a single dose of erythropoietin in the polycythemic mouse—whose spleen is depleted of erythroid elements—pronormoblasts and then normoblasts appear in the spleen during the next few hours. The wave of differentiated cells disappears consecutively from the spleen, giving issue to a peak of reticulocytes after 72 hr (Fig. 10).

Certain more recent observations suggest that erythropoietin also has an action on differentiated erythroid cells. Thus Gallagher *et al.* (1963) and Fischer (1962) have shown that erythropoietin promotes reticulocytosis earlier in normal animals than in transfused animals whose marrow is depleted of normoblasts. Stohlman *et al.* (1963) have found that larger red cells (macrocytes) appear in the blood of normal rats after erythropoietin, but not in transfused rats. If the dose of erythropoietin was divided into two parts, (the second injection being given 24 hr after the first, i.e. when there were differentiated cells in the marrow resulting from the first injection) macrocytes appeared in both normal and transfused animals. Stohlman (1961) has shown that these macrocytes produced by administration of erythropoietin or by the action of endogenous erythro-

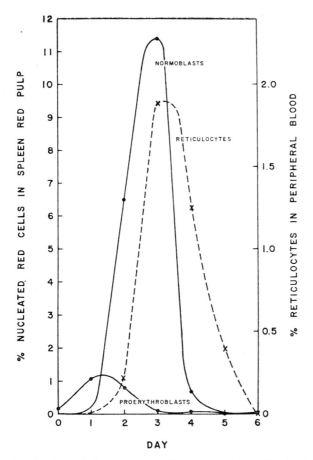

FIG. 10. Erythropoietic response in spleen and peripheral blood after a single injection of erythropoietin in polycythemic mice. (Reproduced by courtesy of *J. lab. clin. Med.*, Filmanowicz *et al.*, (1961)).

poietin (after bleeding, or hemolysis induced by phenylhydrazine) have a shortened life-span. According to this author (Stohlman *et al.*, 1964) erythropoietin induces and controls hemoglobin synthesis: administration of the hormone would accelerate hemoglobin synthesis, until a critical concentration of hemoglobin is reached in the cell and consequently nucleic acid synthesis would be stopped and further division prevented. The number of divisions of the normoblast would thus depend on the rate of hemoglobin synthesis. If it is accelerated, fewer divisions and consequently macrocytes are produced; conversely in the case of reduced synthesis (e.g. in iron deficiency), there are more mitoses, and microcytes appear (Fig. 11).

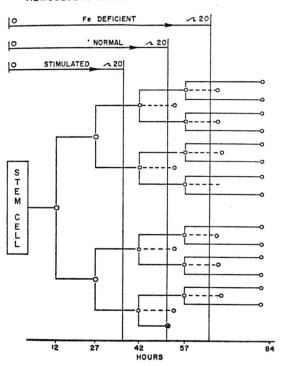

FIG. 11. A model of the kinetics of erythropoiesis in which it is proposed that when a cytoplasmic hemoglobin concentration of 20% is achieved, a negative feedback is initiated which shuts off DNA synthesis and division. (Reproduced by courtesy of *Trans. N.Y. Acad. of Sci.*, Stohlman, (1964)).

As a result of recent studies *in vitro* of hemoglobin (Gallien-Lartigue and Goldwasser, 1965) and of ribonucleic acid (RNA) synthesis (Krantz and Goldwasser, 1965) these authors conclude that the erythropoietic hormone could act by inducing the formation of a messenger RNA responsible for the synthesis of hemoglobin.

VII. METABOLISM OF ERYTHROPOIETIN

If the titer of erythropoietin in the plasma is increased by stimulation (hypoxia, cobalt) or by the administration of exogenous erythropoietin, it falls rapidly in the next few hours. This decrease is due to utilization, inactivation, or urinary excretion of the hormone. Urinary excretion (Weintraub *et al.*, 1964) does not appear to be an important factor in removing erythropoietin from the plasma, since its clearance is only about 1 ml per min.

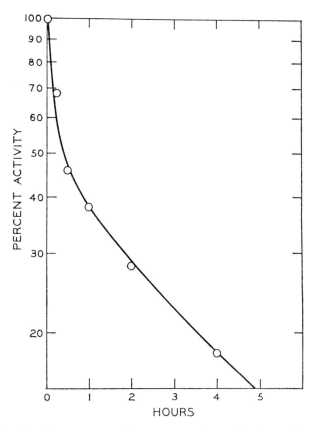

FIG. 12. Disappearance of exogenous erythropoietin from plasma of normal rats. Percentage activity was determined from a dilution curve of human urinary erythropoietin in rat plasma. (Reproduced by courtesy of Grune & Stratton, New York, from *Erythropoiesis*, Stohlman and Howard (1962)).

The rate of disappearance of the hormone from the plasma has been studied either with endogenous or with exogenous erythropoietin. In the first case, erythropoietin plasma level is increased by hypoxia or by injection of cobalt; the hypoxic stimulus is then withdrawn (Stohlman 1959) or the production of erythropoietin in response to cobalt is suppressed by bilateral nephrectomy (Naets and Wittek, 1965). The disappearance of exogenous erythropoietin is studied by following the erythropoietic activity

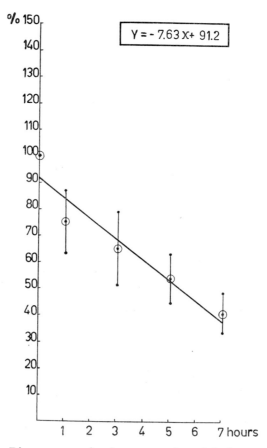

Fig. 13. Disappearance of endogenous erythropoietin from plasma of normal dogs (injected with cobalt) measured 1–7 hr after bilateral nephrectomy (time 0). Erythropoietin titer is expressed in percentage of the titer measured immediately after nephrectomy (0 hr) and considered as 100%. Values are means of 8 experiments ±1 S.E.M. (Reproduced by courtesy of *Acta Haemat.*, Naets and Wittek, in press).

of the plasma after intravenous injection of erythropoietin (Stohlman and Howard, 1962; Weintraub *et al.*, 1964). Stohlman (1958) has shown that in rats subjected for 16 hr to a simulated altitude of 23,000 ft the half-life of erythropoietin, measured after withdrawal of the stimulus, is 3–5 hr. Later this author has shown that human erythropoietin injected in the rat, has a half-life of 2.30 hr (Stohlman and Howard, 1962) (Fig. 12) whereas in the dog the half-life is about 10 hr for exogenous (Weintraub *et al.*, 1964), and 6 hr for endogenous erythropoietin (Naets and Wittek, 1968) (Fig. 13).

A. *Role of the liver*

The metabolism of erythropoietin is not well understood, and its fate in the body is unknown. Several authors regard the liver as the site of inactivation of the erythropoietic factor. Jacobson *et al.* (1956) have shown that after treatment with phenylhydrazine the level of erythropoietin was highest in rabbits with liver damage. They infer that the liver inactivates

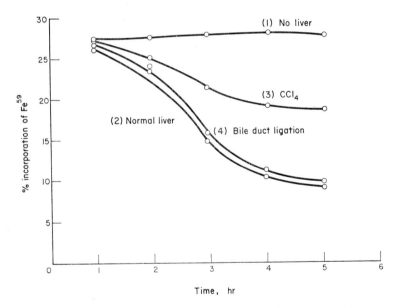

FIG. 14. Metabolism of erythropoietin by the isolated perfused liver. Erythropoietin titer is expressed in ^{59}Fe uptake into red cells of starved injected rats. (Reproduced by courtesy of Grune & Stratton, New York, from *Erythropoiesis*, Burke and Morse (1962)).

erythropoietin, and that damage to the liver by phenylhydrazine reduces this inactivation and thus increases the amount of the hormone in the plasma. Stohlman and Brecher (1957a), however, have not been able to confirm the relation between erythropoietin plasma level and liver damage. Prentice and Mirand (1957) have shown in rats subjected to hypoxia that the plasma level of erythropoietin is higher if the liver is previously injured by carbon tetrachloride. More recently, Burke and Morse (1962) have studied the inactivation of erythropoietin by the liver *in vitro*. During the perfusion of the liver with culture plasma the level of erythropoietin decreases sharply. The ability to inactivate erythropoietin was not impaired by previous ligation of the bile ducts, but was suppressed if the liver had been previously damaged by carbon tetrachloride (Fig. 14). In this kind of experiment, as well as in measures of erythropoietin disappearance rate *in vivo* it seems preferable to utilize erythropoietin from the same species as the recipient animal. It has been shown for instance that rat liver does not inactivate sheep erythropoietin (Fisher and Roheim, 1963).

B. *Role of bone marrow*

A few years ago Stohlman (1959) put forward the hypothesis of bone marrow utilization of erythropoietin, the consumption of the hormone increasing with the number of normoblasts in the marrow. This opinion is based on the fact that the level of erythropoietin is generally higher in anemic patients with medullary aplasia than in those with hemolytic disease and hyperplastic marrow. However, erythropoietin is increased in the serum and urine of patients with hemolytic disorders such as thalassemia, although the marrow has a high percentage of normoblasts (Winkert and Gordon, 1960; Hammond *et al.*, 1962). Stohlman (1959) has shown that the disappearance rate of erythropoietin from the plasma is prolonged in rats whose marrow is depressed by irradiation. Whereas in normal rats the half-life of erythropoietin after hypoxic stimulation averages 3–5 hr, it is 5–10 hr in irradiated rats. In support of this theory, Hammond and Ishikawa (1962) have found that urinary excretion of erythropoietin is suppressed by transfusion for about 36 hr in patients with hemolytic anemia, and for 60–90 hr in those with aplastic anemia. However, this hypothesis has not been confirmed by our recent observation of identical disappearance rate of endogenous erythropoietin in dogs with normal or hyperplastic marrow (Naets and Wittek, 1965, 1968).

VIII. SITE OF PRODUCTION

It seems presently established that the kidney is the main source of erythropoietin. Splenectomy does not affect production of the hormone (Mirand and Prentice, 1957; Piliero, 1959), neither does injury to the bone marrow by irradiation (Linman and Bethell, 1957a) or nitrogen mustard (Erslev and Lavietes, 1954). Excision of 7/8 of the liver, pancreas, stomach, or intestine does not suppress the response to cobalt (Jacobson *et al.*, 1957a). Removal of adrenals, pituitary, thyroid, and gonads does not prevent the response to bleeding (Fried *et al.*, 1956). In fact, only bilateral nephrectomy suppresses the production of erythropoietin (Jacobson *et al.*, 1957a). There is no response to cobalt or hypoxia after bilateral nephrectomy, though ligation of both ureters hardly affects the erythropoietic response to these stimuli. Accordingly, it is concluded that the kidney produces erythropoietin (Goldwasser *et al.*, 1958a). However, the same authors have shown that the plasma of nephrectomized rats subjected to hypoxia

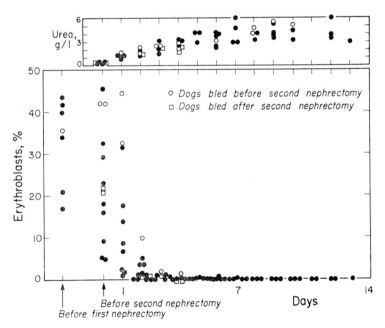

FIG. 15. Disappearance of normoblasts from the bone marrow in dogs after bilateral nephrectomy. At the top are plotted the values of plasma urea before and after nephrectomy. (Reproduced by courtesy of *J. clin. Invest.*, Naets (1960a)).

produced a slight rise in reticulocytes in polycythemic mice; they concluded that if the kidney provided the greater part of the erythropoietin, about 10% of the production might be from some other source (Jacobson *et al.*, 1959). Mirand and Prentice (1957) have obtained contradictory results, showing that nephrectomy does not prevent the increase in erythropoietin titer in response to hypoxic stimulation.

Erslev (1958) found erythropoietin in the plasma of rabbits following bleeding carried out immediately after bilateral nephrectomy. Gallagher *et al.* (1961) reported similar results in nephrectomized rabbits subjected to hypoxia. These experiments suggest also that erythropoietin is produced partly outside the kidney. That the kidney plays an important role in erythropoietin production has been demonstrated in the dog. If a nephrectomized dog is kept alive for 10–14 days by peritoneal dialysis, complete disappearance of normoblasts can be observed as early as 3 days after the operation (Naets, 1958a) (Fig. 15), and ferrokinetic studies confirm that erythropoiesis is abolished (Naets, 1958b) (Fig. 16). However, if the

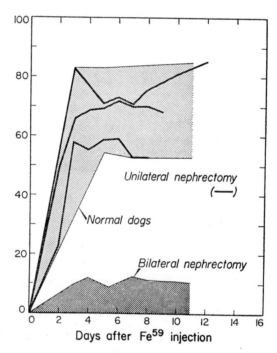

FIG. 16. ^{59}Fe incorporation into red cells of normal dogs and after bilateral and unilateral nephrectomy.

ureters are ligated, erythropoietic function is maintained despite a similar degree of uremic intoxication (Naets, 1958c). These various results, added to the observation that exogenous erythropoietin produces an erythropoietic response in nephrectomized animals (Naets, 1960a; Reissmann *et al.*, 1960; Naets and Heuse, 1964; Kurtides *et al.*, 1965), show that the role of uremia is not essential in the depression of erythropoiesis observed after nephrectomy. It should be emphasized that bilateral nephrectomy causes complete suppression of erythropoiesis in the dog only. In the rat (Reissmann *et al.*, 1960) and the rabbit (Erslev, 1960; Fisher and Friederici, 1961) the formation of red cells is considerably reduced after the operation

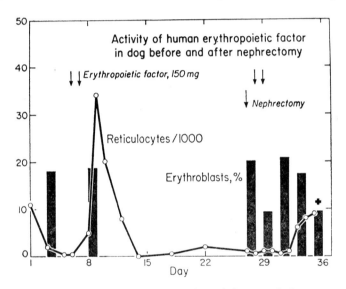

FIG. 17. Effect of human urinary erythropoietin on reticulocytes and bone marrow normoblasts in a dog before and after bilateral nephrectomy. (Reproduced by courtesy of Grune & Stratton, New York, from *Kinetics of Cellular Proliferation*, Naets (1959c).

but not abolished. In man also, erythropoiesis is only depressed by bilateral nephrectomy (Nathan *et al.*, 1964). We have observed 6 anephric patients, kept alive by hemodialysis before renal transplantation, for periods of 1–3 months. In these patients, the normoblasts averaged 14% before operation, fell to 7% in the next 10 days, and recovered after 30 days to an average of 10%, a relatively low value for anemic patients (hematocrit below 25%) (Naets *et al.*, 1968).

In the absence of the kidney, there is no control of erythropoiesis in the dog. After nephrectomy, severe anemia from repeated bleeding no longer produces an erythropoietic response (Naets and Heuse, 1964). Erythropoietin titer, increased by bleeding in the dog, decreases rapidly after bilateral nephrectomy (Fig. 18), but persists after ligation of the ureters

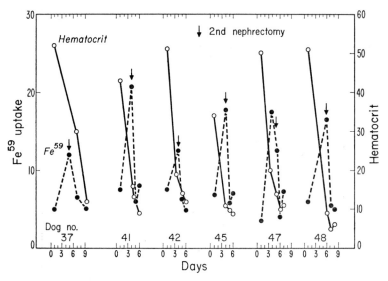

FIG. 18. Erythropoietin plasma level of bled dogs before and after nephrectomy with regard to corresponding hematocrit. Erythropoietic activity is expressed in ^{59}Fe uptake into red cells of starved rats. (Reproduced by courtesy of *Nature, Lond.*, Naets (1959b)).

(Naets, 1960c). Accordingly it seems that nephrectomy abolishes erythropoietic function in the dog by suppressing the production of erythropoietin. Kidney homogenates from bled dogs significantly increased the uptake of ^{59}Fe in fasting rats, in contrast with homogenates of kidneys from normal dogs or of liver or spleen from anemic dogs (Naets, 1960b). These results have recently been confirmed by Contrera *et al.* (1965). Erythropoietic activity has been found in kidneys from rats rendered anemic or subjected to hypoxia; no activity could be demonstrated in extracts of normal kidneys. However, others have reported an erythropoietic response to homogenates of normal kidneys from the rabbit, the rat, and the guinea pig (Lagrue *et al.*, 1960); but extracts of pig, calf, and sheep kidneys have been shown to be inactive (Boivin and Lagrue, 1961). Most authors agree that, apart from the kidney, the extracts of organs tested show no erythropoietic activity (Gordon *et al.*, 1956; Naets, 1960b; Lagrue *et al.*, 1960; Erslev, 1962). *In vitro* studies of renal perfusion have emphasized the importance of the kidney in the production of erythropoietin. Kuratowska *et al.* (1961) and Reissmann and Nomura (1962) have found that blood perfusing an isolated rabbit kidney becomes richer in erythropoietin when the oxygenation of the system is reduced. Fisher and Birdwell (1961) here observed the same phenomenon when perfusing a dog's kidney *in situ* with blood to which cobalt had been added. However, others have not confirmed these observations; thus Erslev *et al.* (1965) did not detect erythropoietin production by a dog's kidney perfused *in vitro* with poorly oxygenated blood.

The exact part of the kidney where erythropoietin is formed is unknown. Osnes (1958) has suggested that the juxtaglomerular apparatus, well known for its association with renin, may be the site of erythropoietin secretion. Hirashima and Takaku (1962) have found a relation between the granularity of the juxtaglomerular apparatus and the amount of erythropoietin in the plasma of rats rendered anemic by bleeding or phenylhydrazine. Constriction of a renal artery also increases the number of granules in the corresponding kidney. Conversely, transfusion polycythemia causes a decrease in the granules of the juxtaglomerular apparatus of the rat. It has therefore been suggested that these granules are an index of erythropoietin production. In all these experiments in which the renal arterial bed is affected, the changes found in the juxtaglomerular apparatus could in fact be related to the production of renin (Tobian, 1962). Moreover, if erythropoietin production is stimulated by hypoxia without changing the blood volume, no increase is found in the number of granulations in the juxtaglomerular apparatus (Goldfarb and Tobian, 1962). Conversely, hyperoxia does not reduce the number of granulations (Goldfarb and Tobian, 1963). It is thus difficult to relate the granularity of the juxtaglomerular apparatus to the production of erythropoietin.

IX. PURIFICATION AND CHEMICAL PROPERTIES

Although erythropoietin has not yet been purified, concentrated material with high biological activity has been obtained from the serum of rabbits (Rambach *et al.*, 1958; Lowy *et al.*, 1959) or sheep (White *et al.*, 1960) rendered anemic with phenylhydrazine, and from the urine of anemic patients. Concentration of the erythropoietic factor in urine is achieved by ultrafiltration (Van Dyke *et al.*, 1957), adsorption on kaolin followed by elution (Gordon, 1960), or alcohol precipitation (Lowy and Borsook, 1962). When plasma is the source of erythropoietin the first step is to remove the bulk of protein by precipitation with ammonium sulphate (Lowy *et al.*, 1958b), chromatography on DEAE columns (White *et al.*, 1960), or simply by boiling. Erythropoietin is in fact known to resist boiling for at least 15 min (Borsook *et al.*, 1954). The later stages of purification require fractionation by alcohol (Lowy *et al.*, 1960), chromatography (White *et al.*, 1950), or gel electrophoresis (Goldwasser *et al.* 1962). These authors have recently achieved a 400,000-fold concentration of the erythropoietic activity of plasma from sheep rendered anemic with phenylhydrazine. This concentrate contained 3000 units per mg of protein, compared to 0.007 units in the original plasma (Goldwasser, 1966). It is not certain that this concentration represents the final stage in the purification of erythropoietin.

Erythropoietin is non dialysable and thermostable, and, if frozen or lyophilized, retains its activity for several months. Chemical studies performed on less concentrated material have lead to the conclusion that erythropoietin is an α-2-glycoprotein, containing variable proportions of carbohydrate, hexosamine, and sialic acid, according to the purity of the preparation (29.2% of carbohydrate, 17.5% of hexosamine, and 13.0% of sialic acid) (Goldwasser *et al.*, 1962). The chemistry of the highly purified material has not yet been performed, and it is probable that the chemical composition ascribed to the less purified material is actually imputable to impurities. The molecular weight of erythropoietic factor extracted from a renal cyst or a cerebellar hemangioblastoma, or concentrated from the urine of anemic patients, estimated indirectly by X-ray inactivation, is of the order of 25,000–30,000 (Rosse *et al.*, 1963a). More recently, determination of the sedimentation coefficient of the highly purified erythropoietin fraction mentioned above, indicates a molecular weight of 60,000–70,000 (Goldwasser, 1966). The biological activity of erythropoietin requires the integrity of the protein molecule. It is abolished by the action of proteolytic enzymes (Lowy *et al.*, 1958a) or neuraminidase, and by substitution reactions such as iodination, acetylation or esterification (Lowy *et al.*, 1960). Garcia and Schooley (1963) have prepared an antibody against erythropoietin by injecting human erythropoietin into rabbits. This antibody is not specific; it neutralizes the erythropoietic activity of plasma from various species—rat, mouse, rabbit, sheep, and man. Rosse and Waldmann (1964) have shown that the antibody neutralizes the activity of plasma from anemic or hypoxic patients as well as erythropoietic factor in fluid from renal cysts or hemangioblastomas. The same authors have found that erythropoietin from these various sources has similar physical and chemical properties. Accordingly it seems that there are no major differences in molecular structure between erythropoietic factors from different sources.

In 1955, Gley and Delor claimed that there were two erythropoietic factors, one fat-soluble and the other water-soluble. Linman and Bethell (1960) have made similar observations. These authors found that a filtrate of boiled plasma from rabbits rendered anemic by phenylhydrazine, when given to rats, stimulated red-cell production and reticulocytosis. But the preparation has no effect on hemoglobin, hematocrit, or ^{59}Fe uptake, the increased red-cell count resulting from microcytosis without modification of hemoglobin synthesis. This thermostable factor is soluble in ether, and appears to have similar properties to batyl alcohol. Besides this factor, these authors consider that there is a second, thermolabile factor able to increase the synthesis of hemoglobin, and resembling erythropoietin. These results are quite different from those reported by other investigators and Borsook (1959) states that he has never been able to demonstrate a lipid factor.

X. CLINICAL ASPECT

In man, measurable amounts of erythropoietin are found in the plasma and urine of most patients with severe anemia (Gordon, 1959). Erythropoietin has also been detected in the amniotic fluid of pregnant women with rhesus incompatibility giving birth to infants suffering from erythroblastosis fetalis (Finne, 1964). Accordingly the anemic fetus seems also to produce erythropoietic hormone, excreted through the urine into the amniotic fluid.

The relation between the levels of erythropoietin and hemoglobin has been studied by several workers (Gurney *et al.*, 1958; Gallagher *et al.*, 1960; Van Dyke *et al.*, 1961; Hammond *et al.*, 1962; Naets and Heuse, 1962). These studies have shown that the hemoglobin must fall below 7 or 8 g per 100 ml before erythropoietin can be measured in man. It has already been pointed out that present methods of assay are not sensitive enough to detect the normal amount of erythropoietin in the plasma, and measure only very high levels. Patients with hemolytic anemia and hyperplastic marrow generally have less erythropoietin than patients with aplastic marrow and the same degree of anemia (Stohlman and Brecher, 1959; Stohlman and Howard, 1962). This difference in behavior between the two groups of patients is not always observed; for instance patients with hemolytic disorders such as thalassemia generally have a high level of erythropoietin in the blood and urine, although the marrow is hyperactive (Winkert and Gordon, 1960; Hammond *et al.*, 1962). One of the highest urinary levels of erythropoietin among the patients studied by Van Dyke *et al.* (1961) was found in a case of paroxysmal nocturnal hemoglobinuria. As has already been mentioned above, Stohlman (1959) has suggested that low levels of erythropoietin generally observed in anemic patients with hyperactive marrow are imputable to utilization of the hormone by the marrow.

The anemia of renal failure excepted, no known anemia appears to depend on deficient production of the hormone. In patients with chronic renal failure, several authors have shown that erythropoietin never rises to a measurable level despite the severity of their anemia (Gurney *et al.*, 1958; Gallagher *et al.*, 1960; Naets and Heuse, 1962) (Fig. 19). Although these clinical findings strongly support the theory of the renal origin of erythropoietin, they are not evidence that the anemia of these patients is due to defective production of the hormone by the diseased kidneys. Other clinical findings also point to the importance of the kidney in erythropoiesis in man, namely the fairly frequent cases of polycythemia associated with renal disorders: malignant tumours (Videbaek, 1950; Herbeval *et al.*, 1957; Damon *et al.*, 1958), hydronephrosis (Cooper and Tuttle, 1957; Ellis, 1961; Gardner and Freymann, 1958), or renal cysts (Cohen, 1960; Jones *et al.*, 1960). In some cases an erythropoietic factor has been shown in the fluid from renal cysts (Gurney, 1960; Nixon *et al.*, 1960; Rosse *et al.*, 1963b), or hydronephroses (Jones *et al.*, 1960), in tumours (Korst *et al.*, 1959; Hewlett *et al.*, 1960; Van Dyke, 1960 Gurney, 1960), and in the plasma of these patients (Donati *et al.*, 1963). In addition to these cases polycythemia has been described secondary to uterine fibroma (Horwitz and McKelway, 1955), hepatoma (McFadzean *et al.*, 1958), pheochromocytoma (Waldmann and Bradley, 1961), and cerebellar hemangioblastoma (Waldmann *et al.*, 1961). The relation between these tumours and the associated polycythemia is established by the remission which follows excision of the tumour. Furthermore, Rosse and Waldmann (1964) have shown that the physical and chemical properties of the erythropoietin extracted from renal cysts and cerebellar hemangioblastomas are similar to those of the erythropoietin which appears in the blood during anemia or hypoxia.

Polycythemia, secondary to hypoxia from respiratory impairment or congenital heart disease, is probably due to excessive production of

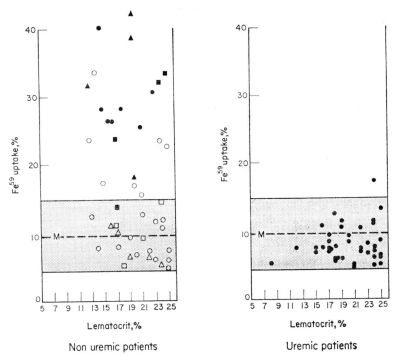

Fig. 19. Erythropoietin plasma level of anemic patients in relation to the degree of anemia, expressed in ^{59}Fe uptake of starved rats. M, mean of ^{59}Fe uptake after injection of normal plasma ± 2 S.D. (Reproduced by courtesy of *J. lab. clin. Med.*, Naets and Heuse (1962)).

erythropoietin. A raised level of erythropoietin has sometimes been found in the plasma of these patients (Linman and Bethell, 1957b; Freedman and Penington, 1963; Boivin *et al.*, 1964; Rosse and Waldmann, 1964). However, others have not found this increase; thus Noyes *et al.* (1962) found a raised level of erythropoietin in such patients after venesection only. The findings in polycythemia vera are also contradictory. Some authors report raised levels of erythropoietin (Linman and Bethell, 1957b; Boivin *et al.*, 1963; Boivin *et al.*, 1964), others have never observed an increase in this disorder, probably due to a dysfunction of cell-proliferation (Noyes *et al.*, 1962; Stohlman, 1962; Gurney, 1965). The doctrinal interest of these observations is obvious, as in secondary polycythemia the erythroid series only is involved, while polycythemia vera appears to be a myeloproliferative disorder affecting usually the different elements of the marrow.

At present no purified erythropoietin is available for clinical use. In˝any case the clinical value of this hormone would appear to be strictly limited, as most anemic patients have a high titer of erythropoietin. It is not impossible that renal anemia might be improved by the erythropoietic hormone. Therapeutic utilization of cobalt, which stimulates erythropoietin production have been unconvincing in clinical practice. Besides, an erythropoietic response to this agent could be expected only in cases where the production of erythropoietin is defective despite the anemia, while the organ elaborating the hormone is still able of increasing its production. Androgens, which appear to act partly by potentiating the effect of erythropoietin, seems to be a better clinical indication (Naets and Wittek, 1964). In children, androgens combined with corticosteroids have been successfully used in a number of cases of pancytopenia (Shahidi and Diamond, 1961). However, in adults, apart from the beneficial effect reported in some cases of myelofibrosis (Gardner and Pringle, 1961), the therapeutic effect of these steroids is disappointing.

REFERENCES

(a) BOOKS, REVIEWS AND MONOGRAPHS

ALPEN, E. L. and CRANMORE, D. (1959). Observations on the regulation of erythropoiesis and cellular dynamics by Fe^{59} autoradiography. In: *The kinetics of cellular proliferation*, pp. 290–300. STOHLMAN, F., Jr. (Ed.). Grune & Stratton, New York.

BANGHAM, D. R. (1962). Biological assay and a standard for "Erythropoietin", pp. 23–28. In: *Erythropoiesis*. JACOBSON, L. O. and DOYLE, M. (Ed.). Grune & Stratton, New York.

BRECHER, G. and STOHLMAN, F., JR., (1959). Humoral factors in erythropoiesis. In: *Progress in Hematology*, pp. 110–32. TOCANTINS, L. M. (Ed.). Grune & Stratton, New York.

BURKE, W. T. and MORSE, B. S. (1962). Studies on the production and metabolism of erythropoietin in rat liver and kidney. In: *Erythropoiesis*, pp. 111–9. JACOBSON, L. O. and DOYLE, M. (Ed.). Grune & Stratton, New York.

ERSLEV, A. J. (1962). Erythropoietin *in vitro*. In: *Erythropoiesis*, pp. 275–85. JACOBSON, L. O. and DOYLE, M. (Ed.). Grune & Stratton, New York.

FISCHER, S. (1962). Studies on the mechanism and site of action of erythropoietin. In: *Erythropoiesis*, pp. 204–15. JACOBSON, L. O. and DOYLE, M. (Ed.). Grune & Stratton, New York.

GOLDWASSER, E. (1966). Biochemical control of erythroid cell development in current topics. In: *Developmental Biology*. MOXONA, A. A. and MONROY, A. (Ed.), pp. 173–211. Academic Press, N.Y., 1966.

GORDON, A. S. (1960). Humoral influences in blood cell formation and release in haemopoiesis. In: *Ciba Foundation Symposium on haemopoiesis*: Cell production and its regulation. WOLSTENHOLME, G. E. and CAMERON, M. P. (Ed.). pp. 325–62. Boston Little, Brown.

HAMMOND, G. D. and ISHIKAWA, A. (1962). The rate of disappearance of erythropoietin following transfusion of severely anemic patients. In: *Erythropoiesis.* JACOBSON, L. O. and DOYLE, M. (Ed.), pp. 128–33. Grune & Stratton, New York.

HAMMOND, G. D., ISHIKAWA, A. and KEIGHLEY, G. (1962). Relationship between erythropoietin and severity of anemia in hypoplastic and hemolytic states. In: *Erythropoiesis*, pp. 351–8. JACOBSON, L. O. and DOYLE, M. (Ed.). Grune & Stratton, New York.

KEIGHLEY, G. (1962). Experiences with assays, units and standards of erythropoietin. In: *Erythropoiesis.* JACOBSON, L. O. and DOYLE, M. (Ed.), pp. 17–22. Grune & Stratton, New York.

LAJTHA, L. G. and OLIVER, R. (1960). Studies on the kinetics of erythropoiesis: A model of the erythron. In: *Ciba Foundation Symposium on Haemopoiesis.* WOLSTENHOLME, G. E. W. and O'CONNOR, M. J. (Ed.), pp. 289–324. J. & A. Churchill, London.

LINMAN, J. W. and BETHELL, F. H. (1960). *Factors controlling erythropoiesis.* Charles C. Thomas, Springfield, U.S.A.

LOWY, P. and BORSOOK, H. (1962). Preparation and properties of erythropoietin concentrates from rabbit plasma and human urine. In: *Erythropoiesis.* JACOBSON, L. O. and DOYLE, M. (Ed.), pp. 33–42. Grune & Stratton, New York.

NAETS, J. P. (1959c). Discussion of identity of erythropoietin and site of production. In: *Kinetics of Cellular Proliferation.* STOHLMAN, F., JR. (Ed.), pp. 359–64. Grune & Stratton, New York.

REISSMANN, K. R. and NOMURA, T. (1962). Erythropoietin formation in isolated kidneys and liver. In: *Erythropoiesis.* JACOBSON, L. O. and DOYLE, M. (Ed.), pp. 71–7. Grune & Stratton, New York.

STOHLMAN, F., JR. and HOWARD, D. (1962). Humoral regulation of erythropoiesis. IX. The rate of disappearance of erythropoietin from the plasma. In: *Erythropoiesis.* JACOBSON, L. O. and DOYLE, M. (Ed.), pp. 120–4. Grune & Stratton, New York.

VAN DYKE, D. C. (1960). Sources and properties of human erythropoietin. In: *Ciba Symposium on Hae $\mathfrak{z}$ opoiesis.* WOLSTENHOLME, G. E. W. and CAMERON, M. P. (Ed.), pp. 397–417. Little, Brown, Boston.

(b) ORIGINAL PAPERS

BARRON, A. G. and BARRON, E. S. G. (1936). Mechanism of cobalt polycythemia. Effect of ascorbic acid. *Proc. Soc. exp. Biol. Med.*, **35**: 407–9.

BERK, L., BURCHENAL, J. H. and CASTLE, W. B. (1949). Erythropoietic effect of cobalt in patients with or without anemia. *New England J. Med.*, **240**: 754–61.

BERT, P. (1882). Sur la richesse en hemoglobine du sang des animaux vivant sur les hauts lieux. *Compt. rend. Acad. Sc.*, **94**: 805–7.

BOIVIN, P. and LAGRUE, G. (1961). Étude sur le facteur érythropoïétique rénal. *Nouv. Rev. franç. Hématol.*, **1**: 518–26.

BOIVIN, P., LAGRUE, G. and FAUVERT, R. (1963). L'activité érythropoïétique du plasma humain au cours de quelques affections hématologiques et autres. *Nouv. Rev. franç. Hématol.*, **3**: 35–50.

BOIVIN, P., LAGRUE, G. and FAUVERT, R. (1964). L'activité érythropoïétique du plasma dans 50 cas de polyglobulie. *Rev. franç. Et. clin. Biol.*, **9**: 170–80.

BORSOOK, H. (1959). A discussion of humoral erythropoietic factors. *Ann. N.Y. Acad. Sci.*, **77**: 725–36.

o

BORSOOK, H., GRAYBIEL, A., KEIGHLEY, G. and WINDSOR, E. (1954). Polycythemic response in normal adult rats to a nonprotein plasma extract from anemic rabbits. *Blood*, 9: 734–42.

CARNOT, P. and DEFLANDRE, C. (1906). Sur l'activité hémopoiétique du sérum au cours de la régénération du sang. *Compt. rend. Acad. sc.*, 143: 384–6.

COHEN, N. R. (1960). Polycythemia associated with bilateral unilocular renal cysts. *Arch. int. Med.*, 105: 301–4.

CONTRERA, J. F., CAMISCOLI, J. F., WEINTRAUB, A. H. and GORDON, A. S. (1965). Extraction of erythropoietin from kidneys of hypoxic and phenylhydrazine treated rats. *Blood*, 25: 809–16.

COOPER, W. M., and TUTTLE, W. B. (1957). Polycythemia associated with a benign kidney lesion: report a case of erythrocytosis with hydronephrosis, with remission of polycythemia following nephrectomy. *Ann. int. Med.*, 47: 1008–15.

COTES, P. M. and BANGHAM, D. R. (1961). Bioassay of erythropoietin in mice made polycythaemic by exposure to air at a reduced pressure. *Nature, Lond.*, 191: 1065–7.

CRAFTS, R. C. (1954). The prevention of anemia in hypophysectomized adult female rats with combined thyroxine and cortisone therapy. *Endocrinology*, 54: 84–92.

CRAFTS, R. C. and MEINEKE, H. A. (1957). Decreased oxygen need as a factor in anemia of hypophysectomized animals. *Proc. Soc. Biol. Med.*, 95: 127–31.

CRONKITE, E. P. (1964). Erythropoietic cell proliferation in man. *Medicine*, 43: 635–7.

DAMON, A., HOLUB, D. A., MELICOW, M. M. and USON, A. C. (1958). Polycythemia and renal carcinoma. *Am. J. Med.*, 25: 182–97.

DANIEL, M., DINGLE, J. T., WEBB, M. and HEATH, J. C. (1963). The biological action of cobalt and other metals. I. The effect of cobalt on the morphology and metabolism of rat fibroblasts *in vitro*. *Brit. J. exp. Path.*, 44: 163–76.

DE GOWIN, R. L., HOFSTRA, D. and GURNEY, C. W. (1962a). A comparison of erythropoietic bioassay. *Proc. Soc. exper. Biol. Med.*, 110: 48–51.

DE GOWIN, R. L., HOFSTRA, D. and GURNEY, C. W. (1962b). The mouse with hypoxia-induced erythremia, an erythropoietin bioassay animal. *J. lab. clin. Med.*, 60: 846–52.

DONATI, R. M., McCARTHY, J. M., LANGE, R. D. and GALLAGHER, N. I. (1963). Erythrocytosis and neoplastic tumors. *Ann. Int. Med.*, 58: 47–55.

ELLIS, H. (1961). Polycythemia due to hydronephrosis. *Proc. R. Soc. Med.*, 54: 157.

ERSLEV, A. J. (1953). Humoral regulation of red cell production. *Blood*, 8: 349–57.

ERSLEV, A. J. (1957). Observations on the nature of the erythropoietic serum factor. II. Erythropoietic activity of serum and bone marrow after time limited exposure to anemic and hypoxic anoxia. *J. lab. clin. Med.*, 50: 543–9.

ERSLEV, A. J. (1958). Erythropoietic function in uremic rabbits. *Arch. int. Med.*, 101: 407–17.

ERSLEV, A. J. (1960). Erythropoietic function in uremic rabbits. II. Effect of nephrectomy on red cell production and iron metabolism. *Acta Haemat.*, 23: 226–35.

ERSLEV, A. J. (1961). Kidney–bone marrow interaction. *Trans. N.Y. Acad. Sci.*, 24: 131–4.

ERSLEV, A. J. and BOISSEVAIN, A. R. (1961). Direct measurements of the early erythropoietic effect of anemia. *Amer. J. Physiol.*, 201: 905–9.

ERSLEV, A. J. and LAVIETES, P. H. (1954). Observations on the nature of the erythropoietic serum factor. *Blood*, 9: 1055–61.

ERSLEV, A. J., SOLIT, R. W., CAMISHION, R. C., AMSEL, S., ILDA, J. and BALLINGER, W. F. (1965). Erythropoietin *in vitro*. III. Perfusion of a lung-kidney preparation. *Amer. J. Physiol.*, 208: 1153–7.

EVANS, E. S., ROSENBERG, L. L. and SIMPSON, M. E. (1961). Erythropoietic response to calorigenic hormones. *Endocrinology*, 68: 517–32.

EVANS, E. S., VAN DYKE, D. C. and ROSENBERG, L. L. (1964). Interaction of the erythrocyte stimulating factor with calorigenic hormones. *Endocrinology*, 75: 758–64.

FILMANOWICZ, E. and GURNEY, C. W. (1961). Studies on erythropoiesis. XVI. Response to a single dose of erythropoietin in polycythemic mouse. *J. lab. clin. Med.*, 57: 65–72.

FINNE, P. H. (1964). Erythropoietin levels in amniotic fluid, particularly in Rh–immunized pregnancies. *Acta Paediat.*, 53: 269–81.

FISHER, J. and FRIEDERICI, L. (1961). Erythropoiese bei bilateral nephrektomierten Kaninchen. *Experientia*, 17: 318–21.

FISHER, J. W. and BIRDWELL, B. J. (1961). The production of an erythropoietic factor by the *in situ* perfused kidney. *Acta Haematol.*, 26: 224–32.

FISHER, S. and ROHEIM, P. S. (1963). Role of the liver in the inactivation of erythropoietin. *Nature, Lond.*, 200: 899–900.

FREEDMAN, B. J. and PENINGTON, D. G. (1963). Erythrocytosis in emphysema. *Brit. J. Haemat.*, 9: 425–30.

FRIED, W., PLZAK, L., JACOBSON, L. O. and GOLDWASSER, E. (1956). *Erythropoiesis*. II. Assay of erythropoietin in hypophysectomized rats. *Proc. Soc. exper. Biol. Med.*, 92: 203–7.

FRIED, W., PLZAK, L. F., JACOBSON, L. O. and GOLDWASSER, E. (1957). Studies on erythropoiesis. III. Factors controlling erythropoietin production. *Proc. Soc. exper. Biol. Med.*, 94: 237–41.

GALLAGHER, N. I., MCCARTHY, J. M. and LANGE, R. D. (1960). Observations on erythropoietic stimulating factor (E.S.F.) in the plasma of uremic and non uremic anemic patients. *Ann. int. Med.*, 52: 1201–12.

GALLAGHER, N. I., MCCARTHY, J. M. and LANGE, R. D. (1961). Erythropoietin production in uremic rabbits. *J. lab. clin. Med.*, 57: 281–9.

GALLAGHER, N. I., SEIFERT, G. L., CALLINAN, J. L., MAES, A. A. and LANGE, R. D. (1963). Influence of erythropoietin on erythropoiesis in polycythemic rats. *J. lab. clin. Med.*, 61: 258–65.

GALLIEN-LARTIGUE, O. and GOLDWASSER, E. (1965). On the mechanism of erythropoietin-induced differentiation. I. The effects of specific inhibition on hemoglobin synthesis. *Biochim. Biophys. Acta*, 103: 319–24.

GARCIA, J. F. (1957). Changes in blood, plasma and red cell volume in the male rat, as a function of age. *Amer. J. Physiol.*, 190: 19–30.

GARCIA, J. F. and SCHOOLEY, J. C. (1963). Immunological neutralization of various erythropoietins. *Proc. Soc. exper. Biol. Med.*, 112: 712–4.

GARCIA, J. F. and VAN DYKE, D. C. (1959). Dose-response relationships of human urinary erythropoietin. *J. appl. Phys.*, 14: 233–6.

GARDNER, F. H. and FREYMANN, J. G. (1958). Erythrocythemia (polycythemia) and hydronephrosis: report of a case with radio-iron studies with recovery after nephrectomy. *New Engl. J. Med.*, 259: 323–7.

GARDNER, F. H. and PRINGLE, J. C., JR. (1961). Androgens and erythropoiesis. II. Treatment of myeloid metaplasia. *New Eng. J. Med.*, 264: 103–11.

GLEY, P. and DELOR, J. (1955). Sur quelques propriétés physicochimiques de l'hématopoiétine. *Compt. rend. Soc. biol.*, 149: 635–7.

GOLDFARB, B. and TOBIAN, L. (1962). The interrelationship of hypoxia, erythropoietin and the renal juxtaglomerular cell. *Proc. Soc. exp. Biol. Med.*, 111: 510–1.

GOLDFARB, B. and TOBIAN, L. (1963). Effect of high oxygen concentration on erythro poietin and the renal juxtaglomerular cell. *Proc. Soc. exp. Biol. Med.*, 113: 35–6.

GOLDWASSER, E., FRIED, W. and JACOBSON, L. O. (1958a). Studies on erythropoiesis. VIII. The effect of nephrectomy in response to hypoxic anoxia. *J. lab. clin. Med.*, 52: 375–8.

GOLDWASSER, E., JACOBSON, L. O., FRIED, W. and PLZAK, L. F. (1958b). Studies on erythropoiesis. V. The effect of cobalt on the production of erythropoietin. *Blood,* **13**: 55–60.

GOLDWASSER, E. and WHITE, W. F. (1959). Purification of sheep erythropoietin. *Fed. Proc.,* **18**: 236.

GOLDWASSER, E., WHITE, W. F. and TAYLOR, K. B. (1962). Further purification of sheep plasma erythropoietin. *Biochim. Biophys. Acta,* **64**: 487–96.

GORDON, A. S. (1954). Endocrine influences upon the formed elements of blood and blood forming organs. *Prog. Hormone Res.,* **10**: 339–94.

GORDON, A. S. (1959). Hemopoietine. *Physiol. Rev.,* **39**: 1–40.

GORDON, A. S., PILIERO, S. J., MEDICI, P. T., SIEGEL, C. D. and TANNENBAUM, M. (1956). Attempts to identify site of production of circulating "erythropoietin". *Proc. exp. Biol. Med.,* **92**: 598–602.

GRANT, W. C. (1955). The influence of anoxia of lactating rats and mice on blood of their normal offspring. *Blood,* **10**: 334–40.

GURNEY, C. W. (1960). Erythremia in renal disease. *Trans. A. Amer. Physicians,* **73**: 103–10.

GURNEY, C. W. (1965). Polycythemia vera and some possible pathogenic mechanisms. *Ann. Rev. Med.,* **16**: 169–86.

GURNEY, C. W. and CHAO PAN (1958). Studies on erythropoiesis. IX. Mechanism of decreased erythropoiesis in experimental polycythemia. *Proc. Soc. exp. Biol. Med.,* **98**: 789–93.

GURNEY, C. W., JACOBSON, L. O. and GOLDWASSER, E. (1958). The physiologic and clinical significance of erythropoietin. *Ann. int. Med.* **49**: 363–70.

HALVORSEN, S. (1964). Effects of hypothalamic lesions on the erythropoietic response to hypoxia in rabbits. *Acta physiol. scand.,* **61**: 1–19.

HERBEUVAL, R., CUNY, G. and LARCAN, A. (1957). Maladie de Vaquez et hypernéphrome. *Presse méd.,* **65**: 132–4.

HEWLETT, J. S., HOFFMAN, G. C., SENHAUSER, D. A. and BATTLE, J. D. (1960). Hypernephroma with erythrocythemia. Report of a case and assay of the tumor for an erythropoietic stimulating substance. *New Engl. J. Med.,* **262**: 1058–62.

HIRASHIMA, K. and TAKAKU, F. (1962). Experimental studies on erythropoietin. II. The relationship between juxtaglomerular cells and erythropoietin. *Blood,* **20**: 1–8.

HODGSON, G., YUDILEVICH, D., HERNANDEZ, P. and TOHA, J. (1957). Effect of plasma from bled and phenylhydrazine treated animals on plasma iron turnover. A test for "Hemopoietine". *Proc. Soc. exper. Biol. Med.,* **96**: 826–9.

HODGSON, G., ESKUCHE, I., FIESCHER, S. and PERRETTA, M. (1960). Effects of urinary hemopoietine on Fe[59] distribution in rats studied while plasma Fe[59] is high. *Proc. Soc. exper. Biol. Med.,* **104**: 441–5.

HORWITZ, A. and MCKELWAY, W. P. (1955). Polycythemia associated with uterine myomas. *J. Amer. Med. Ass.,* **158**: 1360–1.

HUFF, R. L., LAWRENCE, J. H., SIRI, W. E., WASSERMAN, L. R. and HENNESSY, T. G. (1951). Effect of changes in altitude on hematopoietic activity. *Medicine,* **30**: 197–218.

JACOBSON, E. M., DAVIS, A. K. and ALPEN, E. L. (1956). Relative effectiveness of phenylhydrazine treatment and hemorrhage in the production of an erythropoietic factor. *Blood,* **11**: 937–45.

JACOBSON, L. O. and GOLDWASSER, E. (1957). The dynamic equilibrium of erythropoiesis. *Brookhaven Symposia,* **10**: 110–31.

JACOBSON, L. O., GOLDWASSER, E., FRIED, W. and PLZAK, L. (1957a). Role of the kidney in erythropoiesis. *Nature, Lond.,* **179**: 633–4.

JACOBSON, L. O., GOLDWASSER, E., PLZAK, L. F. and FRIED, W. (1957b). Studies on erythropoiesis. IV. Reticulocyte response of hypophysectomized and polycythemic rodents to erythropoietin. *Proc. Soc. Exper. Biol. Med.*, **94**: 243–9.

JACOBSON, L. O., MARKS, E. K., GASTON, E. O. and GOLDWASSER, E. (1959). Studies on erythropoiesis. XI. Reticulocyte response of transfusion-induced polycythemic mice to anemic plasma from nephrectomized mice and to plasma from nephrectomized rats exposed to low oxygen. *Blood*, **14**: 635–43.

JEPSON, J. H. and LOWENSTEIN, L. (1964). Effect of prolactin on erythropoiesis in the mouse. *Blood*, **24**: 726–38.

JEPSON, J. H. and LOWENSTEIN, L. (1965). Erythropoiesis during pregnancy and lactation. I. Effect of various hormones on erythropoiesis during lactation. *Proc. Soc. exp. Biol. Med.*, **120**: 500–4.

JONES, N. F., PAYNE P. W., HYDE, R. D. and PRICE, T. M. (1960). Renal polycythemia. *Lancet*, **i**: 299–303.

KORST, D. R., WHALLEY, B. and BETHELL, F. (1959). Erythropoietic activity of plasma in polycythemia. *J. lab. clin. Med.*, **54**: 916.

KRANTZ, S. B. and GOLDWASSER, E. (1965). 1. On the mechanism of erythropoietin induced differentiation. 2. Effect on RNA synthesis. *Biochim. Biophys. Acta*, **103**: 325–32.

KURATOWSKA, Z., LEWARTOWSKI, B. and MICHALAK, E. (1961). Studies on the production of erythropoietin by isolated perfused organs. *Blood*, **18**: 527–34.

KURTIDES, E. S., RAMBACH, W. A. and ALT, H. L. (1965). Erythropoiesis in rats with acute uremia and the effect of erythropoietin. *Blood*, **25**: 292–8.

LAGRUE, G., BOIVIN, P. and BRANELEC, A. (1960). Activité érythropoiétique d' un extrait rénal. *Rev. franç. Etudes clin. biol.*, **8**: 816–9.

LEVY, H., LEVISON, V. and SCHODE, A. L. (1950). The effect of cobalt on the activity of certain enzymes in homogenates of rat tissue. *Arch. Biochem.*, **27**: 34–40.

LINMAN, J. W. and BETHELL, F. H. (1957a). The effect of irradiation on the plasma erythropoietic stimulating factor. *Blood*, **12**: 123–9.

LINMAN, J. W. and BETHELL, F. H. (1957b). The plasma erythropoietic-stimulating factor in man. Observations on patients with polycythemia vera and secondary polycythemia. *J. lab. clin. Med.*, **49**: 113–27.

LOWY, P. H., KEIGHLEY, G. and BORSOOK, H. (1958a). Isolation of an erythropoietic fraction from the plasma of rabbits made severely anaemic with phenylhydrazine. *Nature, Lond.*, **181**: 1802–3.

LOWY, P. H., KEIGHLEY, G. and BORSOOK, H. (1958b). Question of purity of erythropoietic factor concentrates. *Proc. Soc. exp. Biol. Med.*, **99**: 668–70.

LOWY, P. H., KEIGHLEY, G., BORSOOK, H. and GRAYBIEL, A. (1959). On the erythropoietic principle in the blood of rabbits made severely anemic with phenylhydrazine. *Blood*, **14**: 262–73.

LOWY, P. H., KEIGHLEY, G. and BORSOOK, H. (1960). Inactivation of erythropoietin by neuraminidase and by mild substitution reactions. *Nature, Lond.*, **185**: 102–3.

McFADZEAN, A. J., TODD, D. and TSANG, K. C. (1958). Polycythemia in primary carcinoma of the liver. *Blood*, **13**: 427–35.

MIESCHER, F. (1893). Bemerkungen über eine verbesserte Form der Mischpipette und ihren einfluss auf die Genauigkeit der Blutkörperzahlung. *Cor. Bl. J. Schweiz. Aerzte*, **23**: 830–2.

MIRAND, E. A. and PRENTICE, T. C. (1957). Presence of plasma erythropoietin in hypoxic rats with or without kidney(s) and/or spleen. *Proc. Soc. exper. Biol. Med.*, **96**: 49–51.

MIRAND, E. A., GORDON, A. S. and WENIG, J. (1965). Mechanism of testosterone action in erythropoiesis. *Nature, Lond.*, **206**: 270–2.

MÜLLER, P. TH. (1912). Über die Wirkung des Blutserums anämischer Tiere. *Arch. Hyg.*, **75**: 290–320.

NAETS, J. P. (1958a). Erythropoiesis in nephrectomized dog. *Experientia*, 14: 74–5.
NAETS, J. P. (1958b). Erythropoiesis in nephrectomized dog. *Nature, Lond.*, 181: 1134–5.
NAETS, J. P. (1958c). The kidney and erythropoiesis. *Nature, Lond.*, 182: 1516–7.
NAETS, J. P. (1959a). Erythropoietic activity in plasma and urine of dogs after bleeding. *Proc. Soc. exper. Biol. Med.*, 102: 387–9.
NAETS, J. P. (1959b). Disappearance of the erythropoietic factor from plasma of anaemic dogs after nephrectomy. *Nature, Lond.*, 184: 371–2.
NAETS, J. P. (1960a). The role of the kidney in erythropoiesis. *J. Clin. Invest.*, 39: 102–10.
NAETS, J. P. (1960b). Erythropoietic factor in kidney tissue of anemic dogs. *Proc. Soc. exper. Biol. Med.*, 103: 129–32.
NAETS, J. P. (1960c). The role of the kidney in the production of the erythropoietic factor. *Blood*, 16: 1770–6.
NAETS, J. P. (1963). Relation between erythropoietin plasma level and oxygen requirements. *Proc. Soc. exper. Biol. Med.*, 112; 832–6.
NAETS, J. P. and HEUSE, A. (1962). Measurement of erythropoietic stimulating factor in anemic patients with or without renal disease. *J. lab. clin. Med.*, 60: 365–74.
NAETS, J. P. and HEUSE, A. (1964). Effect of anemic hypoxia on erythropoiesis of normal and uremic dogs with or without kidneys. *J. nucl. Med.*, 5: 471–9.
NAETS, J. P. and WITTEK, M. (1964). Étude du mécanisme d'action des androgènes sur l'érythropoïèse. *C.R. Acad. Sc.(Paris)*, 259: 3371–4.
NAETS, J. P. and WITTEK, M. (1965). Effect of erythroid hyperplasia on utilization of erythropoietin. *Nature, Lond.*, 206: 726–7.
NAETS, J. P. and WITTEK, M. (1966). Mechanism of action of androgens on erythropoiesis. *Amer. J. Physiol.*, 210: 315–20.
NAETS, J. P. and WITTEK, M. (1968). Effect of erythroid hyperplasia on the disappearance rate of erythropoietin in the dog. *Acta Haemat.*, 39: 42–50.
NAETS, J. P., WITTEK, M., TOUSSAINT, C. and VAN GEERTRUYDEN, J. (1968). Erythropoiesis in renal insufficiency and in anephric man. *Ann. N.Y. Acad. Sc.*, 149: 143–50.
NATHAN, D. G., SCHUPAK, E., STOHLMAN, F., JR. and MERRIL, F. (1964). Erythropoiesis in anephric man. *J. clin. Invest.*, 43: 2158–64.
NIXON, R. K., O'ROURKE, W., RUPE, C. and KORST, D. B. (1960). Nephrogenic polycythemia. *Arch. int. Med.*, 106: 797–802.
NOYES, W. D., DOMM, B. M. and WILLIS, L. C. (1962). Regulation of erythropoiesis. I. Erythropoietin assay as a clinical tool. *Blood*, 20: 9–18.
OSNES, S. (1958). An erythropoietic factor produced in the kidney. *Brit. med. J.*, ii: 1387–8.
PILIERO, S. J. (1959). Influence of hypoxic stimuli upon blood formation in endocrine-deficient animals. *Ann. N.Y. Acad. Sci.*, 77: 518–42.
PLZAK, L. F., FRIED, W., JACOBSON, L. O. and BETHARD, W. F. (1955). Demonstration of stimulation of erythropoiesis by plasma from anemic rats using Fe[59]. *J. lab. clin. Med.*, 46: 671–8.
PRENTICE, T. C. and MIRAND, E. A. (1957). Effect of acute liver damage plus hypoxia on plasma erythropoietin content. *Proc. Soc. exper. Biol. Med.*, 95: 231–4.
RAMBACH, W. A., COOPER, J. A. D. and ALT, H. L. (1958). Purification of erythropoietin by ion-exchange chromatography. *Proc. Soc. exper. Biol. Med.*, 98: 602–4.
READ, R. C. (1954). Studies on red-cell volume and turnover using radiochromium. *New Engl. J. Med.*, 250: 1021–7.
REISSMANN, K. R. (1950). Studies on the mechanism of erythropoietic stimulation in parabiotic rats during hypoxia. *Blood*, 6: 372–80.
REISSMANN, K. R., NOMURA, T., GUNN, R. W. and BROSIUS, F. (1960). Erythropoietic response to anemia or erythropoietin injection in anemic rats with or without functioning renal tissue. *Blood*, 16: 1411–23.

ROBINSON, S. H. and SCHMID, R. (1964). The relation of erythropoiesis to bile pigment formation. *Medicine*, **43**: 667–8.

ROSSE, W. F. and WALDMANN, T. A. (1964). A comparison of some physical and chemical properties of erythropoiesis-stimulating factors from different sources. *Blood*, **24**: 739–49.

ROSSE, W. F., BERRY, R. J. and WALDMANN, T. A. (1963a). Some molecular characteristics of erythropoietin from different sources determined by inactivation by ionizing radiation. *J. clin. Invest.*, **42**: 124–9.

ROSSE, W. F., WALDMANN, T. A. and COHEN, P. (1963b). Renal cysts, erythropoietin and polycythemia. *Amer. J. Med.*, **34**: 76–81.

SCHMID, R. and GILBERTSEN, A. S. (1955). Fundamental observations on the production of compensatory polycythemia in a case of patent ductus arteriosus with reversed blood flow. *Blood*, **10**: 247–51.

SCHOOLEY, J. C. and GARCIA, J. F. (1962). Immunologic studies on the mechanism of action on erythropoietin. *Proc. Soc. exper. Biol. Med.*, **110**: 636–41.

SEIP, M., HALVORSEN, S., ANDERSEN, P. and KAADA, B. R. (1961). Effects of hypothalamic stimulation on erythropoiesis in rabbits. *Scand. J. clin. Invest.*, **13**: 553–63.

SHAHIDI, N. T. and DIAMOND, L. K. (1961). Testosterone induced remission in aplastic anemia of both acquired and congenital types. *New Engl. J. Med.*, **264**: 953–67.

STEELE, B. F. (1933). The effects of blood loss and blood destruction upon the erythroid cells in the bone marrow of rabbits. *J. Exp. Med.*, **57**: 881–96.

STOHLMAN, F., JR. (1959). Observations on the physiology of erythropoietin and its role in the regulation of red cell production. *Ann. N.Y. Acad. Sc.*, **77**: 710–24.

STOHLMAN, F., JR. (1961). Humoral regulation of erythropoiesis VII. Shortened survival of erythrocytes produced by erythropoietin or severe anemia. *Proc. Soc. exp. Biol. Med.*, **107**: 884–7.

STOHLMAN, F., JR. (1962). Erythropoiesis. *New Engl. J. Med.*, **267**: 392–9.

STOHLMAN, F., JR. (1964). Humoral regulation of erythropoiesis XIV: A model for abnormal erythropoiesis in thalassemia. *Ann. N.Y. Acad. Sc.*, **119**: 578–85.

STOHLMAN, F., JR. and BRECHER, G. (1956). Stimulation of erythropoiesis in sublethally irradiated rats by a plasma factor. *Proc. Soc. exp. Biol. Med.*, **91**: 1–4.

STOHLMAN, F., JR. and BRECHER, G. (1957a). Humoral regulation of erythropoiesis IV. Relative heat stability of erythropoietin. *Proc. Soc. exp. Biol., Med.*, **95**: 797–800.

STOHLMAN, F., JR. and BRECHER, G. (1957b). Humoral regulation of erythropoiesis III. Effect of exposure to simulated altitude. *J. lab. clin. Med.*, **49**: 890–5.

STOHLMAN, F., JR. and BRECHER, G. (1959). Humoral regulation of erythropoiesis V. Relationship of plasma erythropoietin level to bone marrow activity. *Proc. Soc. exp. Biol. Med.*, **100**: 40–3.

STOHLMAN, F., JR., BELAND, A. and HOWARD, D. (1963). The macrocytic response to erythropoietin. *J. clin. Invest.*, **42**: 984.

STOHLMAN, F., JR., RATH, C. E. and ROSE, J. C. (1954). Evidence for a humoral regulation of erythropoiesis. *Blood*, **9**: 721–33.

STOHLMAN, F., JR., LUCARELLI, G., HOWARD, D., MORSE, B. and LEVENTHAL, B. (1964). Regulation of erythropoiesis. XVI. Cytokinetic patterns in disorders of erythropoiesis. *Medicine*, **43**: 651–60.

TOBIAN, L. (1962). Relationship of juxtaglomerular apparatus to renin and angiotensin. *Circulation*, **25**: 189–92.

TOHA, J., HODGSON, G. and WEASSON, E. (1952). Effecto erythropoyetico de injecciones repetidas de plasma de conejos anemizados por sangria, an conejos normales. *Bol. Soc. Biol. Concepcion (Chile)*, **27**: 69–75.

VAN DYKE, D. C., CONTOPOULOS, A. N., WILLIAMS, B. S., SIMPSON, M. E. and EVANS, H. M. (1954). Hormonal factors influencing erythropoiesis. *Acta Haemat.*, **11**: 203–22.

VAN DYKE, D. C., GARCIA, J. F. and LAWRENCE, J. H. (1957). Concentration of highly potent erythropoietic activity from urine of anemic patients. *Proc. Soc. exper. Biol. Med.*, 96: 541–44.

VAN DYKE, D. C., LAYRISSE, M., LAWRENCE, J. H., GARCIA, J. F. and POLLYCOVE, M. (1961). Relation between severity of anemia and erythropoietin titer in human beings. *Blood*, 18: 187–201.

VIDEBAEK, A. (1950). Polycythaemia vera coexisting with malignant tumors (particularly hypernephroma). *Acta med. scand.*, 138: 239–45.

WALDMANN, T. A. and BRADLEY, J. E. (1961). Polycythemia secondary to a phaeochromocytoma with production of an erythropoiesis stimulating factor by the tumor. *Proc. Soc. exp. Biol. Med.*, 108: 425–7.

WALDMANN, T. A., LEVIN, E. M. and BALDWIN, M. (1961). The association of polycythemia with a cerebellar hemangioblastoma. *Amer. J. Med.*, 31: 318–24.

WEINTRAUB, A. H., GORDON, A. S. and CAMISCOLI, J. F. (1963). Use of the hypoxia-induced polycythemic mouse in the assay and standardization of erythropoietin. *J. lab. clin. Med.*, 62: 743–52.

WEINTRAUB, A. H., GORDON, A. S., BECKER, E. L., CAMISCOLI, J. F. and CONTRERA, J. F. (1964). Plasma and renal clearance of exogenous erythropoietin in the dog. *Amer. J. Physiol.*, 207: 523–9.

WHITE, W. F. and JOSH, G. (1959). Studies on erythropoietin II. Production of high titre plasma in sheep. *Proc. Soc. exp. Biol. Med.*, 102: 686–8.

WHITE, W. F., GURNEY, C. W., GOLDWASSER, E. and JACOBSON, L. O. (1960). Studies on erythropoietin. *Recent prog. Hormone Res.*, 16: 219–62.

WINKERT, J. W. and GORDON, A. S. (1960). Biological assay of human urinary erythropoietic stimulating factor (ESF). *Proc. Soc. exp. Biol. Med.*, 104: 713–6.

AUTHOR INDEX

xiii

SUBJECT INDEX

Date Due

MAY 1 1 1981			